IMMUNOGENETICS

IMMUNOGENETICS

W. H. Hildemann

University of California, Los Angeles

HOLDEN-DAY

San Francisco, Cambridge, London, Amsterdam

To Dorothy,
Lynn, and
Lori

FH

H

PREFACE

So far from being one of his higher or nobler qualities, his individuality shows man nearer kin to mice and goldfish than to the angels; it is not his individuality but only his awareness of it that sets man apart. P. B. Medawar in *The Uniqueness of the Individual,* 1957.

In retrospect, my interest in writing this book began when I taught my first graduate seminar on immunogenetics at the University of California in Los Angeles in the spring of 1961. The eight subject areas I then chose for presentation and discussion for graduate and medical students of heterogeneous backgrounds make up the outline of the chapters of this book. Since there are many interconnecting paths among the subjects considered in the separate chapters, attention is repeatedly called to basic interrelationships, especially when frontier questions are involved. In the past, a student had to cope with a reading list of more than fifty references just to obtain a substantial, introductory overview of the mainstreams of immunogenetics, but even these references dealt mainly with newer results rather than concepts and integrative analyses. Although many excellent reviews of different aspects of immunogenetics have been written over the years, no single source of basic principles and their applications has been available for pedagogic and correlative purposes. The need for such a book has notably increased with rapidly expanding emphasis in the interdisciplinary fields of tissue transplantation, cancer, and the genetic regulation of immune responsiveness.

This book then is intended to emphasize principles and problem-solving rather than to serve as a review of the literature of immunogenetics. Since immunogenetics almost by definition includes those fields where immunology and genetics overlap and subserve each other, the reader should have at least an elementary acquaintance with the concepts of immunology and of genetics. I have tried to provide the necessary background beyond the most elementary level, and the order of presentation was determined by the cumulative complexity of the principles and techniques involved. Those to whom immunogenetics is still largely synonymous with blood-group genetics may be surprised or disappointed that more emphasis is not given to this long-established field. However, given the new breadth of immunogenetics, an effort was made to achieve a stimulating compromise between the usual textbook and the advanced monograph approaches. The level of consideration is intended especially for the

v

new generation of graduate and medical students. Hopefully, the needs of many advanced undergraduates as well as postdoctoral professionals may also be met. This book may also serve to enrich courses in immunology or genetics in the light of recent research and curricular changes.

The introductory chapter, which necessarily includes some difficult material for the novice, is intended as a general foundation upon which later chapters depend in differing degrees. However, since each chapter may be read or used independently, the reader need not necessarily study the chapters sequentially. The figures and tables are meant to be considered in context as an integral part of the presentation. A short list of key references with comments on their focus is given at the end of each chapter. These selected references, which are mostly recent reviews or research articles, contain additional citations of nearly all pertinent earlier work the serious student may wish to pursue in greater detail. Thus, to avoid discouraging him with long bibliographies, which would soon cease to be comprehensive in any event, numerous original and important articles have not been directly cited. I should especially apologize to investigators whose work may have been considered without pausing to assign credits. However, I assume the reader who becomes an active worker will soon discover the identities of the recent contributors to each field with little difficulty.

Generous research support from the U.S. National Institute of Health over the past decade has especially contributed to the advancement of knowledge in immunogenetics which has yielded major benefits for mankind. My own small efforts, especially in preparing this book, have also been notably enhanced by a Lederle Medical Faculty Award. I would acknowledge a special debt to Ray D. Owen and Dan Campbell for inspiring instruction in immunogenetics and immunology during my own graduate student years long ago at the California Institute of Technology. I also appreciate the broadening perspectives gained in later years from collaboration with R. E. Billingham and Peter Medawar at University College London, with George Snell and the immunogenetics group at Bar Harbor, Maine, and with Roy Walford at the University of California, Los Angeles.

Finally, I welcome the opportunity to thank a number of people for much help and encouragement. First, I would mention the lively stimulation of my own graduate students, postdoctoral fellows, and immediate colleagues. For squaring away my reprint collection and typing early drafts, I salute my former technician, Beth Teviotdale. For innumerable days of typing, preparation of illustrations, proof-reading, and enthusiastic attention to other essential details, I salute my secretary, Marlyn Mackey. Lastly, I thank my wife, Dorothy for an uncommon measure of patience and understanding.

Los Angeles, California   W. H. Hildemann
December, 1968

CONTENTS

ONE

FUNDAMENTALS OF IMMUNOGENETICS

Immunogenetics, a term introduced by M. R. Irwin of the University of Wisconsin in the 1930s, originally referred to studies in which immunological methodology was used to explore genetic variation. Immunogenetics may now be more broadly defined to include studies in which the principles and techniques of both genetics and immunology are employed jointly. This interdisciplinary marriage began in the early 1900s with Ehrlich and Morganroth's demonstration of goat blood groups and Landsteiner's discovery of human blood groups. This was about the same time that genetics itself began to revolutionize biology.

Studies of blood groups and other cellular antigens continue to be a major focus of immunogenetics, with important ramifications both in medicine and in molecular genetics. The scope of immunogenetics has been greatly extended during the past decade, however, due to discoveries of fundamental importance in immunology. Almost every facet of modern immunological research and its application involves important genetic considerations. Elucidation of host-parasite relationships depends upon understanding the inheritance of host immune-response capacities as well as antigenic characteristics of particular pathogens. Intraspecific differences are reflected in individual variations in chemical structure of cellular and soluble macromolecules. This intraspecific diversity as revealed in cellular alloantigens and serum allotypes is so great that, except for identical twins or equivalent highly inbred animals, every individual within a species may be regarded as unique. Such uniqueness is best demonstrated by tissue transplantation. Incompatibility leading to eventual graft rejection is the universal rule within vertebrate species—whether fish, mice, or men. A normal, adult recipient reacts against the genetically and antigenetically different tissue of the donor.

One of the most fundamental generalizations in biology is that genes specify and regulate the synthesis of macromolecules required for growth and development. In addition to nucleic acids, which contain the genetic code, the essential macromolecules that distinguish cells as well as individuals of all species are proteins and polysaccharides. The structural complexity and functional specificity of these molecules have only begun to be characterized. It is known, however, that animals dispose of nearly all foreign macromolecules that enter the body. Vertebrates appear to recognize foreignness at the molecular level—whether introduced by a pathogenic microorganism or normal tissue transplant—and respond to such antigens by the formation of antibodies. Antigens then are molecules that will induce an antibody or immune response when innoculated into an animal and will react specifically with the antibodies they have induced. Although antibodies are represented by diverse molecular species, all are found in the globulin fractions of serum or plasma proteins. Antigen-antibody reactions are usually highly specific, and yet single antigens may evoke a multiplicity of antibodies of varying reactivities. A macromolecular "antigen," in the crude sense, is composed of various structural groups or sites, each capable of reacting with antibodies specific for it. Small molecules, even ions, associated with proteins or polysaccharides, may serve as antigenic determinant groups or haptens, but will induce antibodies only when conjugated to a large molecule. In general, antigenic molecules exceed 10,000 in molecular weight and are polyvalent with respect to determinant groups. The combining sites of individual antigens have an estimated size of six or seven sugar residues in polysaccharides and five or six amino acids in proteins. However, single sugars or amino acids within such groups may provide the predominant complementary configuration for specific antibodies. Although nearly all antibodies probably have two identical valence or combining sites per molecule or subunit, antibody molecules formed to a single antigen are not identical. They often have different molecular weights and electrophoretic mobilities as well as different biological effects following combination with the antigen. Thus, antibodies in a particular immune serum may be described as subpopulations of antibody molecules, heterogeneous with respect to various properties, but all able to combine with the inducing antigen. Nevertheless, the essential specificity of antigen-antibody reaction systems is their most noteworthy attribute.

The molecular characteristics of both antigens and antibodies are determined by the genetic constitutions of the cells and of the individuals from which they are derived. In many instances, these characteristics have been identified with particular genes and stages of development, as we shall see in succeeding chapters. The scope of immunogenetics has become increasingly broad. It ranges from intraspecific polymorphisms to the genetics of antibody synthesis and the complexities of transplantation reactions. Despite these many ramifications, a relatively few concepts of genetics and immunology do suffice as a basis for coping with this field.

Gene Concepts and Biosynthesis

The concept of genes as hereditary units of biosynthetic coding has changed and is still changing with the advent of experimental data. A critical history of gene concepts has been compiled recently by Elof Carlson (see key references at the end of this chapter). Let us briefly consider some genetic terms and functions that should already be familiar to many readers. A gene, in the classical sense, was a unit of inheritance that was indivisible structurally or functionally. Genes of diverse species have been characterized in terms of mutation, recombination, and, of course, phenotypic effects. Thus, a *gene* can be defined as: (a) a unit of mutation, (b) a unit of chromosomal structure not divisible by crossing over or breakage, or (c) a unit of morphological or physiological function. As the essential relation between genes and protein synthesis was revealed in the 1940s, George Beadle suggested that the individual gene provides the specificity for a single primary characteristic which is, moreover, generally associated with an enzyme. This equation was revised to "one gene → one polypeptide" when independent genes were found to specify the separate polypeptide chains comprising certain proteins, such as hemoglobins and immunoglobulins.

In this book, the term *gene* will refer generally to distinctive hereditary units located on chromosomes at specific loci in a linear order. *Locus* designates the chromosomal position or site of a gene, as determined by frequency of recombination with separate but linked genes. The term *allele* is defined as an alternate state of the same gene locus. Alleles, then, are regarded as functional alternatives which have not been separated by tests for crossing over. Whether a functional unit is composed of subunits separable by recombination is difficult to ascertain in higher organisms such as mammals, because large numbers of progeny are required to detect rare recombinational events. The question of whether intragenic recombination is universal will certainly continue to concern immunogeneticists, especially those who study mammals.

The gene units of function (i.e., chromosomal loci) in diverse microorganisms are subdivisible into multiple structural elements with a linear arrangement. Supporting this evidence is the fact that gene products (i.e., proteins) are coded from deoxyribonucleic acid (DNA) as a linear sequence of nucleotides subject to recombination. Each gene, according to current dogma, contains the code (i.e., sequence of purine and pyrimidine bases in DNA) for the specific sequence of amino acids in a polypeptide chain. The code or *codon* for each amino acid is probably a triplet of nucleotide bases contained in messenger RNA, which is transcribed from DNA. The primary DNA code then is transcribed into RNA codons which, in turn, are translated into the amino acid sequences of proteins. Several investigations, notably those of C. Yanofsky and his colleagues with the tryptophan synthetase system of *Escherichia coli*, have established that the nucleotide sequences of the gene (genetic map) and the amino acid sequence of the peptide products are colinear. The conventional scheme of gene action in protein synthesis is illustrated in Fig. 1—1.

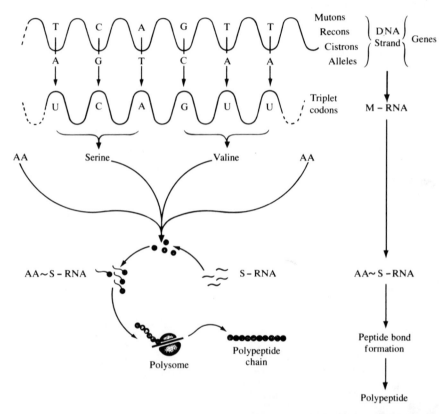

Figure 1—1.   Scheme of gene action in protein synthesis. M—RNA is messenger RNA, S—RNA is soluble RNA, and AA~S—RNA are activated amino acids (AA) brought to ribosomes attached to soluble RNA. Genetic information resides in sequence of contiguous nucleotide pairs which allow differing definitions of genes as units of structure or function.

The terms *muton* for a gene unit of mutation, *recon* for a gene unit of recombination, and *cistron* or *polycistron* for a gene unit of function (the classical gene) have been conveniently used by microbial geneticists, but rarely by immunogeneticists. Unfortunately, useful distinctions among mutons, recons, and cistrons in relation to numbers of nucleotide pairs have not emerged. However, we shall encounter examples of distinctive antigens referable to single amino acid substitutions in immunoglobulin polypeptides governed by allelic genes (Chapter Five).

Why cells of different types, even from the same individual, express only some of the potentialities inherent in their *genome* (i.e., one complete set of genes or the haploid number of chromosomes in higher organisms) is determined by how genes act and interact. Various modifiers, suppressors, mutators, and inhibitors of gene action have been invoked to account for modulations of the genome. The fruitful theory of the operon postulates two classes of genes—the structural gene which codes the structure of a polypeptide, and the regulatory gene which governs the expression of the structural gene through the participation of a repressor or operator. An *operon*, then, is a coordinated unit of expression consisting of an operator (regulatory gene) and the group of structural genes coordinated with it. Although one cannot confidently define given structural genes in relation to a precise number of nucleotide pairs, the units of mutation and recombination may be equated conceptually with a small number of, or even single, nucleotide pairs. Many, but not all, biosynthetic pathways in bacteria are consistent with the operon concept. However, a noncontiguous distribution of genes controlling related biochemical functions appears to be the rule rather than the exception in organisms other than bacteria. The modulation of gene action is almost certainly universal, but the sequential controls, especially in vertebrate classes, are as yet unknown. There is still a tendency to speak of gene interaction when the sequential interaction of separate gene products is really involved. Even *intragenic complementation*, as a test of genetic units of function in microorganisms, is identified by the capacity of two mutant alleles (or partial nonalleles) to yield polypeptide chains which form active (wild-type) enzyme molecules in heterozygotes. Proteins are not directly synthesized on genes, and carbohydrate-containing macromolecules, synthesized by enzymes, are at least one step further removed from the nucleic acids in the chain of action. Most microbial antigens (Chapter Three) and blood group antigens (Chapter Four) belong in the latter category.

First Principles of Immunogenetics

There are two first principles of immunogenetics; the first may be stated as follows:

1. *Every antigen is determined by a dominant gene, i.e., the antigen is present whether the gene is homozygous or heterozygous.*

With few exceptions, this has been a consistent finding. Doubly dominant heterozygotes produce both antigens. Perhaps the best known example of this generalization is the A-B-O series of blood groups in humans. The four main blood groups (phenotypes), O, A, B, and AB, are determined by three multiple alleles. The *O* allele produces no effective antigen, but the *A* and *B* alleles produce their respective antigens in all five possible homozygous or heterozygous genotypes.

The relationship "one dominant allele → one antigen specificity" is not negated by the fact that more than one gene locus may affect an antigen or that a given locus may affect more than one antigen. As a hypothetical example, in the reaction sequence,

$$\text{precursor(s)} \xrightarrow[\text{C enzyme}]{C \text{ gene}} 1 \begin{cases} \xrightarrow[\text{D enzyme}]{D \text{ gene}} 2 \\ \xrightarrow[\text{E enzyme}]{E \text{ gene}} 3 \end{cases}$$

product 2 might always appear to show a one-to-one dependence on the *D* gene even though one or more precursors dependent on other genes such as *C* were required earlier in the sequence. Moreover, antigenic products 2 and 3 could both be said to depend on the *C* gene as well as on the *D* and *E* genes, respectively. A notable example of such gene interaction involves the *Lewis, H,* and *Secretor* genes in man. This and other apparent deviations from simple one-to-one relationships reflected in hybrid antigens or recessively determined antigens will be scrutinized in later chapters.

In a model interaction system using two highly inbred or essentially homozygous but genetically disparate lines of mice, the interstrain cross AA × BB could theoretically yield F_1 hybrids of the uniform constitution AB(C). In other words, C represents an interaction or hybrid antigen(s) dependent on the genes or gene-products of A and B together. We could demonstrate the existence of C by immunizing a rabbit with F_1 cells, then absorbing the resulting antiserum exhaustively with cells from both parental strains and still find unabsorbed antibodies reactive with F_1 cells. Without further experiments involving gene segregants in backcross or F_2 generations, we would not know whether our C antigen was referable to an interallelic or interlocus interaction. Also, additional antiserums produced against the cells of segregant progeny beyond the F_1 generation could reveal more than one hybrid antigen associated with various genotypes.

Despite apparent complexities, the basic one-to-one relationship is meant to indicate that a given antigenic molecule or prosthetic component will be synthesized only when a particular structural gene is present. This conception poses some additional problems, especially in complex blood group systems, where several antigenic factors may be transmitted genetically as a group (*phenogroup*) in apparent association with a single allele. A newer term *haplotype* is equivalent to *phenogroup*. Both terms are used to refer to the product(s) of one of two homologous alleles. Thus, the haplotype or phenogroup corresponds to the product of a single gene dose whereas the total phenotype is controlled by the diploid genotype or both alleles at each genetic locus. In general, the criteria of both genetics and immunology need to be satisfied before an antigen may be attributed to a given gene.

Now we come to the second "first principle" of immunogenetics:

2. *A normal individual possesses or can produce antibodies (or develops immunity) only against those antigens that he or she does not have.*

In the familiar A-B-O system of man, the antibodies against antigens not represented in the individual's cells are normally present in the serum. Thus type O individuals lacking A and B antigens have anti-A and anti-B in the serum whereas type AB individuals produce neither of these antibodies. These relationships are summarized in Table 1–1. Although these naturally occurring

Table 1–1. Immunogenetic Relationships of the A-B-O Blood Group System in Man

Blood Group Phenotype	Possible Genotypes	Reactions Observed with Antibodies		Blood Contains:	
		Anti-A	Anti-B	Erythrocyte Antigens	Serum Antibodies
AB	*A/B*	+	+	A, B	—
A	*A/A, A/O*	+	—	A	anti-B
B	*B/B, B/O*	—	+	B	anti-A
O	*O/O*	—	—	—	anti-A anti-B

antibodies appear to be induced soon after birth by A- and B-like molecules present in foods and intestinal microorganisms, the molecular properties of the antibodies, apart from their specificity, vary according to the genetic constitution of the individual. There are apparently no natural or spontaneously produced antibodies, but only *immune* antibodies resulting from antigenic stimulation. Thus individual animals react with an immune response only to foreign molecules not represented by self-constituents.

Our second principle specifies "normal" individuals because autoimmune diseases reflect exceptions in which an individual reacts against his own tissues. Autoantigenicity is ordinarily but not entirely restricted to those tissue components (e.g., eye lens, thyroid follicle, brain) that are naturally isolated from contact with the lymphatic system and its immunocompetent cells.

A substantial number of immune reactions are wholly or partly dependent upon leukocytes rather than circulating antibodies. Such cellular immunity, as distinct from serum antibody-mediated effects, is decisive in certain infections and tissue transplant rejections, but the mechanisms are poorly understood. In fact, the nature of this cellular immunity is a major unsolved problem of immunology and immunogenetics. For present purposes, it is sufficient to note that most immune reactions involve the participation of both humoral antibodies and immune cells.

Just how an antigen is able to make a heritable impression on stem cells or uncommitted cells from which antibody-producing cells are derived by mitosis or transformation is unknown. In the light of newer understanding of protein biosynthesis, a mutation-like modification of nucleic acid—DNA or RNA—is implicated in antibody induction. This follows because each antibody is a distinctive new protein which would not otherwise have been made. Whether antigens bear instructions for antibody specificity or selectively activate preexisting cell lines or clones that have already arisen by mutation or genetic rearrangements is not yet clear. Much speculation and controversy surround the genetic aspects of antibody responses. Despite a paucity of decisive experimental data in this field of immunogenetics, insights are now forthcoming through studies of serum allotypes or alloantigens (Chapter Five).

The genes that impose distinct antigenic specificities on the polypeptide chains comprising immunoglobulins serve as excellent markers for molecular characterization. In this situation, the concepts of "one gene → one antigen" and "one gene → one polypeptide" may be operationally equivalent. However, the intervening steps in either formulation involve transfer of complex information. If the antigenic determinant is an oligosaccharide, the enzyme product (e.g., a glycosyl transferase) of the gene mediates the functional synthesis yielding the antigen. Except for enzymes, then, all or most antigens are secondary rather than primary gene products.

Antibody Reagents and Absorption Analyses

Serological tests have long provided the central methodology to identify antigenic characteristics. Antibody reagents nicely reveal inherited differences among individuals as well as species. Antibodies easiest to discern are those that give a visible reaction with the antigen in ordinary mediums. Simple, straightforward tests are agglutination of saline-diluted erythrocytes or bacteria in test tubes and precipitation of serum proteins on agar-gel slides. In all such antigenic typing, it is desirable that positive reactions be referable to antibodies of a single specificity. To derive antibody reagents specific for a single antigen, antiserums containing multiple antibody specificities must be absorbed with cells or solutes lacking the particular antigen. In other words, an antiserum containing antibodies against two erythrocyte antigens (e.g., A and B) could be made specific for antigen B following absorption with cells containing antigen A obtained from an individual lacking B. The anti-B reagent produced could then be used to detect the presence of antigen B on the cells of other individuals. Such monospecific or unit reagents are defined by the ability of each reactive cell type to absorb all antibody capable of reacting with any other positive cell, while negative cells remove none of the relevant antibody. Thus, in this example, cells from diverse individuals with the B antigen should absorb out all antibody from the anti-B serum capable of reacting with the cells of *any* other individual of the species. If this does not hold true, as frequently happens, an additional antibody specificity is thereby revealed. Another monospecific reagent may then be prepared to detect the newly discovered antigen.

Antiserums usually contain antibodies of multiple specificities directed against diverse antigenic determinants of the cells or even purified proteins or polysaccharides used in immunization. Monospecific reactions are best detected by cross-absorption analysis using cells or other antigenic preparations obtained from numerous individuals or sources reflecting different genetic constitutions. In a strict sense, one may contend that there is no such thing as a "monospecific" antiserum. Although the methodology of antibody absorption will effectively separate populations and subpopulations of antibodies, the antibodies remaining even after repeated absorptions may never be entirely specific for only one antigenic determinant. This reservation notwithstanding, the term *monospecific* will be used in this book in reference to antiserums which appear to be reactive operationally with only single antigenic specificities. The detailed consideration of absorption analyses to follow may require careful, repeated study by the novice. However, the approaches involved are of fundamental importance and are relevant to all later chapters.

An absorption analysis leading to the recognition of two molecular specificities is illustrated in Table 1–2. Note that the zeros (no reaction) along the diagonal dotted line are essential controls showing all antibodies for the respective absorbing cells were removed during the absorptions.

The column under individual 1 indicates that absorption of this antiserum by these cells removed all antibodies capable of reacting with further number 1 test cells, but left behind antibodies for antigens on the cells of individuals 2, 4, 5, and 6. If the antibodies capable of reacting with the individual antigens in this panel were present in high concentration, several successive absorptions with cells from given individuals might be required to remove all antibodies capable of

Table 1—2.   Absorption Analysis Revealing Two Antigenic Specificities

Test Cells from Individual	Antigenic Symbols Assigned	Antiserum						
		Unabsorbed	Absorbed with Cells of Individual					
			1	2	3	4	5	6
1	A	+	0	+	+	0	+	0
2	B	+	+	0	+	0	0	0
3	—	0	0	0	0	0	0	0
4	AB	+	+	+	+	0	+	0
5	B	+	+	0	+	0	0	0
6	AB	+	+	+	+	0	+	0

giving positive reactions with the absorbing cells. When antibodies are induced in a foreign species (e.g., rabbit anti-rat cell), many are directed toward species-specific antigens. Under these conditions, the unabsorbed immune serum invariably reacts with the cells of all individuals of the donor species. In the example of Table 1—2, which is often found in intraspecies or alloimmune systems, cells of individual 3 failed to react with the unabsorbed serum; this indicates that all the antigens which individual 3 had in common with the donor were also shared by the recipient who produced the antibodies. It also follows (see column under individual 3) that number 3 cells will not absorb out the antibodies capable of reacting with cells from the remaining individuals in the panel. The behavior of each cell source in both the absorption columns and test rows, relative to all other cell sources tested, must be consistent with the antigen symbols designated. A complete cross-absorption analysis of the type illustrated provides a two-dimensional confirmation of the validity of the individual tests.

One may assign symbols to the individual antigens (or antibody subpopulations) detected in Table 1—2 in a systematic way as follows: Beginning with the unabsorbed serum, read down the columns and assign a different letter symbol to the "antigen" detected (positive reactions) in each column. This will be a preliminary or initial assignment of factors to account for the observed reactions.

Individuals	Initial Assignment of Antigen Symbols						
1	A	—	C	D	—	E	—
2	A	B	—	D	—	—	—
3	—	—	—	—	—	—	—
4	A	B	C	D	—	E	—
5	A	B	—	D	—	—	—
6	A	B	C	D	—	E	—

Note the identical configuration of the A and D columns and the C and E columns, i.e., the pairs of letter symbols describe the same pattern of reactions. Deletion of unnecessary symbols may be achieved by reading across and then down the columns of reactions and striking out any symbol that is not required to account for the differences among the individuals tested.

Individuals	Symbols Retained After Deletions		Final Assignment of Symbols
1	–	C	A
2	B	–	B
3	–	–	–
4	B	C	AB
5	B	–	B
6	B	C	AB

The initial columns of symbols A and D are not required because the *differences* among the six individuals are already satisfied by the B and C columns. On the assumption that we are dealing with a previously unknown system, the letters A and B could be used in the final assignment of symbols; the alphabetical sequence would then be continued as new antigens were discovered. If the two antigens assigned are sufficient to account for the individual differences observed, it should follow that absorption of this antiserum with the combined cells of individuals 1 = (A), and 2 = (B) should remove all antibodies capable of reacting with cells of the remaining individuals. Furthermore, one may note that individual 2 reacts with antibodies not absorbed by 1, whereas individual 1 reacts with antibodies not absorbed by 2. These antibodies could be called anti-A and anti-B, thus explaining the whole pattern in these terms. The symbols may stand for stereochemical or fine structural features of either the antigens of their complementary (reciprocal) antibodies. The precise meaning of such symbols often engenders considerable speculation and controversy among immunogeneticists.

The reader may check his understanding of the above analysis by assigning symbols of his own to characterize the pattern of observed reactions. In the final assignment of symbols, the so-called principle of parsimony or Occam's razor should be applied: The least number of symbols that satisfies the observed reactions is to be chosen.

Using the results of an absorption analysis, one may then prepare mono-specific typing reagents by appropriate absorptions. In our example, absorption of the antiserum with cells of individual 1 should remove all anti-A and yield an anti-B reagent which could subsequently be employed to identify the B antigen in any other individual. Supposed monospecific serums on further absorption analysis with antigens of additional individuals will often reveal previously undetected antibody specificities. In other words, absorptions with antigenic preparations from other individuals might reveal additional subpopulations of antibodies, even in what appeared to be monospecific reagents in early tests. In such complex situations, true monospecific reagents are obtained only after further absorptions with antigenic preparations of different types. Absorption analyses of other immune serums would probably reveal additional antigenic types. However, given a standardized and reproducible technique, a battery of monospecific serums can eventually be accumulated that would serve to characterize the antigenic constitution of individuals tested at random. This general approach has proved invaluable in the antigenic characterization of microorganisms (Chapter Three), cellular alloantigens (Chapter Four), and serum allotypes (Chapter Five).

The simple serologic situation where antigen from any positive individuals will absorb the antibodies for all other positive individuals usually reflects a single gene difference. In progeny tests, positive individuals should be either heterozygous or homozygous for an allele producing the antigen, but negative individuals should be homozygous for a different allele at the same gene locus.

The possible results of matings involving one dominant and one recessive or inactive allele are given in Table 1–3. The distribution of the antigen in the progenies is that expected of Mendelian traits. If one or both parents is homozygous dominant, only progeny possessing the antigen should occur. Negative parents should behave as if they were homozygous recessive and produce only progeny lacking the antigen. Although the zygosity of positive parents may be unknown, it can often be deduced after testing of the progeny. Note that negativity in this instance refers only to a given antigen.

In the Table 1–2 example, four phenotypes were found—one possessing only A, one possessing only B, one possessing both A and B, and one possessing

Table 1–3. Expected Proportions of Positive (+) and Negative (−) Individuals in Progenies Involving a Single Antigen Produced by One of Two Alleles

| Type of Mating | Segregation in Progeny | |
| | Proportion | |
	Positive	Negative
+/+ X +/+	1	0
+/+ X +/−	1	0
+/+ X −/−	1	0
+/− X +/−	3	1
+/− X −/−	1	1
−/− X −/−	0	1

neither. Genetically, this result probably reflects either one gene locus with three alleles (*A*, *B*, and *neither*) or two independent loci with two alleles each (*A*, *non-A*, and *B*, *non-B*). Allelism versus independence of the genes producing antigens A and B can be differentiated by antigenic characterization of progeny from matings between parents possessing both A and B and those possessing neither (*AB* × ___). If A and B are determined by alleles, only A and B type progeny should occur, and in essentially equal numbers. If independent genes are involved, then AB progeny will occur and the other possible three types as well, depending on the genotype of the AB parent.

A similar distinction between allelic and nonallelic genes can be made from matings between AB parents: allelic genes could not result in progeny negative for both antigen determinants if there were no alleles able to code for both determinants. The possibility that such alleles exist cannot be excluded. However, extensive progeny testing may be required to distinguish alleles from closely linked genes.

Alleles and Population Structure

Most macromolecules of similar structure and function show antigenic polymorphism traceable to multiple alleles or complex loci. Why such molecular diversity persists is obscure in most instances. The far-ranging implications of the uniqueness of individuals is worth pondering. Long series of multiple alleles distinguishing individuals or subpopulations are commonly found within species ranging from protozoa to man. It should be noted that allelic genes, in general, cause only slight differences in their end products. Substantial differences would presumably destroy the functional integrity of most allelic products. Thus, the human blood-group alleles *A* and *B* appear to differ only in that *A* mediates the addition of an *N*-acetyl-galactosamine and *B*, a D-galactose, to the same precursor glycoprotein. Allelism may be discernable from serologic data alone. When tests reveal that two antigens always occur in individuals alone or together and no individuals lacking both antigens are found, it is highly probable that the determinative genes are alleles. However, appropriate mating tests are usually essential to confirm such findings.

To understand the genetic structure of different populations, one needs to determine the frequencies of known alleles. The following section may prove difficult initially to the reader who has never encountered the concepts of population genetics. It should be helpful to review this material after particular systems in later chapters are studied. Also, the reader might want to consult additional reading concerning genes in populations, as indicated in the general references.

If an allele *A* has a frequency p in a population and its only alternative *B* has a frequency q, $p+q=1$, and the distribution of genotypes in a population breeding at random and in the absence of selection should be $p^2AA + 2pqAB + q^2BB$. In other words, when gametes with chromosomes carrying this gene locus combine in pairs at random, the probability that both will have A is $p \times p = p^2$, and the probability that both will possess B is q^2. The AB heterozygotes then should have a frequency of $pq + pq = 2pq$. This $p^2 + 2pq + q^2$ distribution is equivalent to the binomial $(p + q)^2$. As long as the allele frequencies p and q remain essentially constant, a random-mating population of three genotypes in the proportions $p^2:2pq:q^2$ may be assumed to be in equilibrium, as is usually the case. The formula $p^2AA + 2pqAB + q^2BB$ and its extensions are known as the Hardy-Weinberg Law. The stability and predictability of this relationship depend on: (a) random mating in a large population with all possible genotypes equally fertile, (b) sexes evenly distributed among genotypes in a large population, and (c) individuals compared at similar developmental stages. The last consideration is to avoid being misled by age-dependent antigens.

Genetic drift may often alter an equilibrium, especially when one allele is present in low frequency. Such drift is defined as a random departure from the original gene frequency and is caused by limited interbreeding in a small population. The unusual blood group frequencies found in smaller Eskimo and North American Indian communities are perhaps best explained in terms of genetic drift. Differential mutation or selection favoring one genotype or phenotype may modify allele frequencies in successive generations. Changes in isolated, small populations caused by migrations, as is typical of today's mobile society, also alter the gene frequency significantly. Differences in cultural or behavioral traits, however, often tend to restrict gene exchange between ethnic groups.

Direct demonstration of changes in allele frequencies is achieved only by comparison of successive generations. Bentley Glass studied blood groups in a small community of Dunkers in Pennsylvania. This religious sect was derived from twenty-seven families who came from the German Rhineland to North America in the early 1700s. Their ABO frequencies now differ significantly from those typical of Rhineland Germans as well as from other Americans. The frequency of type A among Dunkers is about 60 per cent, as compared with 40–45 per cent in the other two populations. The B allele is nearly absent among Dunkers. Type O is less common in Dunkers than in Germans or Americans. Although there is no difference in the ABO frequencies of the three current generations of Dunkers, there is a substantial difference in their MN blood groups. The older Dunkers have an M allele frequency of 55 per cent, which is similar to that of German and American populations. The middle-aged group contains 68 per cent of M alleles whereas the frequency in the youngest group has risen to 73 per cent. Since the difference between the oldest and youngest groups is highly significant, the shift in allele frequency among Dunkers can probably be attributed to genetic drift.

Because population immunogenetics often requires gene frequency analysis, one should understand the application of the Hardy-Weinberg principle, at least, to simpler systems like human ABO.* Let p, q and r represent the frequencies of the three major allelic genes A, B, and O, respectively, so $p + q + r = 1$, or 100 per cent. By expansion of the binomial $(p + q + r)^2$, the frequencies of the four phenotypes can be expressed as follows:

Phenotypes	Inclusive Genotypes	Corresponding Phenotype Frequencies
O	OO	r^2
A	$AA + AO$	$p^2 + 2pr$
B	$BB + BO$	$q^2 + 2qr$
AB	AB	$2pq$

If $\bar{O}$, $\bar{A}$, $\bar{B}$, and $\overline{AB}$ symbolize the phenotype frequencies in a population, the gene frequencies may be calculated as follows:

Since

$$r^2 = \bar{O}, \ r = \sqrt{\bar{O}} \tag{1}$$
$$\bar{O} + \bar{A} = p^2 + 2pr + r^2 = (p + r)^2$$

Therefore,

$$p + r = \sqrt{\bar{O} + \bar{A}}$$

So

$$p = \sqrt{\bar{O} + \bar{A}} - \sqrt{\bar{O}} \tag{2a}$$

Similarly,

$$q = \sqrt{\bar{O} + \bar{B}} - \sqrt{\bar{O}} \tag{3a}$$

Since $p + q + r = 1$, $p + r = 1 - q$ and $q + r = 1 - p$, so $1 - q = \sqrt{\bar{O} + \bar{A}}$ and $1 - p = \sqrt{\bar{O} + \bar{B}}$.

$$p = 1 - \sqrt{\bar{O} + \bar{B}} \tag{2b}$$
$$q = 1 - \sqrt{\bar{O} + \bar{A}} \tag{3b}$$

Finally,

$$\sqrt{\bar{O} + \bar{A}} + \sqrt{\bar{O} + \bar{B}} - \sqrt{\bar{O}} = 1 \tag{4}$$

* A. M. Srb, R. D. Owen, and R. S. Edgar, *General Genetics*, 2nd ed. (W. H. Freeman and Co., San Francisco, 1965). Chapter 13 gives a more extensive exposition of genes in populations.

In Caucasian-American populations, blood group frequencies are approximately 45 per cent O, 42 per cent A, 10 per cent B, and 3 per cent AB. By substituting these values in the formulas above, one can determine the respective gene frequencies (1, 2, and 3) and test the validity of the theory of multiple-alleles in this system (formula 4).

Serological Typing Patterns

In animals which cannot be readily bred and tested in captivity, such as large ocean fish or mammals, the genetic basis of antigens distinguishing individuals in wild populations can sometimes be deduced from serological typing patterns alone. Clyde Stormont of the University of California, Davis, has demonstrated the applicability of this approach in blood-typing, a subject we shall consider in depth in Chapter Four. This approach may be illustrated with six serological patterns detected with two or three different antiserums (anti-X, anti-Y, and anti-Z). It is assumed that each antiserum distinguishes individual differences and is reasonably monospecific as ascertained by absorptions.

Antigenic Types	Anti-X	Y
1	+	+
2	+	0
3	0	+
4	0	0

(Pattern a)

This is the classic four-phenotype pattern exhibited by human red cells in tests with anti-A and anti-B. Because this pattern has a maximum expectation for randomly selected pairs of antiserum reagents and because it is typified by the well-known ABO system of blood groups, many students are hardly aware that there could be other patterns. Either the independent pairs of genes X,x and Y,y or the alleles X^x, X^y, and X^0, can explain Pattern a. Independent gene pairs and multiple alleles are usually distinguishable by gene frequency analyses.

Antingenic Types	Anti-X	Y
1	+	0
2	0	+

(Pattern b)

This two-phenotype pattern is rare. About the only good example is in typing certain populations of sheep with anti-O and anti-R reagents. One of the two types is inherited as a recessive. Although this pattern can best be explained by a single pair of alleles with one being dominant, other explanations are not excluded.

| Antigenic | Anti- | |
Types	X	Y
1	+	0
2	0	+	(Pattern c)
3	0	0

This three-phenotype pattern, which is merely an extension of Pattern b to include a "negative" phenotype, is also rarely encountered. It is best exemplified by the reactions of human red cells with anti-Le^a and anti-Le^b, and the reactions of sheep red cells in certain populations with anti-O and anti-R. The patterns of b and c have been invariably associated with serologically reactive, soluble substances elaborated in the tissues and acquired in the plasma by the red cells. Although a single pair of alleles with one being dominant accounts for types 1 and 2, a second locus with epistatic effects is invoked to explain type 3.

| Antigenic | Anti- | |
Types	X	Y
1	+	0
2	0	+	(Pattern d)
3	+	+

There are many examples of this three-phenotype pattern, the classic one being the reactions of human red cells with anti-M and anti-N. This pattern is readily explicable by a pair of codominant alleles, but such systems must often be expanded by invoking more alleles when additional antibodies are considered.

| Antigenic | Anti- | |
Types	X	Y
1	+	+
2	+	0	(Pattern e)
3	0	0

There are also many examples of this three-phenotype pattern. The classic one is the reaction of human red cells with anti-A and anti-A$_1$ serums. Thus, individuals of subgroups A$_1$, A$_2$, and neither may be distinguished, because only unabsorbed anti-A serum reacts with cells having either A$_1$ or A$_2$. This pattern is the simplest of all linear subtyping patterns. Like all linear and nonlinear subtyping relationships, this pattern connotes multiple alleles. Three alleles (X^{xy}, X^x, and X^0) can explain this example.

The final subtyping pattern requires three differential reagents and involves both linear and nonlinear elements.

Antigentic Types	Anti-		
	X	Y	Z
1	+	+	+
2	+	+	0
3	+	0	0
4	0	+	0
5	0	0	0

(Pattern *f*)

This five-phenotype pattern may be regarded as Pattern *a* superimposed on Pattern *e*. Reagents anti-X and anti-Y, when considered independently of anti-Z, exhibit Pattern *a*; whereas each set of pairs, anti-X and anti-Z, and anti-Y and anti-Z, exhibit Pattern *e*. Blood factors X and Y are said to be related through Z as nonlinear subtypes. The classic example of this particular pattern is the reaction of cattle red cells with the reagents, anti-B, anti-G, and anti-K. This pattern can be explained by at least four alleles: X^{xyz}, X^x, X^y, and X^0. An additional X^{xy} allele might also be involved.

Even if the genetic basis of a typing pattern is not deducible with certainty, the relative frequencies of antigenic types in separate breeding populations may differ sufficiently to allow the investigator to identify the source of a population sample. For example, differentiating between American and Asian species of salmon caught in the Pacific ocean has been done in this manner. The potential usefulness of the above typing patterns should become more obvious to the reader when he is familiar with the various systems of cellular alloantigens and serum allotypes detailed in Chapters Four and Five.

Gene-Antigen Relationships Deduced from Phenotype Frequencies

How much genetic information can one derive from phenotype frequencies alone? Two-by-two tables can be useful in distinguishing between allelism and nonallelism based on phenotypes found in random populations of a species. The question of allelism arises regularly in early studies of both cellular and soluble antigens. Although the following problem-solving techniques have been applied mainly to blood group studies, they may be used to advantage in many other systems involving antigenic differences within a species. Here again alleles are considered to be alternate units of a chromosomal locus in contrast to genes at noncontiguous loci. In the usual situation, two antigens X and Y are detectable by anti-X and anti-Y serums in four phenotypic classes: X+Y+, X+Y−, X−Y+, and X−Y−, where the + and − signs indicate presence or absence, respectively, of the antigen. These two antigens are assumed to be derived from either dominant or codominant genes. Also, a total of N random individuals from a population in Hardy-Weinberg equilibrium must have been typed with anti-X and anti-Y. Such data may then be considered in terms of the following hypotheses:

Hypothesis	Number of Loci	Allelic Sets of Genes
A. Nonallelism	2	X, O and Y, O'
B. Three Alleles	1	X, Y, O
C. Four Alleles	1	X, Y, XY, O

A distinction among these genetic hypotheses was attempted especially by Andresen and Baker at Iowa State University using actual data.

Initially a two-by-two table may be constructed as follows, where a, b, c, and d represent the observed number of individuals in each of the four phenotypic classes.

Phenotype	Y+	Y−	Totals
X+	a	b	a + b
X−	c	d	c + d
Totals	a + c	b + d	N

Assuming allelism versus nonallelism where p, q, and $1 - (p + q)$ are the frequencies for genes X, Y, and O, respectively, the expected numbers of phenotypes in these four classes are determined as follows: $1 - (p + q)$ represents the null gene(s) that fails to yield a detectable antigenic product.

Numbers Observed	Numbers Expected	
	Allelism (3 Alleles)	Nonallelism
a(X+Y+)	$N \cdot 2pq$	$(a + b)(a + c)/N$
b(X+Y−)	$N \cdot [p^2 + 2p(1 - p - q)]$	$(a + b)(b + d)/N$
c(X−Y+)	$N \cdot [p^2 + 2q(1 - p - q)]$	$(a + b)(b + d)/N$
d(X−Y−)	$N \cdot (1 - p - q)^2$	$(b + d)(c + d)/N$

Testing of a four-allele hypothesis is more complicated since there are ten genotypes corresponding to the four phenotypes. This requires four additional phenotype frequency formulas in the $a = (X+Y+)$ category, as shown in parentheses below for each relevant genotype.

Phenotypes	Corresponding Genotypes				
X+Y+	X/Y,	XY/O,	XY/X,	XY/Y,	XY/XY
	$(N \cdot 2pq)$	$[N \cdot 2pq(1-p-q)]$	$(N \cdot 2pq \cdot p)$	$(N \cdot 2pq \cdot q)$	$(N \cdot 2pq \cdot 2pq)$
X+Y−	X/X, X/O				
X−Y+	Y/Y, Y/O				
X−Y−	O/O				

For purposes of chi-square analysis of the most probable genetic relationship, the two antigens X and Y must be independent, or referable to three of four alleles. No other possibilities are inherent in the mathematical treatmant of two-by-two tables. Given a total of four phenotypes, p equals $1-\sqrt{(X-Y+)+(X-Y-)/N}$ and q equals $1-\sqrt{(X+Y-)+(X-Y-)/N}$ for purposes of estimating allele frequencies.

Considering a distribution of one hundred phenotypes as 4 X+Y+, 11 X+Y-, 38 X-Y+, and 47 X-Y-, p is calculated to be 0.08 and $q = 0.24$ using the above formulas. The reader's understanding of this approach may be checked by working out the solution to this and subsequent problems. The conventional chi-square formula for testing independence in this situation is $X^2 = (ad - bc)^2 N/(a + b)(c + d)(a + c)(b + d)$. The calculated chi-square value of 1.70 for nonallelism corresponds to $0.10 < P < 0.20$. Expected numbers of phenotypes do not differ significantly from observed numbers, but a hypothesis of allelism fits the observed distribution much better than one of independence at the 5 per cent significance level, as shown in Fig. 1–2. Thus if a straight edge is laid across the p scale at 0.08 parallel to the q scale, the $N = 100$ curve is intersected at q values of 0.39 and 0.92.

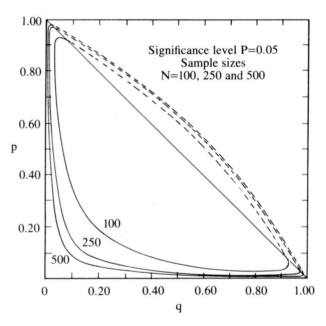

Figure 1–2. Sample sizes required to disprove independent segregation for genes of frequencies p and q by means of the chi-square test and assuming a 3-allelic relationship yielding two identifiable antigens with one null allele. (Adapted from Andresen et al., *Immunogenetics Letter,* Vol. 3: 17, 1963.)

Note, then, that the hypothesis of three alleles for $p = 0.08$ cannot be rejected for $N = 100$ unless $0.39 < q < 0.92$. However, about 250 random individuals would be needed in this instance to disprove independent segregation. Thus, a rather large sample size is required to disprove independence with respect to low gene frequencies. Note that if the chi-square value is not elevated, independence cannot be claimed, because failure to disprove a hypothesis does not constitute proof of the same hypothesis.

If high chi-square and low probability values make both the hypotheses of nonallelism and three alleles unlikely, the four-allele hypothesis should be considered. Such was the case when the phenotype distribution was 133 X+Y+, 136 X+Y-, 88 X-Y+, and 37 X-Y- in a total of 394 random individuals. Here the symbols X and Y actually stand for N and S of the human MNSs blood-group system (Chapter Four) which involves four alleles, as established directly by family data.

Because long series of multiple alleles are commonly responsible for specification of antigens, two-by-two tables often tend to oversimplify reality. To avoid erroneous conclusions, family studies should be undertaken whenever possible. When a codominant locus has more than three alleles in substantial frequencies, family data may involve many possible types of matings. Thus, four alleles represented by ten genotypes may occur in fifty-five different types of matings, while six alleles lead to an impressive twenty-one genotypes and 241 potentially different matings. However, the maximum number of genotypes which can result from any one mating is four, and this would involve unlike heterozygotes. This restriction is being used to advantage in family pedigrees for histocompatibility typing in man (Chapter Eight).

Terminology of Immunogenetics

Thus far in our discussion of antigens and antibodies, special terminology has not been needed to define particular immunogenetic relationships. In the field of comparative immunogenetics and especially tissue transplantation, precise terms are desirable to indicate various donor-recipient relationships. After many years of controversy concerning usage, there is now increasing agreement on terminology. (See summary in Table 1–4.) The preferred prefixes for equivalent nouns and adjectives are: *auto*: self to self, *iso*: between genetically identical individuals, *allo*: between genetically different individuals of same species, and *xeno*: between individuals of different species. The long established terms isoantigen and isoantibody (also, e.g., isoagglutinin and isohemolysin), used especially in blood group studies, denote intraspecific incompatibility or dissimilarity. Unfortunately, the prefix *iso* implies sameness or identity and has this exact connotation in *isogenic* individuals who should *not*, by definition, show any (iso)antigenic disparities. The substitution of alloantigen and alloantibody for isoantigen and isoantibody creates a wholly consistent and etymologically appropriate vocabulary. Nevertheless, the reader should expect to see all of the terms given in Table 1—4 in the literature for quite a while.

Increasing advantage is being taken of inbred strains of animals with a common genetic background except for certain known hereditary differences which may accordingly be studied with greater precision. *Coisogenic strains* are defined as strains identical except for a difference at a single gene locus. Such coisogenicity is presumably achieved only after a mutation occurs in an established inbred strain. *Congenic strains*, now readily available in mice, conveniently approximate the coisogenic state. They have been produced with deliberate selection by continued crossing of a gene from one strain onto the inbred and therefore isogenic background of a different strain. The foreign gene introduced into the established strain is always included in a chromosome segment which contains certain contaminant or additional unwanted genes. As the number of backcross matings to the inbred ("homozygous") strain is increased, however, the number of unselected contaminant genes will decrease until the new strain is nearly coisogenic with the inbred parent strain. Many congenic strains of mice that differ at gene loci governing histocompatibility have been developed in recent years, especially by Dr. George Snell at the Jackson Laboratory, Bar Harbor, Maine. Methods of producing such congenic strains are considered in detail in Chapter Six.

In the most elementary terms, immunogenetics may be defined as the study of gene-antigen-antibody relationships. The "gene → antigen" component involves the elucidation of genetic fine structure and function in relation to structural determinants of macromolecular antigens. "Gene → antibody" relationships may be decisive in controlling immune response capacities because given genes regulate specific antibody responses. The mechanisms and manifestations of "antigen → antibody" reactions are of course central to general immunology as well as immunogenetics.

Complexity and Heterogeneity of Antibodies

The reader should be aware of the major features of antibody structure which will be pertinent in all the chapters to follow. IgG or immunoglobulin gamma, the chief class of antibodies in mammals, is a protein molecule consisting of four polypeptide chains joined together by disulfide (S—S) bonds. There are two light (L) chains and two heavy (H) chains, the members of each pair of chains being identical in a given antibody molecule. A three-dimensional diagram of an IgG globulin molecule is shown in Fig. 1—3. Depending on the source, heavy chains contain about 420 to 440 amino acid units while light chains contain from 210 to 230 amino acids. All known antibodies are found within five major molecular classes of serum immunoglobulins that are distinguished mainly by the different compositions (and antigenicity) of their H chains.

Table 1–4. Terminology of Transplantation and Immunogenetics

Nouns		Adjectives			Immunogenetic Relationship
Preferred	Less Desirable Terms or Synonyms	Preferred	Acceptable Synonyms	Less Desirable Old Terms	
Autograft		Autogeneic	Autogenous Autochthonous	Autoplastic Autologous	Self to self; compatible
Isograft		Isogeneic (Isogenic)	Syngeneic	Isologous	Between genetically identical individuals; compatible
Allograft	Homograft	Allogeneic (Allogenic)		Homologous	Between genetically disparate individuals of same species; usually incompatible
Xenograft	Heterograft	Xenogeneic		Heterologous Heterospecific Heterogeneic	Between different species; incompatible
Allotype Alloantigen Alloantibody	Serum Isoantigen Isoantigen Isoantibody	Allotypic Alloantigenic Alloimmune		Isoantigenic Isoantigenic Isoimmune	Involving genetically disparate individuals of same species; usually incompatible
		Histocompatible	Isohistogenic		Genotype of donor not foreign to host; e.g., inbred strain → F_1 hybrid offspring

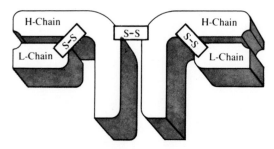

Figure 1—3. Schematic representation of an antibody molecule showing the four polypeptide chains joined by disulfide (S—S) bonds.

These classes in man are most often designated as IgG, IgM, IgA, IgD, and IgE. The first two letters stand for Immunoglobulin and are often interchanged with the gamma (γ) prefix. The predominant antibody classes (i.e., IgG, IgM, and IgA) show striking differences in carbohydrate content, of unknown function, associated with the H chains. The same two types of L chains, designated kappa (K) and lambda (L), are found in nearly all immunoglobulin classes, but both light chains are of the same type in any one molecule. About half of the amino acids of L chains and a lesser fraction of H chains are constant or invariant; the remainder of both H and L chains, including the antibody combining sites, are highly variable in their amino acid sequences. Studies with separate H and L chain fractions from known purified antibodies strongly suggest that both chains are involved in the specific combining sites of the usual bivalent molecules. At least several amino acids are contained in antibody combining sites, but the critical number responsible for complementariness toward an antigen continues to be an exasperating unknown.

Since antibodies of any specificity whatsoever may be found in any molecular class, there is no general correlation between class and specificity. Moreover, no chemical or physical property has yet been found that can distinguish among diverse antibody populations of different specificity. The only method available for the separation of such antibody populations is selective absorption, as previously discussed. Although an individual animal may fail to respond, or respond poorly, to a given antigen, no limit is known to the number of specific antibodies that any one species—whether mouse or man—can synthesize.

The genetic control of antibody structure is under much speculation. Is one species potentially capable of synthesizing an infinite number of antibodies or only a large, but hereditarily limited number of specificities? Both the biological (i.e., functional) and molecular heterogeneity of antibodies are formidable, especially from a genetic standpoint. In addition to subclasses showing substantial H-chain differences and allelic variants leading to separate modifications of both H and L chains, there is "idiotypic complexity." Thus, individual animals may produce seemingly unique antibodies distinct from those inducible in other individuals of the same species. Little is known yet about the relationship of idiotypic alterations to heavy or light chain composition. These different levels of complexity are illustrated schematically in Fig. 1–4.

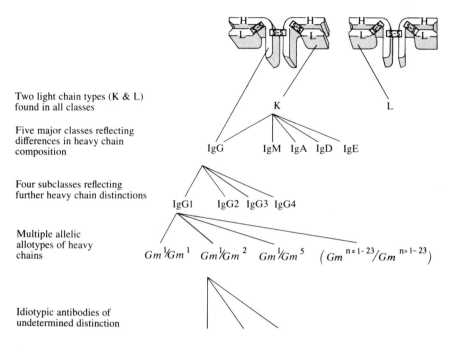

Two light chain types (K & L) found in all classes

Five major classes reflecting differences in heavy chain composition

Four subclasses reflecting further heavy chain distinctions

Multiple allelic allotypes of heavy chains

Idiotypic antibodies of undetermined distinction

K   L

IgG   IgM IgA IgD IgE

IgG1   IgG2 IgG3 IgG4

Gm^{1}/Gm^{1} Gm^{1}/Gm^{2} Gm^{1}/Gm^{5} $\left(Gm^{n=1-23}/Gm^{n=1-23}\right)$

Figure 1–4.   Complexity and heterogeneity of antibodies is manifested at several levels. Subdivisions of human immunoglobulins are shown here for just one branch at each level. Differences in genes at various loci are probably responsible for idiotypic specificities. (See Chapter Five for detailed consideration of immunoglobulin classes and allotypes.)

The specific configuration of the antibody-combining site is in the variable section of the molecule and is determined presumably by the amino acid sequence. Given the present understanding of the nature of protein synthesis, most immunogeneticists assume that antigens select for or "turn-on" preexisting "gene → antibody" potentialities. They reject the alternative that antigens serve merely as templates to impress complementary configurations on "normal" immunoglobulins at the polysome level of terminal synthesis (Chapter Two).

According to one hypothesis, there may be a single gene coding for the stable section of each chain and many genes (hundreds of thousands?), equivalent to the individual's repertoire of antibody possibilities, coding for the variable sections. The immunocyte would also need a regulatory gene or enzyme to fuse the stable and variable sections into complete molecules. However, heavy and light chains appear to be synthesized continuously from the amino- to the carboxyl- end without intermediates. This could argue against separate synthesis and later union of the constant and variable portions of the chains.

Another concept involves genetic recombination during ontogeny: several complex loci might be divided into stable and variable regions with sufficient interchange of nucleotides in the variable region during cell division to allow coding for a large, potential spectrum of antibodies.

Hypermutation hypotheses must account for limitation of the variability to only part of the light and heavy polypeptide chains. Mutation would presumably have to be controlled in such a way that changes in single nucleotides did not occur. Otherwise the reading frame for the constant part of the gene would be displaced because the variable parts of the polypeptide chains in the N-terminal halves are synthesized first.

Still another idea envisages a recognition point in each complex locus for heavy or light chain synthesis. Enzymatic splitting or other types of modulation of the gene in the portion that codes for the variable section, followed by repair, could conceivably lead to codon rearrangements or repression.

At this time, several theories which favor somatic recombination as the principal basis for antibody diversity are receiving much attention, but the evidence is not compelling. Whatever the answer, the extensive constant and variable sections in both heavy and light chains evidently require complex genetic-control mechanisms. In the broadest sense, the characteristics of "gene → antigen → antibody" interactions encompass diverse molecular, developmental and physiological events. The initial section of Chapter Five dealing with classes and properties of immunoglobulins may also be consulted for further amplification of this subject.

Antibody-Specificity Relationships

Even in this introduction, the reader should become alert to the more difficult interpretive issues in relating symbolism for antigen-antibody reactions to the genes that control antigenic molecules. We shall return to this theme in later chapters in connection with *Salmonella* somatic antigens, complex blood group systems such as Rh in man, and immunoglobulin allotype systems. Most genes which behave as Mendelian alleles have many antigenic determinants associated with their individual macromolecular products, but few or none of the antigenic units may be unique to any one allele. Of the thirty-three antigenic specificities associated with the twenty alleles of the *H-2* system of mice, for example, all but seven occur in conjunction with at least three different alleles. Indeed, specificity 5 recurs some thirteen times (see Chapter Four, page 100). In this and most other instances, the chemical identity of the individual antigenic components in relation to intramolecular localization is unknown.

There are two disparate views of the relationship between a specific antiserum that defines a given antigen and the antigenic molecule or submolecule with which it reacts. According to one view, each distinctive specificity (e.g., numbers 1–33 in the *H-2* system cited) represents a distinct antigen or subunit, such as a given amino acid in a polypeptide chain. The other view holds that a single antigenic unit or site may elicit the production of heterogeneous antibodies which are all directed, at least partially, to the one site. Moreover, single known sugars in antigens like those of *Salmonella* somatic polysaccharides may determine several different antigenic specificities, depending on the adjacent molecular attachments. Whenever there are subpopulations of distinctive antibodies reactive with different stereochemical features of the same antigen, cross-reactions with similar antigens are expected. Elimination of cross-reactive antibodies lacking precise specificity may be accomplished by absorptions and absorption analyses as discussed earlier (page 8).

It is axiomatic that not all antibodies are uniquely complementary to the antigens which evoked them. Karl Landsteiner's numerous studies with conjugated antigens involving chemically defined haptens made it clear long ago that "antibodies react most strongly upon the homologous antigen, but also regularly, with graded affinity, on chemically related substances." An absorbed antiserum may retain certain cross-reactive antibodies, just as a number of similar keys may fit a lock more-or-less well. The actual structure of the lock (antigen) is characterized, *reciprocally*, of course, by the three-dimensional pattern of the best-fitting key(s) (antibody).

In a molecular sense, an antigen and its complementary antibody must be defined reciprocally. From the viewpoint which equates a distinct antigen with a well-defined serological specificity, designation of an antigenic unit as R should indicate a certain chemical entity, irrespective of the possible molecular heterogeneity of antibodies that may possess anti-R combining sites. The contending viewpoint would define R less precisely as a symbol of capacity to react with a subpopulation of similar antibodies having the specificity anti-R. In other words, R may be thought merely to symbolize a subpopulation of antibodies (i.e., an antibody reagent) of anti-R specificity.

Still another approach focuses attention on R as a precise molecular unit on the one hand, and on anti-R as a defined, but imprecise, identifying reagent on the other. Antigen in the singular sense of a defined portion of a macromolecule (e.g., an oligosaccharide or certain amino acid or acids) is often referred to as an antigenic specificity, determinant, site, or unit. The choice of term need not imply a certain degree of complementariness or affinity for the corresponding antibodies. Although antibodies may conform differentially to very small substituent groups or haptens such as $COOH$, SO_3H, and AsO_3H_2 on aminobenzene rings, and may even distinguish ortho-, meta-, and para-positions of the same group, the total area of an antibody-combining site is ordinarily sufficient to include many additional molecular groups nearby.

In the case of the ABH and Lewis antigens of man (Chapter Four), the antigenic symbols can be related to known sugars and their linkages. It is not certain whether all antigen symbols may eventually be interpreted in terms of known small molecules. In this respect, one may dare to hope that the tyranny of antibody heterogeneity may yet be overcome as well as understood.

Diversity of Immunogenetic Approaches

In addition to well-established serologic systems, there are many new immunogenetic approaches ranging from tissue transplantation tests to mixed cell culture techniques now serving to elucidate reactivities which are often subtle. Special techniques of serotyping are now employed for ever finer resolution of cellular alloantigens and for a more precise definition of the antibodies responsible for disease than was possible before. Transfusion reactions to blood cells and maternal-fetal immunization, as in hemolytic disease of the newborn (Chapter Four), are important in this connection.

Recent investigations indicate that specific tolerance (Chapter Seven) permits the uninhibited growth of certain tumors in experimental animals. The question arises whether cancer in humans develops only in individuals with impaired or defective immune responses. The consistent occurrence of specific and usually weak tumor antigens in diverse experimental systems (Chapter Three) supports the belief that techniques for stimulating or augmenting specific immune responses may prove important in cancer therapy. On the other hand, successful human organ transplantation requires not only approximate antigenic matching of donors and recipients, but cautious use of immunosuppressive drugs to prevent early graft rejection due to some, seemingly inevitable, mismatching (Chapter Eight). Weak antigenic disparities and promotion of allograft tolerance are sought in this connection as being most promising. Many of these problems, however, are more easily stated than solved.

The scope of the subject of immunogenetics may be epitomized by a triangle as follows:

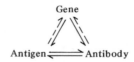

Reciprocal arrows are meant to indicate all possible biosynthetic or regulatory interactions among specific genes, antigens, and antibodies. Relationships suggested by solid arrows are well established in many areas, but those indicated by broken arrows are little understood.

KEY REFERENCES

1. ANDRESEN, E., and L. N. BAKER. "Distinguishing Between Various Genetic Theories Using Random Population Material." *Immunogenetics Letter*, Vol. 3: 95–99, 1964. Details usefulness and limitations of two-by-two tables and chi-square analysis in distinguishing between allelism and nonallelism in random-breeding populations.

2. *ANTIBODIES*. Cold Spring Harbor Symp. Quant. Biol., Vol. 32, 1968. The section on evolution and genetics of antibodies, pp. 133–172, focuses on theories and possible mechanisms of antibody variability in terms of the genetic code.

3. CARLSON, E. A. *The Gene: A Critical History*. W. B. Saunders Co., Phila. and London, 1966. Traces and incisively evaluates classical and modern concepts of genes and their interactions.

4. HILDEMANN, W. H. "Immunogenetic Studies of Poikilothermic Animals". *Amer. Naturalist*, Vol. 96: 195–204, 1962. Considers immunological competence as a primary genetic attribute; also discusses independent approaches to immunogenetic characterization of populations of vertebrate species.

5. *ISOANTIGENS AND CELL INTERACTIONS* Wistar Institute Symp. Monogr. No. 3, Wistar Institute Press Phila., 1965. Considers various cellular and antigenic interactions, especially among inbred strains of mice.

6. LANDSTEINER, K. *The Specificity of Serological Reactions*, rev. ed. Harvard Univ. Press, Cambridge, 1947. A classic monograph, still well worth careful study, by a great pioneer.

7. OWEN, R. D. "Immunogenetics," in *Proc. X Internatl. Congr. Genet.*, Vol. 1, Univ. of Toronto Press, pp. 364–374, 1959. An excellent review of the fundamentals of immunogenetics as understood through the decade of the 1950s.

8. ———. "Methods in Mammalian Immunogenetics," in *Methodology in Mammalian Genetics*, Holden-Day, Inc., San Francisco, pp. 347–377, 1963. Summarizes diverse immunogenetic methods and discusses their limitations.

9. PORTER, R. R. "The Structure of Antibodies." *Scientific American*, Vol. 217: 81–90, 1967. Interprets concisely current knowledge of antibody structure and heterogeneity in relation to possible genetic controls of antibody specificity.

10. RUSSELL, P. S., and A. P. MONACO. *The Biology of Tissue Transplantation*. Little, Brown & Co., Boston, 1965. Covers the fundamentals of transplantation biology in a concise and readable way.

11. SHREFFLER, D. C. "Molecular Aspects of Immunogenetics," in *Ann. Rev. Genet.,* Vol. 1: 163–184, 1967. Briefly reviews various immunogenetic systems and their applications with emphasis on the genetic control of alloantigen biosynthesis.

12. SRB, A. M., R. D. OWEN, and R. S. EDGAR. *General Genetics,* 2nd ed. W. H. Freeman and Co., San Francisco, 1965. Recommended reading for those whose knowledge of basic genetics is rudimentary or rusty.

TWO

INHERITANCE OF IMMUNE RESPONSE CAPACITIES

The capacity to resist or withstand infection and to dispose of foreign substances that enter the tissues is essential to the survival of all species—ranging from microorganisms to man. The staphylococci must cope with virulent phages and antibiotics just as man himself must be able to cope with the staphylococci. Specific immunological competence or memory has appeared, until quite recently, to be characteristic only of vertebrates. The adaptive immunity of vertebrates is generally associated in ontogeny, and phylogeny with the development of lymphocytic cells, a thymus gland, and the ability to produce serum antibodies. The available evidence suggests that invertebrates, microorganisms, and plants have more generalized or, in some classes, perhaps more specialized phagocytic or molecular mechanisms to dispose of pathogens. Beyond nonspecific phagocytosis, little is yet known about the seemingly versatile defense mechanisms of invertebrates.

Exciting recent work of E. L. Cooper reveals the occurrence of specific transplantation immunity in annelid worms. Concomitant immunological memory is also evident, but any potential for circulating antibody production remains to be detected. Although a variety of agglutinating, bactericidal, and lytic substances has been described in invertebrates, humoral antibodies with vertebrate properties have not been identified. Serum components comparable to vertebrate globulins are conspicuously lacking in most if not all invertebrate serums. On the other hand, immune responses in vertebrates have become increasingly well defined at both cellular and humoral (immunoglobulin) levels.

Instruction Versus Selection for Antibody Specificity

Understanding of the mechanisms of immune responses must depend upon knowledge of the genetic control of specific immune reactions. Two contrasting conceptions of the instigation of antibody production—instructive and select-ive—with many variations have been proposed. Put as a question, do antigens merely select certain competent cell lines that arise by mutation or differentia-tion, or do they transmit instructions for antibody specificity? Increasing evidence that antibody specificity is determined by the primary amino acid sequence of the constituent H and L chains negates older instructive theories proposing that antigens serve as templates which imprint specific complemen-tarity into the secondary and tertiary structure of immunoglobulins. Instruction could conceivably derive from the combination of antigenic determinants with nucleic acids which in turn mediate specific changes in polypeptide structure. On this basis, antigens could be presumed to modify RNA codons at the level of translation of genetic information into amino acid sequences.

Selective theories, on the other hand, postulate that the information required to make any given antibody is already present in the individual prior to antigenic stimulation. Antigen then functions to stimulate synthesis or increased produc-tion of antibodies by appropriate clones or cell lines. A high rate of spontaneous somatic mutation or genetic recombination may be invoked for selection alone to be operative while comparable induced changes in nucleotide sequences are required for instruction alone. In either event, a cell making a given antibody should have a correspondingly unique sequence of nucleotides for globulin synthesis. An imposing amount of genetic information is required to account for the large number of known antibodies and tolerant states on any basis. Further speculation concerning instructive and selective components of specific respon-siveness is not warranted because critical evidence is insufficient at this time.

Immune Responses to Infectious Agents

It has long been recognized that diverse stocks or strains of domestic animals, from honey bees to horses, show profound differences in genetic resistance to particular pathogens. Such resistance often has a multigenic basis, as might be expected from the complex sequence of events involved in most immune or resistance responses. In a number of instances, genetically determined host resistance to infection appears to depend primarily upon the specific immune reponse. For example, several strains of mice, selectively inbred by Gowen, each show a characteristic degree of resistance to a cloned strain of *Salmonella typhimurium.* As shown in Fig. 2–1, the range, measured as per cent animals surviving infection, is from nearly complete resistance to practically complete susceptibility. It should be noted that the same host genotypes capable of

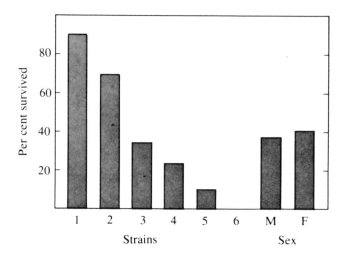

Figure 2–1. Resistance of different strains and sexes of inbred mice to a cloned line of *Salmonella typhimurium*; measured with respect to survival twenty-one days after infection with 2×10^5 bacteria. (Adapted from Gowen, *Bact. Revs.*, Vol. 24: 192, 1960.)

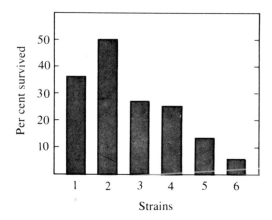

Figure 2–2. Resistance acquired by the same inbred strains of mice indicated in Fig. 2–1 following immunization with heat-killed *S. typhimurium*. The immunized mice were challenged with a large dose of 5×10^7 virulent bacteria and were scored as before. Note that specific immunity acquired by host genotypes after vaccination is generally similar in degree to that found in the absence of prior immunization. (Adapted from Gowen, *Bact. Revs.*, Vol. 24: 192, 1960.)

surviving infection were likewise able, in similar degrees, to develop and utilize the specific immunity induced by a killed vaccine of this *Salmonella* strain (Fig. 2–2). Dominance of most genes facilitating resistance or immunity was indicated in these extensive studies. Females were generally found to be more resistant than males. In various other studies, females have also been found to give stronger antibody responses than males.

The relative specificity of immunogenetic resistance to disease is demonstrated by the finding that a high degree of resistance to one pathogen may often exist alongside of low resistance to an unrelated pathogen. Thus, one of Gowen's strains most resistant to mouse typhoid proved highly susceptible to pseudorabies virus. Moreover, two strains similarly resistant to pseudorabies showed a disparate vulnerability to ricin, the toxic protein of the castor bean.

Resistance or susceptibility to infectious agents usually involves complex interactions between host and parasites. Indeed, under certain circumstances, the host's immune response may be only of secondary importance. In sickle-cell anemia, for example, substitution of a valine residue for a glutamic acid in the globin (i.e., beta-chain) portion of hemoglobin is the molecular basis of the disease. Patients with sickle-cell anemia are unusually susceptible to *Salmonella* infections with concomitant osteomyelitis. However, heterozygous individuals with the sickle-cell trait are partially resistant to falciparum malaria or to its cerebral manifestations. It is apparent that the otherwise deleterious sickle-cell gene represents a selective advantage in malarious regions such as tropical Africa. However, the reason for the special vulnerability of homozygous recessive individuals to osteomyelitic Salmonellosis is obscure. The fungus disease, disseminated coccidiomycosis, is markedly more frequent in Filipinos and American Negroes than in Caucasians. Here susceptibility is associated with dark pigmented skin and the specific immune response is not decisive. Although hereditary constitution is universally recognized as important in determining the relative susceptibility of the individual to infection, the particular genes responsible for this predisposition are unknown in most instances. Familial tendency to certain infectious diseases such as leprosy or tuberculosis may often be attributed to prolonged or intimate contact with the pathogen and exposure to high dosages.

Even a normally adequate immune response capacity may be circumvented by genetic changes in virulence of the pathogen. The potential virulence of pneumoccoci is known to be determined by the amount of specific capsular polysaccharide synthesized because the polysaccharide has substantial antiphagocytic effects. Similarly, the virulence of streptococci depends on the presence and amount of type-specific M protein on the bacterial surface because the protein also inhibits phagocytosis. Efficient phagocytosis leading to enzymatic digestion of complex particulate antigens is usually an essential prerequisite for antibody production.

A variety of hereditary defects associated with impaired immune responses to infectious agents in man are outlined in Table 2–1. Fundamental aberrations in serum globulin production restrict the individual's ability to produce specific opsonins essential for prompt phagocytosis. Such abnormalities range from almost complete absence of antibody synthesis (hypogammaglobulinemia) to excessive production of one or more classes of immunoglobulins that fail to facilitate leukocytic destruction of virulent bacteria. Recent data suggest that lack of ability to respond to specific antigens is the cause rather than the result of the deficiency in plasma cells in most types of hypogammaglobulinemia. The so-called Swiss type of profound agammaglobulinemia is mainly an autosomal recessive trait (but occasionally X-linked) which leads to a failure of embryonic differentiation of the thymus gland. This entity is now commonly designated as hereditary thymic aplasia. No chromosomal abnormality has been found in affected children. The sex-linked recessive determination of congenital hypo-gammaglobulinemia has been repeatedly confirmed by its diagnosis in boys whose normal sisters subsequently had sons with the disease. Heterozygous female carriers of the gene are not detectable by currently available methods. The incidence of this gene is unknown; it appears to be rather closely linked to the $Xg(a)$ blood group locus, but its relation to other X-linked loci remains to be determined. Although at least several genetic loci are probably involved in different hypergammaglobulinemias, particular loci probably determine given defects in class-specific polypeptide chains. These questions are now under intensive investigation.

Genetic defects in the production of normal granulocytes lead to hyper-susceptibility to bacterial infections. This leukocyte type then is essential for the immune destruction of bacteria in man. The Chediak-Higashi syndrome, inherited as an autosomal recessive trait, was first described in man in 1943 by Beguez-Cesar and was later discovered in mink and cattle. Affected individuals of all three species are notably susceptible to bacterial infections, and additionally in mink to a slow viral disease known as Aleutian disease. Blood granulocytes and monocytes of affected individuals, which are defective in phagocytosis, contain enlarged granules. Presumably homologous genes are involved in all three species.

In many other hereditary diseases, such as diabetes mellitus, the relationship between the primary abnormality and defective immune responsiveness is unknown. Although diabetes mellitus is attributable to a single recessive gene, the well-known association between obesity and diabetes implicates other genetic and environmental factors as well. It should be noted that these serum globulin and leukocyte abnormalities do not generally impair the immune response to viruses. Except in infants with hereditary thymic aplasia, which also engenders susceptibility to viral infections, the capacity for cellular hyper-sensitivity reactions and for allograft rejection remains intact. Why these

Table 2–1. Some Hereditary Defects Associated with Impaired Immune Responses to Infectious Agents in Man

Hereditary Disease	Aberration or Phenotypic Manifestation	Associated Infection	Genetic Basis	Reliability of Genetic Evidence
A. *Serum globulin abnormality*				
1. Hypogammaglobulinemia	Deficiency of lymphoid cells producing serum antibody; absence of γM and γA; low levels of γG	Bacterial infections; viral hepatitis	Sex-linked recessive	Convincing
2. Agammaglobulinemia (hereditary thymic aplasia)	General failure of immunoglobulin production associated with atrophy of all lymphoid tissues	Bacterial infections; viral hepatitis	Autosomal recessive	Convincing
3. Hypergammaglobulinemia	Abnormal and excessive production of γG, γA, *or* γM immunoglobulins	Chronic bacterial infections	Polygenic	Suggestive
B. *Leukocyte abnormality*				
1. Familial neutropenia	Deficiency of granulocytes	Bacterial infections	Dominant	Suggestive
2. Chediak-Higashi	Abnormal granulocytes with diminished phagocytic ability	Bacterial infections	Autosomal recessive	Suggestive
C. *Unknown relationship to immune responsiveness*				
1. Sickle-cell anemia	Abnormal hemoglobin	Salmonellosis, esp., osteomyelitis	Autosomal recessive	Convincing
2. Diabetes mellitus	Abnormal insulin metabolism	Staphylococcal skin infections; pyelonephritis; tuberculosis	Autosomal recessive	Suggestive
3. None	Dark pigmented skin	Disseminated coccidioidomycosis	Dominant (variable expression)	Convincing

fundamental dissociations in some immune responses occur is little understood and invites further study.

Mutations in antigenic type may allow a pathogen to infect populations that lack immunologic memory or preexisting immunity against the new strain. The cyclic epidemics and pandemics of influenza are attributable to such mutations. The complex cause-and-effect relationships between host and pathogen genotypes defy unequivocal analysis unless each of the variables is evaluated in controlled experiments.

Genetic influences on resistance of sheep, mice, and chickens to certain animal parasites have received some experimental attention. With malarial or helminth parasites, for example, the genotype of the pathogen as well as the host must be considered. It is doubtful whether the specific immune responses of the host to most animal parasites decisively influence the outcome. Metazoan parasites, in particular, often persist in the face of acquired immunity demonstrable by high titers of humoral antibodies. When strains of mice with substantially different survival patterns to the malarial protozoan (*Plasmodium berghei*) are crossed, the challenged hybrids often live longer than either parent. Such heterosis may be attributed to the interaction of many genes or gene products favorable to survival. The fact that F_2 hybrids failed to show simple Mendelian segregation of genes affecting parasitemia supports polygenic determination. F_1 hybrids from certain crosses showed mean survival times similar to those of the more resistant parent whereas those from other crosses reacted like the less resistant parent strain. In general, males survived several days longer than females. Susceptibility of mice to malaria is not correlated with genetically different hemoglobin types.

The differential resistance of inbred mice to enteric nematode worms (*Nematospiroides dubius*) is also revealing. By using mortality, LD50/30 values, worm burdens, infectivity of the third-stage larvae, and longevity of adult worms as criteria, S.-K. Liu established that the C3H strain is more susceptible than the A, CF1, C57 and Webster strains. Webster mice were much more resistant than C3H mice in relation to all experimental criteria. Thus, about two and one-half times as many larvae were required to kill 50 per cent of adult Webster mice within thirty days as compared to C3H mice. Yet F_1 hybrids of these two strains were even more resistant to the nematode than the resistant parent strain. Only one unselected strain of mouse nematode was tested, and no backcross or F_2 data are available for comparison. Ideally, one would also like to know the effect of attempted preimmunization of the host mice in such experimental systems.

Levels of Experimental Definition of Heritability of Immune Responses

Immunologists have long been aware of the wide variability in antibody reponses of mammalian species to any given antigen. For example, when a group of random-bred rabbits is immunized in the same way with xenogeneic protein, some will produce much antibody, some may produce little or no detectable antibody, and many give intermediate amounts. Because most immunologic studies are best served by potent immune serums, animals which are poor responders to a particular antigen are usually disposed of without further study. Although many investigators have intuitively recognized the probable genetic control of the ability to produce antibodies, decisive immunogenetic evidence is surprisingly scanty. As we proceed to consider the known and probable relationships between host genotypes and specific immune responses at progressive levels of experimental definition, four major variables must be taken into account.

1. *Genotypes of Experimental Animals.* A random population in Hardy-Weinberg equilibrium would be most heterogeneous, or least defined, and could be expected to show a broad range of immune responses to nearly all antigens. Selected coisogenic or congenic strains differing at only one known gene locus would be best defined because significant differences in any measured immune response could be associated with one gene locus unmodified by other genetic differences. Intermediate between these extremes would be animals selected for certain phenotypic traits or particular genotypes, but otherwise heterogeneous, or inbred strains with multiple interstrain genetic differences on homozygous backgrounds.

2. *Complex versus Chemically Defined Antigens.* Although a species of *Salmonella* or blood cells from an individual are sometimes termed *the* antigen when used for immunization, a complex mixture of many antigens is really involved. Many distinct and overlapping immune or antibody responses are induced in the immunized animal under these conditions. When clones of a given microorganism or homogeneous subpopulations of cells are employed, one is still dealing with complex antigens with many determinant groups, but the source is better defined and the antigenic polymorphism is reduced considerably. Much better definition is achieved when highly purified or homogeneous preparations of proteins or polysaccharides are used for immunization, even though multiple antigenic determinants are still involved. One obtains greater sophistication when chemically defined haptens are conjugated to purified macromolecules. Theoretically, maximal definition is achieved when a hapten is conjugated to the responding animal's own macromolecules. Single allelic or mutational variants of known macromolecules or alloantigens in inbred strains also represent optimally defined sources.

3. *Assays of Specific Immunity or Antibody Responses.* In conventional serology, the antibody response in commonly measured in whole serum titers assayed by agglutination, precipitation, or complement fixation. Although such tests are useful in the diagnosis of immune responsiveness to infectious agents, they are complex because heterogeneous populations of antibodies with divergent

reactivities contribute to the overall reaction. The heterogeneity of antibodies even to a single antigen has long been recognized. Precipitating versus nonprecipitating antibody or saline-agglutinating versus blocking antibodies to blood group antigens constitute heterogeneities with opposing effects. Neutralization or cytotoxicity assays of antibody give better definition to the extent that functional activity is being determined. Increased functional immunity or hypersensitivity measured in vivo can be well defined if cellular or antibody heterogeneity is predetermined and controlled. Similar qualifications apply to measurements of rate of immune elimination of labeled antigen. Given the distinctive properties of the five major classes of mammalian immunoglobulins, any study in depth should take into account the antibody response with respect to each immunoglobulin class. The highest level of definition is obtained when purified or fractionated antibodies of given molecular classes are measured by the most sensitive and reproducible techniques available.

4. *Tactics of Immunization and Testing.* Every specific immune response is substantially influenced by the tactics and timing of immunization. The chief variables, in addition to the species selected for immunization, are dosage of antigen, route of inoculation, the schedule of immunization, and the external environment. The effective dosage of antigen depends on the inherent adjuvanticity or persistance of the preparation as well as the route of inoculation. For the induction of transplantation immunity, a skin graft is much more effective than an equivalent number of dissociated spleen or lymph node cells. Bovine serum albumin in a water-in-oil emulsion containing killed Mycobacteria (Freund's adjuvant) is a potent immunogen when inoculated into mice, but the same soluble protein is ineffective if administered in a physiological saline solution. A single injection of a low dosage of specific pneumococcal polysaccharide preparation may be sufficient to produce in a mouse or a man a maximal, lifelong immunity with persistent antibody synthesis. On the other hand, multiple injections of certain histocompatibility or blood-group alloantigens may be necessary to obtain a detectable antibody response which is often of short duration. These are just a few of the many examples of wide disparities in immune responsiveness that are closely dependent upon the tactics of immunization.

Environmental conditions sufficient to maintain normal health will usually assure a full immune potential in mammalian and avian species. Lower vertebrates and invertebrates which are ectothermic or poikilothermic are much more influenced by the external environment. With aquatic species, water chemistry as well as temperature are major variables. Thus, to characterize an immune response as a function of genetic constitution, *variable* dosage, route, schedule and/or environment is less desirable than *constant* dosage, route, schedule and environment. The latter approach would yield the highest level of experimental definition if each factor is predetermined to provide maximal sensitivity for the assays employed. These relationships are given in Table 2–2.

Table 2–2 Levels of Experimental Definition of Major Variables Involved in Measurement of Inheritance of Specific Immune Responsiveness

	Responders	Antigens	Antibodies or Immunity	Tactics of Immunization and Testing
Least defined	Random population	Complex: Species of microorganisms; heterogeneous mixtures of cell types; different macromolecules such as whole serum or cell extracts	Ab titer of whole serum measured by agglutination, precipitation, or complement fixation	Variable dosage, route, schedule and/or environment
Partially defined	Selected for certain phenotypic traits	Complex: Clones of microorganisms; homogeneous subpopulations of cells; macromolecules of one general type such as serum albumin fraction	Immune elimination of labeled antigen. Increased functional immunity or hypersensitivity. Ab response measured in terms of particular immunoglobulin classes; neutralization or cytotoxity assays of Ab produced	Constant dosage, route, schedule and environment
Well-defined	Selection according to particular genotypes	Highly purified or homogeneous preparations of proteins or polysaccharides		Constant dosage, route, schedule and environment
Maximally defined	Inbred strains or equivalent homozygotes. Selected coisogenic or congenic strains	Haptens conjugated to purified macromolecules or responders own macromolecules; synthetic poly-amino acids; single allelic or mutational variants of defined macromolecules or cells	Purified or fractionated Ab of given molecular classes measured by most sensitive and reproducible techniques available	Constant dosage, route, schedule and environment, each predetermined to provide maximal sensitivity for assays employed

Genetic Control of Defined Antibody Responses

Let us now consider available evidence for the genetic control of ability to produce antibodies. In one study, families of rabbits from random-bred stock were divided into "weak," "medium," and "strong" antibody producers to the antigens of whole human serum. The rabbits were classified according to titers from interfacial precipitin tests following ten intravenous injections of 0.1 ml human serum at two-day intervals. F_1 progenies were obtained and the most revealing crosses are shown in Fig. 2–3.

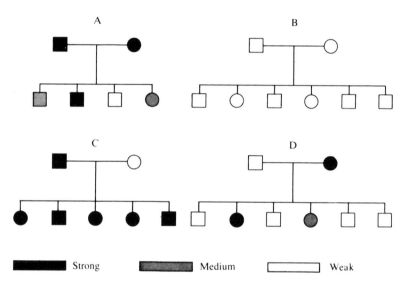

Figure 2–3. Results of tests of precipitin production in F_1 rabbits from crosses of strong X strong (A), weak X weak (B) and strong X weak (C and D) reactors. (After Kleczkowska and Kleczkowski, *Ztchr. Immunitätsforsch.*, Vol. 95: 218–226, 1939.)

It was found that "strong" serums contained antibodies to both globulin and albumin fractions whereas "weak" serums contained antibodies only to globulin determinants. From numerous crosses of the types indicated, the inability to respond to albumin determinants could be attributed to a single, autosomal recessive gene. Crosses of type A could lead one to assume a dominant allele mediating competence to respond to albumin with the "medium" or intermediate antibody producers representing heterozygous individuals. However, the results of crosses of types C and D revealed a more complex genetic control since only "medium" and "weak" reactors should occur in the progeny if a single dominant and recessive pair of alleles were involved. Backcross or F_2 progenies would have to be evaluated to decide whether additional "strong" alleles, other genetic loci, or both determine the classes of reactivity observed. In terms of major experimental variables, these early experiments leave much to be desired at all levels of definition.

Better experimental definition has been achieved in attempts to inbreed guinea pigs selectively both for and against the ability to produce antitoxins to diphtheria toxoid. Such experiments are illustrated in Figs. 2–4 and 2–5. Parental guinea pigs were initially selected from random-bred stock on the basis of substantial antitoxin production or no measurable antitoxin production to a single, subcutaneous injection of toxoid administered under standardized conditions. Although this antigen is a complex, xenogeneic protein, the test system measured only neutralization of the toxic components of the macromolecule by a limited spectrum of the induced antibodies on intracutaneous titration in normal rabbits. The first generation selected for antitoxin production yielded 90–100 per cent responders in three sublines. However, some nonproducers still appeared after continued selection for six successive generations of sib matings. With comparable selection against responsiveness to toxoid, it took five generations to obtain a high percentage of nonproducing progeny. This conclusion must be qualified by the fact that the number of progeny tested in the F_4 and F_5 generations was small.

There was no sex difference in either the distribution of producers and nonproducers or the antitoxin titers in these experiments. This data suggests that capacity for antitoxin production is mediated mainly by dominant genes at multiple autosomal loci. The analysis could be carried much further. About twenty generations of brother-sister inbreeding with separate selection for producers and nonproducers would be required to assure near homozygosity. Test crosses between producers and nonproducers and their hybrid progeny could then establish dominant versus recessive determination and provide an estimate of the number of loci involved. Concurrent determination of neutralization titers with respect to particular immunoglobulin classes, allotypes, or other genetic markers could lead to further dissection of gene-antibody relationships. To the extent that numerous gene loci control different steps leading to the biosynthesis of antitoxin, systems of this type could be quite difficult to analyze at the molecular level.

Several investigators have found significant seasonal variation in diphtheria antitoxin production by guinea pigs. Antitoxin production is often weaker in animals immunized in the winter and spring than in animals immunized in summer and autumn, Since vitamin supplementation does not compensate for the difference, other environmental factors such as the length of the day may be involved. Thus, seemingly inconsequential environmental variables may be important and should not be ignored in the design of long-term experiments.

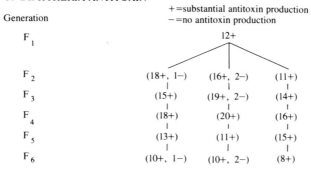

SELECTION FOR PRODUCTION
OF DIPHTHERIA ANTITOXIN

Generation

+ =substantial antitoxin production
− =no antitoxin production

F_1 12+

F_2 (18+, 1−)   (16+, 2−)   (11+)

F_3 (15+)   (19+, 2−)   (14+)

F_4 (18+)   (20+)   (16+)

F_5 (13+)   (11+)   (15+)

F_6 (10+, 1−)   (10+, 2−)   (8+)

Figure 2—4. Results of selection (+ X + matings) for heightened capacity of guinea pigs to produce diphtheria antitoxin in successive generations of sib matings. The numbers of adult guinea pigs in each of three sublines responding to a single subcutaneous injection of 1 ml. diphtheria toxoid containing 10 Fl. U. after four weeks are indicated in parentheses. (Adapted from Scheibel, *Acta Path. Microbiol. Scand.*, Vol. 20: 464—484, 1943.)

SELECTION AGAINST PRODUCTION
OF DIPHTHERIA ANTITOXIN

Generation

+ =substantial antitoxin production
− =no antitoxin production

F_1 (14+, 9−)

F_2 (12+, 3−)   (3+, 13−)   (7+, 7−)

F_3 (8+, 14−)   (3−)   (3+, 3−)

F_4 (3+, 4−)   (5+, 3−)

F_5 (2−)   (1+, 6−)

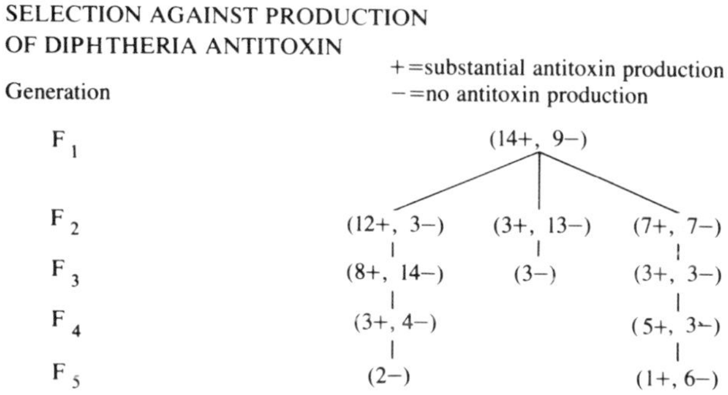

Figure 2—5. Results of selection (− X − matings) against capacity of guinea pigs to produce diphtheria antitoxin in successive generations of sib matings. The same experimental protocols as in Fig. 2—4. (Adapted from Scheibel, *Acta Path. Microbiol. Scand.*, Vol. 20: 464—484, 1943.)

The quantitative inheritance of specific antibody responsiveness to complex soluble and particulate antigens has been extensively studied by W. A. Sobey of Australia in random-bred stocks of rabbits and mice. The previously described studies dealt only with the ability or inability to produce a certain antibody. Additional questions may now be raised. To what extent is the level or rate of antibody production in primary and secondary responses under genetic control? Is there a positive correlation in degree of antibody responsiveness to related antigens or to antigens of certain molecular properties? Is the measurement of the overall antibody response to a complex antigen greatly affected by the individual antigenic determinants? In such experiments, analyses of frequency distributions of antibody responses and their 95 per cent confidence limits are required. Moreover, calculation of correlation coefficients of primary and secondary responses to various antigens allows identification of related and unrelated responses.

The ability of two random-bred, but genetically distinctive, strains of Flemish Giant and Ermine Rex rabbits to produce antibodies to tobacco mosaic virus (TMV) was found by Sobey to be highly heritable as evidenced by parent-offspring comparisons. Although the mean frequency distributions of secondary responses to routine injection of TMV in the two populations of rabbits were not significantly different, the regression of the mean secondary response of offspring on the mean secondary response of parents gave a high estimated heritability ($h^2 = 0.876 \pm 0.09$). This value indicates that nearly 90 per cent of the variability in this population is genetically determined; heritability is the percentage of the total measured variance attributable to additive genetic variance. Antibody responses to this antigen of high molecular weight were measured as a function of precipitation in the equivalence zone, using an arbitrary scale that reflected the logarithmic production of antibody. With the moderate immunization employed, agar double diffusion tests suggested that TMV was eliciting only a single specific antibody response. Had a greater antigenic stimulus been routinely used, the single measurements obtained would have included more than one antibody response. Precipitin assays might then have yielded a low or nonsignificant measure of heritability.

This assumption was supported by a comparable study of the secondary response to bovine plasma albumin (BPA) in the same populations of rabbits. No substantial heritability ($h^2 = 0.09$) of the overall response to this complex antigen could be demonstrated. Agar immunodiffusion tests showed that this BPA preparation had at least seven antigenic subfractions, two of which were globulin contaminants. Under these conditions, substantial heritability might be found if the response were directed mainly toward one major or strong antigen, or if the test system measured each distinctive antigen-antibody reaction separately. The heritability of the hemolysin response of random-bred mice to sheep red cells was also low, but varied according to when the immune serum was collected. The full meaning of these results is not clear because of the minimal definition of major variables (Table 2–2).

Ideally, components of variance such as the effect of age, dose, route of administration, and schedule of immunoglobulin determinations should be separately appraised. Appropriate characterization of individual antibody responses in different immunoglobulin classes could reveal the extent to which each is under genetic control, provided immunogenic competition or synergism of component antigens is minimal. Recent experiments have shown significantly different 19S (IgM) immune hemolysin responses to sheep erythrocytes by spleen cells from various inbred strains of mice, including certain pairs of congenic strains, as measured by standardized and sensitive plaque assay techniques. Variation between the strains was found to be much greater than variation within the strains.

The following experiments, as described in recent literature, indicate that different immunoglobulin classes represented in specific antibody responses are under separate genetic control. Some strains of inbred mice show both electrophoretically fast ($7S\gamma_1$) and slow ($7S\gamma_2$) gamma globulin classes of antibody toward ovalbumin three months after initial sensitization; other strains show only $7S\gamma_1$ antibody under the same conditions.

Specificity of Genetic Regulation

Some of the rabbits studied by Sobey produced no detectable antibodies to BPA (bovine plasma albumin) even after heavy or prolonged immunization. These animals retained antigen in their circulation for long periods, but even after disappearance of circulating antigen, failed to produce antibodies. By contrast, responders showed antibody as soon as the antigen was cleared from the circulation. The nonresponders to BPA did respond normally to other antigens tested, however. A central immunogenetic or enzymatic block in immune induction toward bovine plasma protein is suggested. The clear implication is that certain genes may control more than one immune response without affecting antibody responses in general.

At least some forms of specific immunological unresponsiveness can be demonstrated to be under genetic control. Certain rabbits and mice which failed to respond to immunogenic doses of bovine serum albumin also yielded proportions of "negative" progeny in test-crosses. This is consistent with the supposition that two or three gene loci contributed to the unresponsiveness. The "negative" animals gave normal antibody responses to other antigens including chicken egg albumin. In these experiments, Sobey and co-workers were aware that apparent absence of an antibody response could be misleading because they could not distinguish between a "negative" and a very weak responder. However, most "negative" animals at the fifth generation of selection failed to develop

BSA antibodies even after repeated booster injections and showed persistent circulating BSA instead. Genetic control governing the failure to produce antibodies to synthetic antigens has also been demonstrated in guinea pigs and in mice. These situations suggest unresponsiveness at an early stage of potential antigen processing.

We may now consider whether genetic regulation of responsiveness is restricted to particular classes of related antigens. In other words, are responses to quite different antigens determined by independent loci or is there a tendency for individuals of certain genotypes to respond well or poorly to all antigenic stimuli? Here again, the available evidence is inconclusive, coming primarily from experiments with complex antigens and random-bred recipients.

High or low degrees of primary and secondary responsiveness of rabbits to diphtheria toxoid were found to be positively correlated, as were primary responses to diphtheria and tetanus toxoids. However, such positive correlations were also demonstrated between responses to TMV and diphtheria toxoid, and between TMV and bovine red cells. No correlations were apparent for responses to tetanus toxoid, *Shigella shiga*, human red cells or Bushy Stunt virus. Apart from the anomalous correlations involving TMV, it appears that genes at many loci independently regulate different antibody responses. Nevertheless, individual rabbits tested with all these antigens tended to give either good or poor responses. In the absence of progeny tests and careful control of sex, age, nutrition, and other factors, a general predisposition to respond at an inherent level to all antigenic stimuli remains doubtful. It should be noted that generalized immunologic hyperreactivity has been found in human patients with diseases such as rheumatic fever and sarcoidosis, but the cause-and-effect relationships are obscure.

Additional comparative correlations of antibody responses of random-bred mice and rabbits to various antigens are given in Table 2–3. Strongly positive correlations between responses to two strains of influenza virus were found while weak or negative correlations characterized the responses to unrelated antigens with the exception of tobacco mosaic virus. Comparisons of responses of inbred or congenic strains and their hybrid progenies to antigens of similar protein composition, molecular weight, or of the same species origin would be a promising extension of this line of investigation.

Although immunogenetic studies of resistance to infectious agents must necessarily involve complex antigens with multiple determinants, the use of highly inbred host strains and selectively cloned stocks of pathogens limits the complexity in a most desirable way. To evaluate a given host-parasite relationship, the investigator must initially find at least two host strains that are relatively resistant and susceptible to the pathogen in an appropriate test system. Resistance of the all-or-none type to a virulent pathogen is uncommon. In other words, a host strain highly resistant to a pathogen at low dosage will often show

Table 2–3. Correlation of Antibody Responses to Various Related and Unrelated Antigens in Mice and Rabbits from Random-Bred Colonies (Adapted from Adams and Sobey, *Aust. J. Biol. Sci.*, Vol. 14: 594–597, 1961)

Antigen Responses Correlated*	Correlation Coefficient**	Degree of Correlation	Antigen Responses Correlated*	Correlation Coefficient***	Degree of Correlation
	MICE			RABBITS	
MEL(N)-LEE(N)	0.51	Strong	TMV-PXV	0.35	Moderate
MEL(A)-LEE(A)	0.32	Moderate	TMV-MEL	0.53	Strong
MEL(N)-MEL(A)	0.59	Strong	TMV–LEE	0.62	Strong
LEE(N)-LEE(A)	0.71	Strong	PXV-MEL	−0.17	Negative
MEL(N)-LEE(A)	0.47	Strong	PXV-LEE	−0.09	Negative
MEL(A)-LEE(N)	0.29	Moderate	MEL-LEE	0.97	Strong
O-Vi	0.34	Moderate	MEL–VV	0.14	Weak
O-MEL(N)	−0.09	Negative	LEE–VV	0.14	Weak
O-MEL(A)	−0.10	Negative	TMV–VV	0.21	Moderate
O-LEE(N)	−0.04	Negative	PXV-VV	−0.21	Negative
O-LEE(A)	0.10	Weak			
Vi-MEL(N)	−0.02	Negative			
Vi-MEL(A)	−0.04	Negative			
Vi-LEE(N)	−0.01	Negative			
Vi-LEE(A)	−0.03	Negative			

* MEL, LEE = influenza virus strains; O, Vi = *Rhizobium meliloti* antigens; TMV = tobacco mosaic virus; PXV = potato X virus; VV = vaccinia virus; N = neutralization titer; A = hemagglutination-inhibition titer.
** S.E. = 0.14; degrees of freedom = 194–256
*** S.E. = 0.16; degrees of freedom = 50

increasing susceptibility as dosages are increased. Resistance itself, frequently multifactorial in nature, may often be subdivided and evaluated with respect to different pathogenic components. These assertions may now be considered in some detail.

Inheritance of Susceptibility to Tumor Viruses

Certain tumor viruses furnish a unique opportunity for concurrent study of the genetic basis of susceptibility to infection as well as to cancer or tumor development. Chang and Hildemann investigated the mode of inheritance of susceptibility to polyoma virus in neonatal F_1 hybrids and reciprocal backcross progeny of the highly susceptible AKR/J and relatively resistant C57BL/6J strains of mice. The experimental virus stock, after cultivation on AKR mouse embryo cell cultures, was purified three times by the plaque technique. The following criteria were used to measure susceptibility to the virus after neonatal inoculation: incidence of runting and/or tumor development, spectrum and multiplicity of tumors, latent period before the appearance of gross tumors, and capacity of virus to multiply with cytopathic effect in cell cultures of various host genotypes.

Susceptibility to tumorigenesis appeared to be determined by a single autosomal gene with incomplete dominance. Consistently high but apparently submaximal susceptibility of (AKR $\times$ C57BL/C) F_1 hybrids was found at both low and high virus dosages. The recessive resistance of the C57BL/6 strain was largely overcome by neonatal infection with polyoma virus in high dosage. High susceptibility of albino AKR mice to a distinctive runting syndrome, characterized as a specific acute or subacute manifestation of polyoma disease, was recessively inherited. The greatly increased susceptibility to runting of albino as compared with black progeny of the F_1 female $\times$ AKR male backcross was highly significant at both virus dosages tested. These results are summarized in Tables 2–4 and 2–5. Quantitative genetic analysis of the segregation data showed that susceptibility to runting was effected by interaction of the albino gene, or a gene closely linked to it, and another independently segregating recessive gene also carried by the AKR strain. Thus at least three independently segregating gene loci must be invoked to account for the overall evidence of susceptibility. Polyoma tumors frequently developed in the absence of runting, but long-surviving runts always developed tumors. Among other qualifications attached to the genetic analysis, the incomplete dominance ascribed to the two genes governing susceptibility to tumorigenesis and resistance to runting might really reflect modifying effects of additional genes. This means that other genes not directly associated with the inherited susceptibility may operate in the developent of polyoma virus-induced disease. Describing inherited susceptibilities solely in terms of host genotypes assumes a uniform pathogen genotype and a uniform experimental environment.

Table 2–4 Incidence of Runting and Tumors in Mice Inoculated with 1.4 × 10³ Plaque-Forming Units (PFU) of Polyoma Virus (*Low Dosage*) by Intracardiac Route Within Twenty-Four Hours After Birth (After Chang and Hildemann, *J. Nat. Cancer Inst.*, Vol. 33: 303–313, 1964)

Mouse Strains and Progenies	Number of Mice Infected	Runted Mice*		Mice with Tumor**		Mice Runted and/or Developing Tumor		Latent Period for Tumor Induction (Weeks)	
		No.	%	No.	%	No.	%	Average	Range
AKR	67	64	95.5	21	31.3	67	100.0	8.00	6–9
C57BL/6	52	4	7.7	13	25.0	16	30.8	16.15	7–26
(C57BL/6 ♀ × AKR ♂) F₁	85	8	9.4	70	82.4	75	88.2	11.04	7–20
F₁ ♀ × AKR ♂ (backcross)									
Albino	89	35	39.3	64	71.9	87	97.8	8.27	6–13
Black	77	9	11.7	70	90.9	72	93.5	8.88	6–21
Total	166	44	26.5	134	80.7	159	95.8	8.59	6–21
C57BL/6 ♀ × F₁ ♂ (backcross)	50	8	16.0	27	54.0	34	68.0	13.67	10–25

* Incidence of naturally occurring runts was consistently less than 2 per cent in control litters of all progenies tested.
** This indicates the total number of infected mice that subsequently developed tumors irrespective of presence of runting. Numerous runted mice died before tumors were detectable, but long-surviving runts always developed tumors.

Table 2–5. Incidence of Runting and Tumors in Mice Inoculated with 1.4×10^5 Plaque-Forming Units (PFU) of Polyoma Virus *(High Dosage)* by Intracardiac Route Within Twenty-Four Hours After Birth (After Chang and Hildemann, *J. Nat. Cancer Inst.*, Vol. 33: 303–313, 1964)

Mouse Strains and Progenies	Number of Mice Infected	Runted Mice*		Mice with Tumor**		Mice Runted and/or Developing Tumor		Latent Period for Tumor Induction (Weeks)	
		No.	%	No.	%	No.	%	Average	Range
AKR	48	48	100.0	0	0	48	100.0	–	–
C57BL/6	38	11	28.9	19	50.0	30	78.9	12.68	10–19
(C57BL/6 ♀ × AKR ♂) F$_1$	52	23	44.2	34	65.4	48	92.3	8.00	6–16
F$_1$ ♀ × AKR ♂ (backcross)									
Albino	36	30	83.3	14	38.9	36	100.0	7.79	6–11
Black	29	17	58.6	17	58.6	29	100.0	9.12	6–20
Total	65	47	72.3	31	47.7	65	100.0	8.52	6–20
C57BL/6 ♀ × F$_1$ ♂ (backcross)	54	19	35.2	35	64.8	50	92.6	9.34	7–14

* Incidence of naturally occurring runts was consistently less than 2 per cent in control litters of all progenies tested.
** This indicates the total number of infected mice that subsequently developed tumors irrespective of presence of runting.

Uniform susceptibility of cell cultures to the multiplication and cytopathic effect of polyoma virus, irrespective of host genotype, revealed that host resistance in vivo did not depend on the absence of cells subject to continuing infection. Additional evidence suggests that early, efficient maturation of the immune response capacity is a major component of the genetic resistance to malignant infection associated with the C57BL genotype. Increased susceptibility to malignancy reflected either in runting disease or tumorigenesis was positively correlated with reduction in the average latent period for tumor development. The resistance of C57BL mice to tumorigenesis was associated with a strong tendency for tumors to develop only in the salivary glands whereas AKR mice and their susceptible albino backcross progeny developed multiple tumors with significantly greater frequency.

These observed differences in resistance among infected progenies are compared statistically in Table 2–6. Among the criteria of susceptibility evaluated, the incidence of the runting syndrome was most sensitive, followed by the average latent period for appearance of tumors, overall incidence of runting and/or tumors, the incidence of mice with more than one type of tumor, and the incidence of mice with tumor. The least sensitive indicator was the incidence of mice with tumors other than those of salivary glands. Far more significant ($P < 0.05$) and highly significant ($P > 0.01$) differences are revealed in the comparisons involving the low dosage of polyoma virus. It is probable that at very high virus dosage, genetic resistance to tumorigenesis could be entirely obscured under these experimental conditions.

Although sex of host did not modify susceptibility to polyoma virus, males were found to be at least twice as resistant as females to a virus-induced murine leukemia. In this instance, castration diminished the natural resistance of males while testosterone administration greatly increased the resistance of females. In most cases, female mice give better immune responses than males of the same strains (cf. also Chapter Six).

Susceptibility to Gross leukemia virus in mice has also been analyzed by Lilly by means of crosses of virus-susceptible and virus-resistant inbred strains. For instance, with resistance simply dominant in (C3H × C57BL/6) F_1 hybrids, the proportion of resistant animals among backcross progeny should be $\frac{1}{2}^n$ and in the F_2 generation, $\frac{3}{4}^n$, where n is the number of independent genes (loci) involved. The segregation of resistant and susceptible mice observed in backcross and F_2 progenies suggested that two independent loci are determinative. In several strain combinations, the virus-resistant phenotype appears to have been caused by a dominant allele for resistance at each of these loci. Conversely, either one of the alternative, recessive genes (homozygous) led to Gross virus susceptibility in animals injected at birth. One of these loci (Rgv-1) appears to be closely linked to the H-2 histocompatibility locus in the ninth linkage group. The H-2 cellular alloantigens (cf. Chapters Four and Six) were identified in

Table 2–6. Significance of Differences in Incidences of Runted Mice and Mice with Various Tumors, and in Average Latent Periods for Tumor Induction Among Progenies Infected with Polyoma Virus* (From Chang and Hildemann, *J. Nat. Cancer Inst.*, Vol. 33: 303–313, 1964)

Any two lines of mice may be compared by reference to the square lying at the crossing position of corresponding column and row. Upper half of table lying above diagonal line represents results with high dosage and lower half results with low dose of virus.**

	AKR	C57BL/6	(C57BL ♀ × AKR ♂) F₁	F₁ ♀ × AKR ♂ (Backcross) Albino	F₁ ♀ × AKR ♂ (Backcross) Black	F₁ ♀ × AKR ♂ (Backcross) Total	C57BL/6 ♀ × F₁ ♂ (Backcross)
AKR		HS HS HS HS – –	HS – HS S – –	HS – HS X X X	HS – HS X X X	HS – HS X X X	HS – S – – –
C57BL/6	HS – HS HS HS S		X X HS HS X X	HS HS HS HS X X	X HS HS HS X X	HS HS HS HS X X	X X X HS X X
(C57BL ♀ × AKR ♂) F₁	HS – HS HS HS HS	X HS HS HS X X		HS – X X X X	S – X X X X	HS – S X X S	X X X S X X
F₁ ♀ × AKR ♂ Albino	HS – X X HS S	HS HS HS HS X X	HS – X X X X		HS – S X X X	HS S HS HS X X	HS – X HS X X
F₁ ♀ × AKR ♂ Black	HS – S HS HS HS	X HS HS HS X X	HS – S HS X X	S – X X X X		X HS HS HS X X	S X X X X X
F₁ ♀ × AKR ♂ Total	HS – X S HS HS	HS HS HS HS X X	HS – S X X S	HS S HS HS X X	X HS HS HS X X		HS X S X X X
C57BL/6 ♀ × F₁ ♂	HS – HS HS HS HS	X HS HS X X X	X HS S X X X	HS S HS HS X X	X HS HS HS X X	X HS HS HS X X	

* HS: Highly significant ($P < 0.01$); S: Significant ($0.01 < P < 0.05$); X: Nonsignificant ($P > 0.05$); –: Omitted because of the interfering effect by the high incidence of runted mice.

** Each square contains information as follows:

a	b
c	d
e	f

where:

a = incidences of runted mice.
b = incidences of mice with tumor.
c = incidences of mice runted and/or developing tumor.
d = average latent periods for tumor induction.
e = incidences of mice with tumors other than those of salivary glands.
f = incidences of mice with more than one kind of tumor.

individuals derived from crosses by hemagglutination tests using specific antiserums. As illustrated in Fig. 2–6, the high susceptibility of H-2^k/H-2^k segregants indicates the presence of a recessive gene for susceptibility in the C3H genome linked to H-2. Lilly interprets the failure of about 10 per cent of H-2^k/H-2^k segregants to develop leukemia within the ten-month observation period to mean that either (a) the Rgv-1 locus is situated about ten map units away from H-2 allowing for about 10 per cent recombination to occur, or (b) susceptibility is determined by part or all of the H-2 locus itself, but with a penetrance of only 90 per cent.

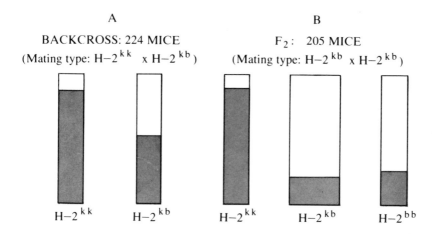

A	B
BACKCROSS: 224 MICE	F_2: 205 MICE
(Mating type: H-2^{kk} x H-2^{kb})	(Mating type: H-2^{kb} x H-2^{kb})

H-2^{kk} H-2^{kb} H-2^{kk} H-2^{kb} H-2^{bb}

Figure 2–6. Final incidence of Gros virus-induced leukemia in backcross (A) and in F_2 (B) generations, segregating for H-2 alleles, from crosses of C3Hf/Bi (H–2) and C57BL/6 (H–2^k). The shaded area of each bar represents the fraction of mice injected at birth which subsequently developed leukemia. (From Lilly, *Genetics*, Vol. 53: 533, 1966.)

Among the many such genes studied, only the Rgv-1 locus and the linkage group *I* locus responsible for the runting effects of polyoma virus have been located on the linkage map. It appears significant that different alleles of the H-2 locus of the mouse, so critical for histocompatibility in general, should greatly influence host responses to leukemogenic viruses as well. Histocompatibility genotypes might also explain provocative differences in inheritance of resistance to polyoma tumorigenesis found in certain strains of mice.

Simple Versus Complex Genetic Bases of Disease Susceptibility

Genetically determined host susceptibility to particular viruses and bacteria may be attributed to single, autosomal, dominant or recessive genes. As one might expect, multiple genes are more commonly implicated. Some examples from published studies are indicated in Table 2—7.

Table 2—7. Principal Genetic Basis of Host Susceptibility Determined for Various Infectious Agents

| Pathogen | Host Species | Genetic Susceptibility (+) | | |
		Single Dominant Gene	Recessive Gene	Polygenic
Hepatitis virus	Mouse	+		
Friend leukemia virus	Mouse	+ (?)		
Rous Sarcoma virus	Chicken	+		
Arbo B viruses	Mouse		+	
Ectromelia virus	Mouse		+	
Erythroblastosis virus	Chicken		+	
Gross leukemia virus	Mouse			+ (2 loci)
Polyoma virus	Mouse			+ (3 loci)
Mammary tumor virus	Mouse			+
Salmonella	Chicken			+
	Mouse			+

In the case of Friend leukemia virus (FV), genetic susceptibility may depend on the *virus* genotype. Thus, susceptibility of (C57BL/6 $\times$ DBA/2) F_1 mice, as measured by spleen lesions and ability to sustain virus proliferation upon serial passage, is dominant toward one strain of virus, but recessive toward another. As adults, the C57BL/6 parental strain is highly resistant and the DBA/2 highly susceptible to both strains of virus. Either a "one locus-three allele" or a "two independent loci-two alleles each" hypothesis could explain these results in the absence of tests on backcross and F_2 progeny. In other experiments by Axelrad utilizing highly susceptible SIM mice, (SIM $\times$ C57BL/6) F_1 hybrids exhibited intermediate susceptibility to FV. Data on spleen focus formation in F_2 hybrids and in reciprocal backcross progeny were consistent with the hypothesis that FV susceptibility is controlled primarily by a single autosomal gene locus. In successive backcrosses to either parental strain, the relevant alleles continued to function as predicted without apparent "dilution." Note, however, that the latter investigation dealt with only a single strain of FV.

Where progeny tests have yielded segregation ratios suggesting simple Mendelian alternatives for susceptibility versus resistance, additional genetic loci may be involved in the complex process of immune elimination. To prove that only a single-gene locus is determinative would require testing susceptible and resistant congenic strains and their hybrid progenies. To my knowledge, no such experiments have ever been performed. A recent study by Tennant and Snell of genetic influence on viral leukemogenesis did compare allelic substitutions at several histocompatibility loci in congenic strains of mice. Although different degrees of resistance to leukemogenesis were found, the histocompatibility differences alone were not sufficient to account for the results. It is entirely possible that the absence of a single enzyme in host macrophages could prevent digestion of a given pathogen following phagocytosis. Indeed, the macrophages of different strains of mice are responsible for the apparent genetic difference in susceptibility to hepatitis and Arbo B viruses.

Several strains of mice were found to be either completely susceptible or resistant as neonates when inoculated intraperitoneally with virulent mouse hepatitis virus. Crosses between susceptible inbred Pr mice and resistant inbred C3H mice gave F_1 progeny that were entirely susceptible like the Pr parent strain. The proportion of susceptible progeny in the F_2 and backcross to C3H generations was sufficiently close to 75 per cent and 50 per cent susceptibility, respectively, to support the assumption of a single dominant gene for susceptibility. Moreover, the same genetic differences in susceptibility of these strains and their hybrid progenies showed up in tissue culture tests of macrophage susceptibility. Cultures from resistant strains of mice showed no destruction of macrophages by virus whereas susceptible mice yielded macrophages that were destroyed within two to three days in culture. The cytopathic effect of the virus was selective in that fibroblasts and epithelial cells from susceptible mice were not affected. Thus, genetic susceptibility depends on the selective destruction of macrophages that normally prevent viremia. The importance of phagocytosis by the reticuloendothelial system in curtailing infections is well established. Extensive studies by Goodman and Koprowski indicate that histiocytic-macrophage cell types enforce the dominant resistance of mice to the antigenically similar, arthropod-borne (Arbo B) viruses responsible for encephalitides in man. The effect of the recessive allele in morphologically similar cells of susceptible mice is to allow virus multiplication and invasion. Note, however, that the same dominant gene produced resistance to the several distinctive Arbo B viruses tested.

The striking difference in response to yellow fever virus by susceptible C3H mice and resistant PRI mice is illustrated in Fig. 2–7. The transient viremia in C3H mice at eight days after infection was associated with high concentrations of virus in the brain tissue. In contrast, no living virus was detectable in either the blood or brains of the virus-resistant PRI mice at any time.

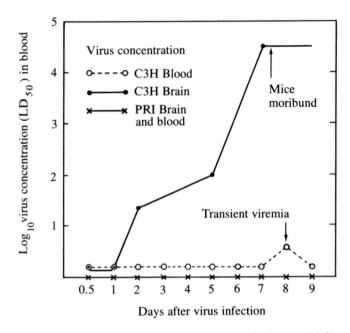

Figure 2–7. Comparison of yellow fever (17D strain) virus multiplication and viremia in susceptible C3H mice and resistant PRI mice following intracerebral inoculation. No living virus persisted in either the blood or brain tissue of PRI mice. (Adapted from Goodman and Koprowski, *J. Cell. Physiol.*, Vol. 59: 344, 1962.)

Destruction of ingested microbes by phagocytes appears to be notably specific with respect to different pathogens. This is not surprising, since different genes are associated with resistance to different pathogens. By suitable selection and inbreeding, Webster developed strains of mice that were bacteria-resistant (BR) and bacteria-susceptible (BS) to certain species of *Salmonella*. When these mice were tested for resistance to louping ill virus, some of the BS mice were resistant to virus infection, but BR mice were susceptible. Inbred strains of BRVS and BSVR mice were then produced. Subsequent crossbreeding with selection for susceptibility to certain bacteria and viruses also yielded bacteria- and virus-resistant (BRVR) as well as bacteria- and virus-susceptible (BSVS) inbred lines. Thus, all four possible combinations of susceptibility and resistance to *Salmonella* species and Arbo B viruses were obtained. Simple, independent Mendelian inheritance of these separate traits was apparent. More extensive investigation of specificity in terms of additional, unrelated pathogens was not undertaken.

Resistance to infectious disease cannot be underestimated in terms of population survival, as is especially true of wild animals in captivity. I have observed this frequently in my work with diverse species of tropical fish. Thus, a whole school of Cardinal Neon Tetras (*Cheirodon axelrodi*), thriving under near optimal conditions in a large aquarium, may become heavily infected with a common protozoan parasite such as *Ichthyophthirius* introduced with food or plants. If untreated, at least 90 per cent of the fish will die, but the survivors usually retain a substantial immunity to this pathogen. An analogous historical example was the great human influenza pandemic of 1918–1919. J. B. S. Haldane long ago stressed the significance of resistance to disease for natural selection and evolution. Darwinian fitness in terms of immunological competence may often be more important among vertebrates than considerations of predation or food resources.

Genetic differences in immune responsiveness also affect the incidence of experimentally induced, autoimmune disease. Mice of the BSVS strain are much more vulnerable to experimental allergic encephalomyelitis than many other strains. Likewise, guinea pigs of the Hartley strain develop encephalomyelitis in response to a dosage of central nervous tissue antigen that does not cause disease in several other strains. Random-bred Hartley strain animals also show a much higher incidence of experimental allergic thyroiditis than inbred-strain-13 animals after intradermal inoculation of low doses of guinea-pig thyroid extract. In other experiments, Swiss mice were more susceptible to allergic thyroiditis than C57BL mice. Whether these strain differences reflect primary differences in immune responsiveness or secondary manifestations of target-tissue damage remains to be determined.

Genetic Control of Naturally Occurring Antibodies

The natural occurrence of serum alloantibodies or isoantibodies long ago raised the issue whether such antibodies were spontaneous genetic products or induced by antigens always present in the environment. In the case of anti-A and anti-B in man, or similar antibodies in other mammals, the evidence favors the latter assumption. Nevertheless, the relevant genotype of the responder often determines the quality of antibody produced.

With respect to human ABO blood-group genotypes, homozygous A_1A_1 individuals produce anti-B of about 300,000 molecular weight ($S_{20} \sim 11.0$). Group OO individuals have anti-B with a weight of about 170,000 ($S_{20} \sim 6.5$), but A_1O heterozygotes yield a macroglobulin anti-B ($S_{20} \sim 15.5$) rather than a mixture of the smaller antibodies characteristic of homozygotes. However, group O serums show additional heterogeneity in the specificities and cross-reactions of their anti-B agglutinins. At least one subpopulation of B antibodies, cross-reactive with A cells, is present in many O serums but absent from A serums. The quantitative ability of group O persons to produce anti-A_1 and anti-B appears to be largely under genetic control since the correlation between the titers of either parent and those of the children approximates the theoretical 0.5 expected under complete genetic control for levels of both types of antibodies.

Although uncontrolled immunization probably accounts for most naturally occurring antibodies, there are some possible examples of true, natural antibodies normally elaborated by direct gene action. The soluble, specific blood-group substances J and Oc present in certain cattle give rise to four phenotypes—J, JOc, Oc, and the absence of both. Cattle lacking both antigens are found not only in the class having both anti-J and anti-Oc, but in classes containing anti-J alone, anti-Oc alone, or lacking both antibodies (Table 2—8).

Table 2—8. Classification of 453 Hereford Cattle According to Anti-J and Anti-Oc Antibodies and J and Oc Soluble Antigens Found in Their Serums (After Sprague, *Genetics*, Vol. 43: 913—918, 1958)

Phenotypic Class	No. of Cattle	No. with Anti-J and Anti-Oc	No. with Anti-J Alone	No. with Anti-Oc Alone	No. Lacking Both Antibodies
J, Oc	29	0	0	0	29
J	93	0	0	0	93
Oc	58	0	33	0	25
Neither J or Oc	273	17	60	111	85

There is no reason to suspect that either anti-J or anti-Oc in these animals is associated with irregular immunization. Neither J-positive nor Oc-positive animals exhibit the phenotype anti-Oc. The capacity to produce anti-Oc is attributable to a single dominant gene. The Oc antigen, related both serologically and genetically to J, is unusual in being inherited as a recessive character.

In certain guinea pigs, a natural state of delayed allo- or iso-hypersensitivity exists toward a heritable component in the serum of other normal guinea pigs. This serum factor is determined by an autosomal dominant gene. Other examples such as the statistical evidence indicating the genetic control of production of natural agglutinins for sheep erythrocytes in inbred strains of mice leave open the question of spontaneous immunization with heterogenetic antigens like the Forssman hapten which is widely distributed in nature. The question of natural antibodies is of great theoretical interest since selective theories of antibody production propose that all antibodies may be elaborated normally and that an antigen merely selects complementary ones for increased synthesis.

Chemically Defined Antigens

Until recently, little experimental advantage has been taken of haptens or chemically defined, antigenic determinants. The now classic studies of Landsteiner showed that a large variety of small molecules or even ions, incapable of inducing antibody production by themselves, could provoke specific antibodies when conjugated to proteins or polysaccharides. When the genetic basis of such hapten antibody responses is studied, one can minimize the problem of multiple antibodies, each perhaps under separate genetic control, formed against the many different determinants found even in purified macromolecular antigens. If both the hapten and carrier macromolecule are foreign to the animal, absorptions with the carrier are needed to remove antibodies directed against determinants other than the hapten alone. This step can theoretically be circumvented if the hapten is coupled to the responders' own macromolecules. However, much less defined experiments have yielded some meaningful insights.

Random-bred rabbits were divided into three groups according to their responses to bovine serum albumin coupled by azolinkage to two haptens, sulfanic acid and p-aminobenzoic acid. Most of the rabbits produced antibodies either very well or very poorly to both haptens, but the third group reacted well to only one of the two haptens. Since the carrier protein was the same, the different response of the third group must have depended on a mechanism other than enzymatic competence to process the carrier macromolecule.

Haptens lightly coupled to polyamino acids, or polyamino acids alone, may serve as effective, chemically defined antigens. Random-bred guinea pigs of the Hartley strain, immunized with several different haptens conjugated to poly-L-lysine, either made antibodies specific for each hapten or showed no immune response to any of them. In other words, guinea pigs capable of responding immunologically to one hapten-polylysine conjugate can respond also to polylysine conjugates of the other haptens. The haptens included dimethylaminonapthalenesulfonyl, dinitrophenyl, p-toluenesulfonyl, and benzylpenicilloyl molecules. Strong hypersensitivity of both the Arthus and delayed types, and a high concentration of hapten antibodies occurred in the responders whereas nonresponders showed no evidence of specific responsiveness when given sensitizing injections in complete adjuvant plus repeated booster injections. Inbred guinea pigs of strain 2 were all responders while strain 13 animals were entirely unresponsive.

Among the random-bred animals tested by Levine and Benacerraf with dinitrophenylpoly-L-lysine, matings between nonresponders yielded only unresponsive progeny whereas more than three-fourths of the progeny from matings between responders behaved like their parents. Of 31 progeny from numerous matings of nonresponders with heterozygous responders, 14 were responders. There was no evidence of sex-linkage from reciprocal test-crosses.

Thus, it is apparent that the ability of guinea pigs to aquire immunity to dinitrophenylpoly-L-lysine conjugates is determined by an autosomal dominant gene. This responsiveness is presumably referable to the poly-L-lysine since various hapten substitutions made no difference in the all-or-none responses observed. A minimum of 7-8 lysyl residues in hapten conjugates of oligo-L-lysines is required for immunization of responsive guinea pigs and for evocation of delayed hypersensitivity reactions in these animals. At an analogous level of discrimination, antibodies elicited toward different antigenic determinants on purified bovine insulin molecules have been demonstrated to be under genetic control in inbred strains 2 and 13 guinea pigs.

A series of amino acid polymers, made by introducing 5 to 60 molecules of alanine into glutamic acid$_{60}$-lysine$_{40}$ (GLA$_5$-GLA$_{60}$), gave the following per cent responders as measured by passive hemagglutination, among presumably random-bred Swiss mice: GLA$_5$—45 per cent; GLA$_{10}$—85 per cent; GLA$_{20}$—90 per cent; GLA$_{30-60}$—100 per cent. When the adult progeny of responders and nonresponders to GLA$_5$ were immunized with GLA$_5$, the results suggested that the ability to respond might be referable to a single, autosomal dominant gene. However, greater immunogenetic complexity may be inferred because highly inbred strains of mice showed either all-or-none responses to GLA$_5$ and GLA$_{10}$ in contrast to the heterogeneous Swiss animals.

In related investigations by McDevitt and Sela, CBA and C57 mice responded to controlled immunization with a synthetic polypeptide, poly (tyr, glu)-poly DL-ala-poly lys, [(T,G)-A—L], in Freund's complete adjuvant, with a tenfold or greater difference in antigen-binding capacities of their serums. These two strains responded equally well to bovine serum albumin, employed as an unrelated, complex antigen. F$_1$ hybrid mice responded like the superior antibody-producing C57 parent strain to [(T,G)-A—L] whereas F$_1$ × CBA backcross mice showed a bimodal distribution of phenotypes. In the latter case, the proportions were nearly 1:1, which was consistent with a single locus, dominant versus recessive allele control. Moreover, F$_1$ × C57 backcross mice all gave heightened immune responses, many even better than those of C57 animals (Fig. 2—8). Antibody responses among segregating hybrid progeny exceeded the two phenotype ranges of the parental strains. This indicates the participation of multiple genes affecting the quantity of antibodies produced. Also, a tenfold lower dose of antigen yielded an intermediate response in F$_1$ hybrids. This suggests a gene-dose or interaction-effect in heterozygotes. Polygenic regulation appears inescapable, despite some imprecision in the assay method. Immunization of CBA and C57 mice with [(H,G)-A—L], a synthetic polypeptide in which histidine was substituted for tyrosine, reversed the relative responsiveness of the two strains. Indeed, C57 mice failed to respond at all. Thus, it appears that the genetic control of the response to [(T,G)-A—L] is specific for an antigenic combination of tyrosine and glutamic acid.

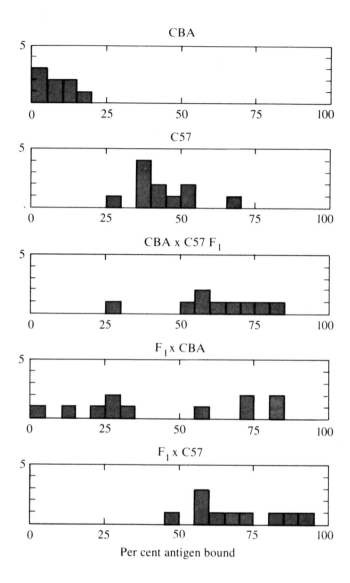

Figure 2—8. Immune responses of CBA and C57 mice, their F_1 hybrids, and reciprocal backcross progeny given 100 µg of (T,G)–A––L 509 in complete Freund's adjuvant, and boosted with 100 µg of the same antigen in saline. Bimodal distribution of phenotypes in $F_1 \times$ CBA backcross progeny suggests a primarily single gene locus affecting the quantity of antibodies produced. Otherwise, occurrence of antibody responses outside the two phenotype ranges of the parental strains among hybrid progenies suggests participation of multiple genes. (Adapted from McDevitt and Sela, *J. Exp. Med.,* Vol. 122: 523, 1965.)

Beyond polygenic, dominant responsiveness, separate systems of genetic control for different antigenic determinants on similar carrier molecules are apparent from these studies. Note, however, that we are still dealing with potentially complex haptens rather than single antigenic determinants. Also, the titering system used measures only antigen-binding capacity and not necessarily the actual antibody protein present in the test serums. Adult animals of the same age (two to three months at the outset) and of both sexes were used in all these experiments. No sex differences in responsiveness were noted.

Why the same hapten may provoke specific antibody production when attached to a protein, but not when conjugated to certain synthetic polypeptides is still a mystery. The elusive quality of macromolecular complexity is somehow involved. Again with two inbred strains of guinea pigs, linear and branched copolymers containing lysine were immunogenic in all animals of strain 2, but none of strain 13. The opposite situation occurred with a linear copolymer of tyrosine and glutamic acid. Yet a copolymer of glutamic acid, tyrosine, and alanine was just as immunogenic in both strains and their F_1 hybrids. The immune response or lack of it in F_1 hybrids corresponded to that of strain 2, suggesting dominance of the determining genes in strain 2. Although gene-controlled enzymatic competence at the macrophage level may often be important to distinguish between immune responders and nonresponders, this can hardly account for all the genetic differences in responsiveness already observed.

In congenic strains of mice, the antibody response to 2,4,6-trinitrophenyl mouse serum albumin (MSA) appears to be regulated primarily by products of the *H-2* locus. Following immunization with TNP_{11}-MSA, mice from each of five strains and their hybrid progenies representing congenic pairs differing at the *H-2* and *H-3* loci were recently tested by Rathbun and Hildemann. Note that the hapten was conjugated to the recipient strain's own protein as a carrier. Individual antiserum samples were collected at seven to twenty-eight days after primary and secondary injections and were titered using an antigen binding capacity test with ^{125}I labeled TNP_5 bovine serum albumin. The A/J (H-2^a) strain gave a low antibody response while its congenic partner A.BY (H-2^b) produced a significantly higher response ($p = 0.001$) at all times tested. Similarly, strain B10.A (H-2^a) gave a lower response than its H-2^b partner C57BL/10. The response of both (A/J $\times$ A.BY) F_1 and (C57BL/10 $\times$ B10.A) F_1 was not significantly different from the low responding parental strains ($p = 0.5$). The response of F_2 mice was consistent with the expected 1/4 H-2^a/H-2^a (low responders): 1/2 H-2^a/H-2^b (low responders): 1/4 H-2^b/H-2^b (high responders). The response of strain B10.LP-a was not significantly different from its *H-3* disparate partner C57BL/10. All strains tested produced substantial and very similar levels of antibody to two other haptens, 2,4-dinitrophenyl and arsanilic acid—also conjugated to mouse albumin derived from the immunized strains. These results support the hypothesis that the low antibody response to the TNP hapten is determined by the *H-2*[a] allele as a dominant trait whereas homozygosity for the *H-2*[b] allele leads to high responsiveness even on diverse strain backgrounds.

Of the many aspects of inherited immune responsiveness, only the more elementary relationships between relevant genes and specific antibodies have been considered so far. Maximal definition of all experimental variables, as outlined in Table 2–2, has yet to be accomplished in a test system. Since all biosynthetic processes are ultimately gene-controlled, it probably follows that every immune response must be under precise genetic control. Nevertheless, there is an obvious paucity of detailed evidence and much scope for further investigation.

KEY REFERENCES

1. ADAMS, K. M., and W. R. SOBEY. "Inheritance of Antibody Response. V. Correlated Antibody Responses to Various Related and Unrelated Antigens." *Aust. J. Biol. Sci.*, Vol. 14: 594–597, 1961. One of a series evaluating genetic control of antibody responses in rabbits and mice.

2. BANG, F. B., and A. WARWICK. "Mouse Macrophages as Host Cells for the Mouse Hepatitis Virus and the Genetic Basis of Their Susceptibility." *Proc. Nat. Acad. Sci.*, Vol. 46: 1065–1075, 1960. Tests of hybrids between resistant and susceptible strains revealed genetic segregation of susceptibility and resistance in the F_2 and backcross generations. Similar susceptibilities occurred both in mice and in macrophage cultures derived from them.

3. BATTISTO, J. R. "Genetic Control of a Guinea Pig Serum Factor Toward Which Natural Delayed Iso-Hypersensitivity Occurs." *Nature*, Vol. 198: 598–599, 1963. Presense in certain strains of guinea pigs of normal serum factor toward which natural hypersensitivity exists in other strains found to be controlled mainly by an autosomal dominant gene.

4. BEN-EFRAIM, S., S. FUCHS, and M. SELA. "Differences in Immune Response to Synthetic Antigens in Two Inbred Strains of Guinea Pigs." *Immunology*, Vol. 12: 573–581, 1967. Investigation of various types of immune response to some linear and branched synthetic polypeptides extended to inbred strains of guinea pigs and their hybrids.

5. CHANG, S. S., and W. H. HILDEMANN. "Inheritance of Susceptibility to Polyoma Virus In Mice." *J. Nat. Cancer Inst.*, Vol. 33: 303–313, 1964. Invokes at least three independently segregating gene loci to account for overall evidence of susceptibility. Early and efficient maturation of immune response found to be major component of genetic resistance. See also later paper in *J. Nat. Cancer Inst.*, Vol. 40: 363–375, 1968.

6. COX, R. P., and C. MACLEOD. "Relation Between Genetic Abnormalities in Man and Susceptibility to Infectious Disease," in *Methodology in Human Genetics*. Ed. W. J. Burdette, Holden-Day, Inc., San Francisco, pp.156–185, 1962. Summarizes hereditary defects in man associated with impaired immune responses to infectious agents.

7. FILITTI-WURMSER, S., Y. JACQUOT-ARMAND, G. AUBEL-LESURE, and R. WURMSER. "Physiochemical Study of Human Isohaemagglutination." *Ann. Eugen.*, Vol. 18: 183–202, 1954. Determines that ABO genotype of individual determines quality of corresponding antibodies present in serum.

8. GOODMAN, G. T., and H. KOPROWSKI. "Study of the Mechanism of Innate Resistance to Virus Infection." *J. Cell. Compar. Physiol.*, Vol. 59: 333–373, 1962. Shows that resistance to Arbo B virus infection in mice is dependent on a dominant gene affecting ability of macrophages to destroy virus.

9. GOWEN J. W. "Genetic Effects in Nonspecific Resistance to Infectious Disease." *Bact. Rev.*, Vol. 24: 192–200, 1960. Summarizes many years of author's work revealing polygenic determination of degrees of resistance of mice to *Salmonella typhimurium* and the importance of specific immunity.

10. LEVINE, B. B., and B. BENACERRAF. "Genetic Control in Guinea Pigs of Immune Response to Conjugates of Haptens and Poly-L-lysine." *Science*, Vol. 147: 517–518, 1965. Shows that development of immune response to poly-L-lysine in guinea pigs depends on a single, autosomal dominant gene probably affecting antigen catabolism.

11. LILLY, F. "The Inheritance of Susceptibility to the Gross Leukemia Virus in Mice. *Genetics*, Vol. 53: 529–539, 1966. Two independent loci appear to govern susceptibility to this virus, one locus being closely linked to *H-2* in the ninth linkage group.

12. LIU, S.-K. "Genetic Influence on Resistance of Mice to *Nematospiroides dubius.*" *Exp. Parasit.*, Vol. 18: 311–319, 1966. Heritability of differences in resistance among various strains of mice to infection with nematode larvae is deduced from multiple criteria. This article reveals complexity inherent in immunogenetic studies with animal parasites.

13. MCDEVITT, H. O., and M. SELA. "Genetic Control of the Antibody Response. I. Demonstration of Determinant-Specific Differences in Response to Synthetic Polypeptide Antigens in Two Strains of Inbred Mice." *J. Exp. Med.*, Vol. 122: 517–531, 1965. See also follow-up study by these authors in *J. Exp. Med.*, Vol. 126: 969–978, 1967. Two articles reflect the design, execution, and control of meaningful experiments involving chemically defined antigens.

14. PADGETT, G. A., R. W. LEADER, J. R. GORHAM, and C. C. O'MARY. "The Familial Occurrence of the Chediak-Higashi Syndrome in Mink and Cattle." *Genetics*, Vol. 49: 505–512, 1964. Leukocyte abnormalities associated with increased susceptibility to infectious diseases found to be determined mainly by an autosomal, recessive gene in mink, cattle, and man.

15. SOBEY, W. R., J. M. MAGRATH, and A. H. REISNER. "Genetically Controlled Specific Immunological Unresponsiveness." *Immunology*, Vol. 11: 511–513, 1966. Multiple gene loci appear to contribute to specific unresponsiveness in mice and rabbits. Consistently unresponsive animals obtainable by selective breeding.

16. SPRAGUE, L. M. "On the Distribution and Inheritance of a Natural Antibody in Cattle." *Genetics,* Vol. 43: 913–918, 1958. The origin of a natural antibody in cattle designated anti-Oc is ascribed to the action of a dominant gene, but the occurrence of this antibody also depends on the J-Oc system of soluble cattle blood groups.

17. Symposium on Defense Reactions in Invertebrates. *Fed. Proc.,* Vol. 26: 1664–1715, 1967. Far-ranging evidence concerning both cellular and humoral "immune" responses is reviewed by several contemporary workers.

18. WEBSTER, L. T. "Inheritance of Resistance of Mice to Enteric Bacterial and Neurotropic Virus Infections." *J. Exp. Med.,* Vol. 65: 261–286, 1937. A clsssic contribution in which all four possible combinations of susceptibility and resistance to *Salmonella* species and Arbo B viruses were produced by selection and inbreeding of mice.

THREE

CHARACTERIZATION OF MICROORGANISMS

Thus far we have emphasized the exquisite capacity of vertebrates to produce specific antibodies and to develop immunity toward the diverse antigenic determinants of cells and their products. There are many theoretical and practical reasons for continuing interest in the antigenic specificities of microorganisms. Our focus in this chapter, consequently, will range from gene-macromolecular product relationships to fundamentals of diagnostic microbiology.

In the realm of infection and disease, survival of pathogenic microorganisms depends on their ability to circumvent or override the host response to their foreignness or antigenicity. The identification of pathogenic bacteria or viruses and the preparation of vaccines often require the characterization of both species- and strain-specific antigens. Subtle but important differences in cellular or viral constituents may often be discerned only by appropriate antigen-antibody reactions. Living microorganisms, like cells in general, contain many specific antigens, some of which are effective and others poor inducers of antibody production. However, it is noteworthy that the virulence of a pathogenic organism is usually referable to a certain class of antigen. The capsular polysaccharides of the pneumococci, for example, are type specific as well as essential for the virulence of the organism. In this species, polymers of basic sugar units are combined in various sequences to give nearly one hundred distinct serologic types. The virulence-determining antigens of microorganisms include polysaccharides, proteins, carbohydrate-protein conjugates and polysaccharide-lipid-protein complexes, the last found in many Gram-negative bacteria located in the intestinal tract.

In diagnostic microbiology and epidemiology, serologic typing is often the principal tool for identification of etiologic agents. Spontaneous mutations in antigenicity are known to yield new strains of bacteria and viruses which then possess a selective advantage to the extent that potential hosts lack preexisting immunity to the antigens of the new strains.

Immunogenetic characterization of microorganisms poses special problems because many novel patterns of sexual and asexual reproduction substantially complicate genetic analyses. Many fungi and protozoa, as well as bacteria and viruses, are haploid or contain only one complete set of genes. When zygotes or sexual products are formed, they soon undergo division to yield haploid forms again, including recombinants. Under these circumstances, and also in asexually dividing cells, mutations will be expressed immediately and exposed to environmental selection.

In many species of fungi and protozoa, sexual reproduction occurs only between individuals of different mating types. Such compatibility patterns, which we shall consider in some detail, are heritable and involve antigenic surface constituents that may be characterized as serotypes. Comparable sexuality occurs in many bacterial species in the form of a conjugation mechanism in which genetic recombination is effected by the one-way transfer of genes from donor to recipient bacteria. Donor bacteria in conjugation possess an episomal sex factor which is readily transmitted along with part of the donor bacterial chromosome to recipient cells lacking the factor. However, the donor bacteria generally transfer only part of their genome to recipients with the consequent formation of incomplete zygotes.

It is now clear that episomes are infectious genetic determinants present in addition to the normal cellular genome. Episomes are thought to include all elements capable of independent replication and transfer which show genetic interaction with the genomes of microbial host species. They may have alternative cytoplasmic and chromosomally integrated states. Three types of episomes or "conjugons" involved in direct cell-to-cell, sexual exchange have so far been described: the F (fertility) factors, the Cf (colicinogenic) factors and the RTF (resistance transfer) factor. In genetic transfers involving transduction, bacteriophages of low virulence act as episomal carriers of one gene or a few closely linked genes. This parasexual phenomenon is common in Gram-negative bacillary species. Elevated mutability in bacteria may be caused by mutator genes and by interaction between chromosomal genes and episomes. Mutator genes are known in *Salmonella typhimurium, Escherichia coli,* and *Neisseria meningitidis.*

Finally, there is the process of transformation, probably uncommon in nature, in which single donor genes in the form of unencumbered deoxyribonucleic acid may induce homologous hereditary changes upon assimilation by recipient bacteria. The essential peculiarity of sexual reproduction of all kinds in bacteria is the unequal genetic contribution of the two parents. Further details concerning mechanisms of genetic transfer may be found in the excellent volumes by Hayes and by Braun. It is sufficient for present purposes to realize that the genetic determination of antigenic macromolecules in microorganisms often involves unusual events beyond the scope of Mendelian inheritance as applied to higher animals.

Since our purpose is to emphasize principles rather than detailed histories of many species of microorganisms, only certain illustrative studies will be considered in depth. Serotype systems in protozoans have received much deserved attention, notwithstanding complex mating types and unusual nucleocytoplasmic interactions. Antigenic determinants and serotype patterns in bacteria will be considered next, with special emphasis on the cell wall polysaccharide and flagellar protein antigens of *Salmonella* species. Finally, we shall cope with the relatively new and difficult fields of oncogenic viruses and tumor-specific antigens.

Ciliary Antigens and Serotype Systems in Protozoa

Unlike most microorganisms, the ciliates are diploid or polyploid at the somatic level. During periods of fission (i.e., asexual reproduction) in the most extensively studied species, *Paramecium aurelia*, individuals possess two diploid micronuclei and a single macronucleus containing forty or more diploid sets of chromosomes. Although the phenotype is determined by the genes in the macronucleus, macronuclei in successive sexual generations are derived anew from germinal micronuclei. There is reciprocal fertilization during sexual conjugation which yields exconjugants containing identical diploid nuclei derived by fusion of haploid nuclei from each mate. Thus the genotypes of any two exconjugant clones are identical although such cells may of course be heterozygous at many loci. A variable exchange of cytoplasmic constituents also occurs during conjugation. The essential features of conjugation are illustrated in Fig. 3–1. A self-fertilization process, known as autogamy, involving meiosis usually occurs at intervals after many asexual generations. Autogamy results in the internal fusion of two genetically identical haploid nuclei. After autogamy a given clone may yield a population of diverse genotypes as a consequence of Mendelian segregation, but each ex-autogamous clone is found to be completely homozygous. Although ciliates possess unusual life cycles from a cytogenetic standpoint, nearly all of their traits appear to be inherited in conventional Mendelian fashion. It should be noted that even dominant mutations occurring in the polyploid macronucleus may not be revealed amid the mass of unchanged genomes. On the other hand, mutations in micronuclear genes may be detected after one or two sexual generations.

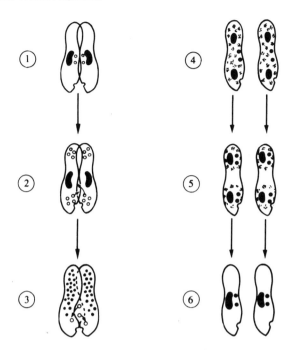

Figure 3—1. Essential features of sexual conjugation in ciliates of compatible mating types. (1) Fusion of two parental organisms of opposite mating type, each with one macronucleus and two diploid macronuclei. (2) Production of eight haploid nuclei from the germinal micronuclei of each conjugant. Seven of these nuclei disappear and the remaining nucleus in each conjugant passes into the paroral cone. (3) The nuclei in the paroral cones divide mitotically, forming 'male' and 'female' gamete nuclei. The female gamete nuclei enter the cytoplasm of the parental animals and fusion of male and female gamete nuclei from opposite mates then occurs, followed by two mitotic nuclear divisions. The old macronuclei disintegrate. (4) Two products of each fusion nucleus differentiate into new macronuclear anlagen, while the other two become new micronuclei. Old macronuclear fragments gradually disappear. (5—6) Asexual fission yields typical organisms with two micronuclei and one macronucleus.

Perhaps most remarkably, the breeding relations in ciliates involve systems of mating types or multiple sexes. Different stocks or clones, i.e., progenies of single individuals, may be assigned to groups such that all stocks of the same group interbreed freely while different groups of stocks are incompatible and do not mate successfully. Each variety or syngen represented by diverse clones contains one or usually two mating types that will agglutinate and conjugate when mixed. Thus, conjugation requires contact between two individuals of complementary mating types. A partial summary of the extensive mating reaction relationships in *P. aurelia* is shown in table 3–1. This brief resume of the main features of the life cycle is given to facilitate understanding of subsequent immunogenetic studies. In recent studies, the terms *clone* and *syngen* have been used in preference to *stock* and *variety*, respectively. The differentiation of mating type systems shows remarkable similarities to the serotype systems of ciliary antigens which may now be considered in some detail.

The extensive polymorphism of ciliary antigens in *Paramecium aurelia* and *Tetrahymena pyriformis* provides scope for increased understanding of gene-antigen relationships as well as nuclear-cytoplasmic interactions. Each individual of any one clone has the macronuclear genetic potential for the expression of a series of different alternative ciliary antigens or serotypes. Ciliates of each serotype may be immobilized by dilute homologous antiserum, but not by antiserum against other serotypes. The antiserum is usually prepared by repeated immunization of a rabbit. The serotype specificity resides in a single, soluble protein localized primarily in the cilia and body wall. One such immobilization antigen designated A in stock 51 of *P. aurelia* has been characterized by Preer at the University of Pennsylvania as a large protein with a molecular weight of about 2.5×10^5. After appropriate isolation, immobilization antigens may also be compared by immunodiffusion tests in agar gels.

The frontiers of molecular biology have been extended by serotype inheritance studies initiated in the 1940s by Sonneborn at the University of Indiana and continued by such scientists as Beale, Finger, Nanney, and Preer. Although multiple alleles at many different loci are associated with diverse immobilization antigens in *P. aurelia*, each antigen is usually referable to a single gene or cistron. Normally only one of these antigens is detectably present at any one time in a single organism. However, two allelic serotypes may be simultaneously expressed in heterozygous exconjugants until one of the alleles is eliminated by autogamy. Since individual cells generally show only one serotype at a time, it follows that only one genetic locus is active under given conditions. This is the unusual phenomenon of mutual exclusion among nonallelic ciliary antigens. Changes in environmental factors such as temperature and growth rate, without any change in genotype, commonly lead to transformations from one serotype to another. Even cell-free culture fluid from one serotype can cause transformation of cells of another serotype. This may be regarded as an example of induced gene expression since donor and recipient cells of identical genotypes can promote such transformation.

During the short period of transition involving only one or two fissions, it is possible to detect both the disappearing initial serotype and the newly developing serotype concurrently. As a rule, this is the only time that two different antigens determined by nonallelic genes can be found concomitantly in single cells. However, there are other exceptions to the mutual exclusion principle. One is that heterozygotes regularly express both allelic serotypes. In

Table 3–1. Partial Summary of Mating Reactions in *Paramecium aurelia* (Adapted from Sonneborn, Personal Communication)*

Group A comprises Syngens 1 (mating types I, II), 3 (V, VI), 5 (IX, X), and 9 (XVII, XVIII).
Group B comprises Syngens 2 (III, IV), 4 (VII, VIII), 6 (XI, XII), and 8 (XV, XVI).

Mating Type	I	II	V	VI	IX	X	XVII	XVIII	III	IV	VII	VIII	XI	XII	XV	XVI
I	–	+	–	–	–	40	–	–								
II	–	–	–	–	40	–	–	–								
V	–	–	–	+	–	–	–	–								
VI	–	–	+	–	–	–	–	–								
IX	–	–	–	–	–	+	–	–								
X	–	–	–	–	+	–	–	–								
XVII	–	–	–	–	–	–	–	+								
XVIII	–	–	–	–	–	–	+	–								
III									–	+	–	–	–	–	–	–
IV									–	–	–	–	–	–	–	–
VII									–	–	–	+	–	–	–	–
VIII									–	–	+	–	–	–	–	–
XI									–	–	–	–	–	+	–	–
XII									–	–	–	–	+	–	–	–
XV									–	–	–	–	–	–	–	+
XVI									–	–	–	–	–	–	+	–

* A plus (+) entry indicates normal conjugation followed by formation of fertile progeny while a minus (–) entry indicates no conjugation or occurrence of mating which yields no viable progeny. Otherwise, maximum percentages of conjugant pairs formed in tests among mating type combinations are indicated. There are actually 6 syngens known in group A, 7 syngens in group B, and 1 in group C (not shown) representing a total of 28 mating types. The different pairs of mating types within each syngen are always compatible.

addition, Margolin found a persistent phenotype in *P. aurelia* in which two nonallelic serotypes D and M are simultaneously expressed. The dual phenotype was maintained through many reproductive cycles when the organisms were grown at maximal fission rate at 27–35°C. Whereas serotype D occurred as a single antigen under other conditions, the M antigen was found only in the presence of D. Similar dependent relationships have also been found among certain mammalian blood group antigens. These will be considered in the following chapter.

A competitive relationship in the biosynthesis of D and M is suggested by the finding that an increase in the quantity of one antigen in any one stock is correlated with a decrease in the other. Moreover, the manifestation of the dual phenotype is associated with a particular *M* allele. Only one type of antigen is normally detected per clone, even from clones capable of synthesizing several types of hybrid antigens. The novel phenomena of *mutual exclusion* and of *serotype transformation* of ciliary antigens have been repeatedly confirmed.

An example of the inheritance of allelic serotypes in *P. aurelia* from the work of Beale at Edinburgh University is shown in Fig. 3–2. Each of two clones designated 60 and 90 in syngen 1 may exhibit three serotypes—type S at low temperatures, type G at intermediate temperatures, and type D at high temperatures. The G and D antigens were found to be clone-specific as evidenced by immobilization reactions in appropriate antiserums. At a constant temperature of about 25°C, conjugation between 90G and 60G yielded F_1 hybrids with both G serotypes expressed simultaneously. The hybrid phenotype was detectable only after about five fissions. Prior to this stage, the hybrid clones showed only the serotype of the parent from which the cytoplasm was derived. Evidently, the proteins resulting from the new F_1 macronucleus replace the preexisting ciliary protein gradually as required during sequential cell divisions. The dual hybrid phenotype persisted through many fissions until about five fissions after autogamy. The F_2 progeny then showed only the 90G or 60G serotype in a 1:1 ratio. All the F_2 clones were like the original parents with no other G serotypes evident. Since no recombinant classes were obtained, it may be concluded that the distinctive G antigens in these two clones are determined by a pair of codominant alleles. It should be noted that the coexistence of both antigens in the F_1 generation was revealed by immobilization in the presence of either anti-90G or anti-60G serums. Moreover, rabbit anti-F_1 serum possessed both antibody specificities which could be completely removed after separate absorptions with homozygous 90G and 60G organisms. The latter finding, incidentally, indicates that no additional hybrid or interaction antigen was produced in the F_1's. Otherwise the respective parental cells would not have removed all antibodies capable of reacting with the F_1 progeny. A probable gene dosage effect is suggested by the finding that higher antiserum concentrations were necessary to immobilize the F_1 than were needed for the parental types.

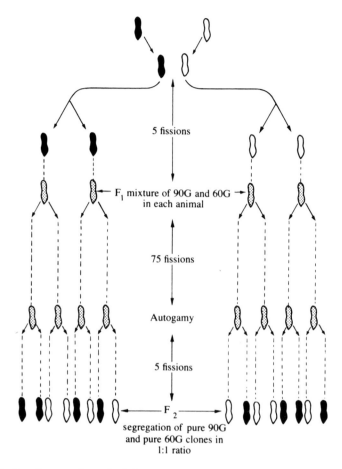

Figure 3—2. Segregation of allelic antigenic types 90G and 60G in F_1 and F_2 progeny. (Modified after Beale, 1954.)

When the same two clones were transformed to their distinctive D serotypes in culture at 30°C, matings again yielded F_1's with a mixture of both D antigens which subsequently segregated in 1:1 ratios in the F_2 generation. However, F_2 subcultures maintained at both 25°C and 30°C revealed four antigenic classes in about equal proportions—the two parental classes and two recombinant classes with respect to the four possible G and D antigens. This evidence indicates that the genetic loci for G and D are independent or not closely linked.

In general, antigenic cross-reactivity reflecting shared sequences of amino acids is notably lacking among the nonallelic serotypes detectable in particular clones. This finding is rather surprising inasmuch as a structural protein of specialized function is involved. Early chromatographic analyses of tryptic peptides from five immobilization antigens of *P. aurelia*, syngen 4, provided so-called fingerprint patterns amenable to detailed comparisons. Although no detectable differences in patterns were found for antigens under the control of these alleles, the nonallelic antigens exhibited quite different fingerprints. However, no two of nine allelic D types were chemically identical in a later study, although five were indistinguishable by immunological criteria. I. G. Jones found considerable variation among peptide maps of allelic types, but the differences were far less extensive than those associated with nonallelic types. A close correlation was shown between similarity of peptide maps and degree of serological cross-reactivity. Structurally, purified antigenic protein may consist of two identical half-molecules joined by disulphide bonds. It is apparent then that the process of serotype transformation requires the synthesis of polypeptides with quite different amino acid sequences to replace the protein characteristic of the previous ciliary antigen. On the other hand, it is evident that allelic genes determine structurally similar proteins which may be expected to share antigenic determinants in common. The allelic D antigens of syngen 1, for example, are partially cross-reactive with specific antiserums and chromatographically separable as well. The consistent genetic evidence of a one allele → one ciliary protein relationship suggests that the entire protein (i.e., polypeptide sequence) is specified by a single gene locus in contrast, for example, with vertebrate immunoglobulins or hemoglobins where the constituent polypeptide chains are specified by independent gene loci. However, this assumption bears further scrutiny because the actual manifestation of a specific antigen in a particular clone or strain is the result of a complex interaction of genes, cytoplasm, and environment.

Beyond the Mendelian modes of genetic transmission thus far considered, ciliary antigen phenotypes appear to be controlled at least partly by cytoplasmic components. As noted earlier, the dual expression of allelic serotypes in F_1 progeny requires several fissions following conjugation. Immediately after conjugation the serotype of the parental cytoplasm is retained. When matings involve different nonallelic serotypes, the original parental serotypes usually persist in the two conjugant clones. However, under conditions of massive cytoplasmic exchange during conjugation between clones of different serotype, the exconjugants usually yield clones of identical serotype with the serotype expressed depending on the conditions of the cross. Such clones also show the same mating type; again the type expressed is determined by the environmental conditions during conjugation.

In essence then, the traits of the progeny tend to be indistinguishable when cytoplasmic mixing occurs during mating. Otherwise, the traits remain distinct and segregate predictably. It is clear that different cytoplasmic states can become established in ciliates with identical genotypes. Crosses between strains of identical genotype but different serotypes reveal that the cytoplasm plays a decisive role in the maintenance of serotypic phenotypes. Considering the life cycle as a whole, there can be little doubt that the primary flow of genetic information is from micronucleus to macronucleus to cytoplasm. The system of genetic control of serotypes in *P. caudatum* is essentially identical to that found in *P. aurelia*. Differences among homologous serotypes from crosses of various stocks are governed by multiple alleles whereas crosses involving nonhomologous or nonallelic serotypes show cytoplasmic control of gene expression. The extent to which autonomous or semi-autonomous cytoplasmic episomes may influence differentiation or contribute hereditary information in ciliates is still largely unknown.

The serotype systems in *Paramecium* and *Tetrahymena* both show many similarities and also significant differences. In both species, single clones can differentiate or can be transformed into a variety of serotypes, albeit a particular cell normally expresses only one antigen at a time. However, in *Tetrahymena* the mutual exclusion of distinctive serotypes in heterozygotes generally occurs with allelic genes as well as nonallelic genes. All heterozygous combinations though derived from homozygous parents yield sublines showing considerable variability in phenotype. Although these sublines eventually express one allele or the other, a minority of intermediate phenotypes showing both antigens in different degrees may persist through many fissions.

The particular allelic combination established in a heterozygote determines the direction of allelic repression. The interallelic exclusion of the most studied H locus antigens in *Tetrahymena* appears to be strictly under nuclear control. Repression of alleles in the *H* serotype system has not proved modifiable by temperature, by antiserum, or by exposure to cell breis or RNA extracts from different serotypes. Cytoplasmic transmission of serotype from one generation to the next has not been found. The results of various $F_1 \times F_1$ and $F_1 \times$ parental clone crosses show that the phenotypes of the heterozygotes do not influence the phenotypes of the next generation. In other words, the micronuclear genotype is not modified when a heterozygote undergoes serotype transformation.

The distribution of mating types and serotypes among progeny of a contrasting pair indicates that differences in both traits in cells of identical genotype are associated with macronuclear differentiation. Despite initial variability, all clones produce pure phenotypes in both systems at the same rate, calculated by Nanney to be 0.0113/cell division. Nevertheless, the *H* serotype and mating type systems are attributable to independent genetic loci. No positive correlation is found between the serotypes and mating types of mature cultures involving genotypes that allow both forms of differentiation. Similar but separate mechanisms must regulate the phenotypic expression of the two systems. Nanney and Dubert postulated from collaborative work at the

California Institute of Technology that the asexual assortment of mating types and serotypes had the following cytogenetic basis.

1. The macronucleus consists of a population of diploid subnuclei.
2. These subnuclei become differentiated by suppression of one allele of each pair in each subnucleus.
3. These differentiations, once established, are perpetuated in further subnuclear replications.
4. Pure clones are produced by random assortment of differentiated subnuclei.

Although the evidence for intact diploid genomes is indirect, newer findings favor the view that phenotypic variants reflect subnuclear differentiation and epigenetic allelic repression rather than genetic recombination.

A new T serotype system different from the H serotypes found at lower temperatures is expressed in *Tetrahymena pyriformis*, syngen 1, grown at 40°C. Three T phenotypes are determined by three alleles at a locus not closely linked to other known loci. There is a sharp discontinuity between the expression of H and T serotypes as determined by immobilization tests with specific rabbit antiserums; cells reactive with both antiserums were found only in cultures maintained at 36–37°C. R. B. Phillips detected the distinctive serotypes of both parents in T heterozygotes initially, but cellular multiplication of clones subsequently yielded only one of the two types in nearly equal proportions. Such T serotype differentiation occurred within about thirty fissions after conjugation at 25°C–in the previous absence of T antigen expression. The kinetics of stabilization were similar to those found for H serotypes and unstable mating types. All these loci involve codominant alleles, and their respective, alternative expression is analogous to allotypic immunoglobulins (Chapter Five) produced by heterozygous mammalian lymphoid cells. The presumed directive or suppressive roles of RNA or protein "messengers" or episomes in determining the functional state of protozoan macronuclei invite further investigation.

Antigenic Determinants and Serotype Patterns in Bacteria

Antigenic variation in bacteria has long been studied intensively to facilitate classification of species and diagnosis of infection. Large numbers of distinctive serotypes, often reflecting subtle differences in the structure of cell surface lipopolysaccharides and proteins, may be identified among otherwise similar bacteria by use of appropriately absorbed antiserums. A consideration of serotype patterns in the *Salmonella* group of intestinal pathogens is instructive from both genetic and immunologic standpoints. More than 700 "species" have now been classified in the genus *Salmonella* on the basis of differences in serotypes. Two major genetic systems of serotypes, designated O for the somatic or cell wall polysaccharides and H for the flagellar protein antigens, are found in

Salmonella species. Nearly eighty serotypes, dubiously classified as separate species, are distinguishable on the basis of the O antigens alone. Despite the great diversity of antigenic polysaccharides, a simplified classification is possible because many clones or serotypes show strong cross-reactions and thus must possess similar antigenic determinants. The finding of major common determinants has led to the grouping of species or serotypes together in classes. In the scheme devised by Kauffman and White (Table 3–2), major groups are designated by capital letter, and individual O determinants, as defined by exhaustive cross-reaction and cross-absorption tests with antibodies obtained by immunizing rabbits, are distinguished by number.

Table 3–2   Illustrations of Kauffmann-White Scheme of Serological Classification of *Salmonellae*

Group	Serotype	O Antigen	H Antigen Phase 1**	Phase 2
A	*S. paratyphi A*	1, 2, 12	a	—
B	*S. abortus-equi*	4, 12	—	e, n, x
	S. paratyphi B	1, 4, 5, 12	b	1, 2
	S. stanley	4, 5, 12	d	1, 2
	S. bredeney	1, 4, 12, 27	l, v	1, 7
C1	*S. paratyphi C*	6, 7, Vi	c	1, 5
	S. montevideo	6, 7	g, m, s	—
C2	*S. newport*	6, 8	e, h	1, 2
C3	*S. kentucky*	(8)*, 20	i	Z_6
D	*S. sendai*	1, 9, 12	a	1, 5
	S. typhi	9, 12, Vi	d	—
	S. enteritidis	1, 9, 12	g, m	—
	S. panama	1, 9, 12	l, v	1, 5
E1	*S. london*	3, 10	l, v	1, 6
E2	*S. newington*	3, 15	e, h	1, 6
E3	*S. minneapolis*	(3), (15), 34	e, h	1, 6
E4	*S. senftenberg*	1, 3, 19	g, s, t	—

*A parenthesis is used to indicate that this serotype possesses only part of the somatic antigen designated within the bracket.
**These antigens have already illustrated the limitations of an alphabetical notation by exceeding twenty-six in number.

Over 95 per cent of strains isolated from natural sources fall into one of five groups, A through E. Each group shares a common somatic antigen. Where two or more somatic antigens are present, one determines the group to which the strain is assigned. Thus, group B consists of those serotypes carrying O antigen 4, and group D serotypes share O antigen 9. Several groups are divided into subgroups whose members each possess a second antigen in common. Groups A, B, and D_1 have almost identical factors 12 in common; all are also sensitive to phages P22 and 27, and a common antigen appears in the three groups after conversion by these phages. The H or flagellar antigens may exist in two alternative forms, designated phase 1 and 2. The determinants of the specific phase 1 are either peculiar to a given serotype or are shared by only a few other serotypes. However, the group phase 2 components are shared by many other O types. A culture of a given diphasic strain may consist entirely of bacilli in either the specific phase or the group phase, or may include representatives of both phases. However, the two sets of flagellar antigens do not exist as mixtures in the same, individual bacteria. A clone usually remains in one phase for many generations but retains the capability of transforming into the alternative phase. Certain species such as *S. paratyphi A* and *S. abortus-equi* are monophasic, i.e., apparently capable of exhibiting only one set of flagellar antigens. It may be noted in Table 3—2 that H antigenic complexes in both phases 1 and 2 are also found within the major O groups. The combined use of small letters and Arabic numerals in designating H antigens is unfortunately confusing and should be revised.

Many of the antigenic specificities identified by a single numeral or letter in the Kauffman-White scheme are themselves complex, consisting of several distinctive determinants. Thus the antigenic constitution of most serotypes is far more complex than is suggested by the notations given in the table. Because of "minor" somatic or flagellar antigens, cross-agglutination may occur between serotypes which appear to have no common antigens in terms of the current K-W scheme. Only "major" antigens of differential diagnostic importance have been regularly recorded.

Apart from diagnostic considerations of Salmonellosis, the chemical attributes and genetic control of the antigenic macromolecules of *Salmonella* are of fundamental interest. The determinants of specificity in the O antigens reside wholly in the polysaccharide moiety of the cell wall lipopolysaccharides. The lipopolysaccharide is highly antigenic and is an integral component of the endotoxin, a protein-lipid-lipopolysaccharide complex which is responsible for the fever, diarrhea, edema, and internal hemorrhage produced by injection of heat-killed bacteria. The polysaccharide portion, which can be isolated from the complex by mild acid hydrolysis, carries the complete O-antigen specificity of the microorganism and is nontoxic. All O-antigen specificities of a given serotype are located in a single polysaccharide molecule and the constituent determinants are referable to certain monosaccharide or oligosaccharide groupings. Purified oligosaccharides of low molecular weight have been characterized for their haptenic specificity by a variety of inhibition tests with rabbit antibodies directed against the intact lipopolysaccharides. This represents the basic immunologic methodology employed in the identification of these antigenic determinants. Certain mutations lead to complete loss of O-antigen specificity and the altered surface structure of these so-called "rough" mutants is associated with a loss of virulence.

Recent studies indicate that *Salmonella* lipopolysaccharides contain as many as eight different sugars. The substantial degree of antigenic specificity involved points to equivalent specificity in the sequence and linkage of these sugars. Analyses of mutants of *Salmonella typhimurium* in which biosynthesis of specific lipopolysaccharide precursors is blocked reveals the probable structure of the lipopolysaccharide as shown in Fig. 3–3. The whole macromolecule

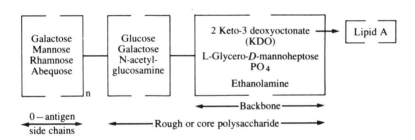

Figure 3–3. Postulated structure of the lipopolysaccharide of *Salmonella typhimurium*. (Modified from Osborn and Weiner, *Federation Proc.*, Vol. 26: 71, 1967.)

consists of a complex heteropolysaccharide covalently linked to a specific lipid, lipid A. The outer portion of the polysaccharide carries the O-antigen determinants in long side chains. O-antigen chains are linked in an unknown manner to the internal core. Although the structure and composition of the O-antigen chains vary extensively among *Salmonella* species, the core structure is similar throughout the genus. The mutant unable to synthesize uridine diphosphate glucose makes only the backbone structure containing keto-deoxyoctonate, heptose, and phosphate. The core molecule with additional side chains of glucose, galactose, and *N*-acetylglucosamine is synthesized in the rough strain and the guanosine diphosphate mannose-deficient mutant. Only the wild type strains produce the O-antigenic side chains of repeating units of rhamnose, mannose, galactose, and abequose joined to the core molecule. Osborn and co-workers at the Albert Einstein College of Medicine suggest that the "rough" phenotype may arise from mutation either at the level of nucleotide sugar synthesis or at a stage in the assembly or attachment of O-antigenic side chains.

A recent conception of the overall biosynthesis of O-antigens is illustrated in Fig. 3–4. The first step involves transfer of galactose-1-P of UDP-galactose to an

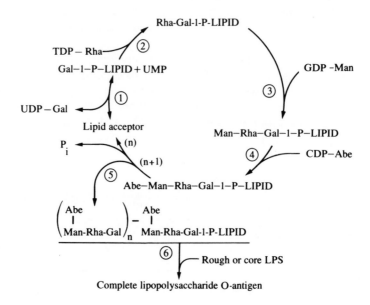

Figure 3–4.   Postulated pathway of biosynthesis of O-antigens in *Salmonella* species. (Modified after Osborn and Weiner, *Federation Proc.,* Vol. 26: 71, 1967.)

endogenous lipid acceptor. The lipid participates directly in the transfer of glycosyl units. Sequential addition of rhamnose and mannose to form the di- and trisaccharide-phospholipid intermediates follows. The complete tetrasaccharide repeating unit is then formed in the presence of CDP-abequose, and coupled to yield a lipid-linked O-antigen polymer.

Only the wild types possessing the entire antigenic side chains are pathogenic. Yet loss of the side chains or even part of the core molecule appears to have little effect on the ability of mutant strains to multiply in vitro. Presumably the complete lipopolysaccharide facilitates host invasion and inhibits phagocytosis. As previously noted, the capsular polysaccharides of the pneumococci are known to confer resistance to phagocytic digestion. No mutant *Salmonella* are known to lack the backbone or lipid portions of the lipopolysaccharide, which suggests that these components are indispensable.

Since all of the major antigens of the A through E groups, with the exception of C_1 contain galactose, mannose and rhamnose, Robbins and Uchida suggested that distinctive O antigens could depend upon one or more of the following modifications of the basic galactosyl-mannosyl-rhamnose pattern: (1) change of position of linkage or anomeric configuration within the basic trisaccharide sequence; (2) attachment of a dideoxyhexose or other monosaccharide such as glucose at specific points on the repeating trisaccharide structure; and (3) deletion of one of the three basic monosaccharides or substitution of another monosaccharide for one of the basic three. The 3,6-dideoxyhexoses associated with many *Salmonella* O antigens have been shown to serve as strong antigenic determinants. However, less than half of the O antigens contain dideoxyhexoses and the other monosaccharides constitute important haptens even in polysaccharides that do carry dideoxyhexoses. Sugars responsible for the specificity of some O-antigens of *Salmonella* are shown schematically in Fig. 3–5. These

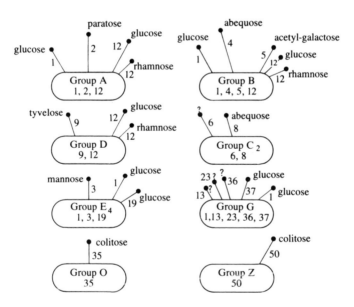

Figure 3–5.   Schematic representation of sugars responsible for the specificity of some O-antigens of *Salmonella* as determined by serological inhibition studies. The group-specific O determinants of the Kauffman-White scheme are shown within the soma (e.g., 1, 2, 12 in Group A). The "immunodominant" sugars, terminal or otherwise, which possess the highest affinity for the corresponding antibodies are shown at the ends of lines projecting from the soma. Note that O-antigens containing the same sugars may still belong to different serogroups: e.g., antigens 4 and 8, or 35 and 50, contain terminal abequose and colitose, respectively, but each numbered determinant is serologically distinct.

sugars need not be structurally terminal. The individual O specificities of a *Salmonella* serotype are carried by one and the same lipopolysaccharide molecule and are not separable as small molecules by chemical or serological fractionation. Various soluble blood-group substances in man are also known to derive their specificity from oligosaccharide units (see Chapter Four).

Transduction experiments reveal that the genes governing the O-specific part of the lipopolysaccharide are located in a cluster or a complex *O* locus. There appears to be one large *O* operon containing genes for all the enzymes, including transferases, involved in the synthesis and assembly of the nucleoside-phosphate forms of the special sugars. The genes for O-antigens 2, 4, and 9 occupy the same *O* locus in *S. paratyphi A, S. typhimurium,* and *S. typhosa,* respectively, and are probably allelic because of their mutual replacement in transduced hybrids in the absence of detectible recombinants. Although *O* alleles of different groups may yield substantially different serotypes, many alleles apparently determine slight differences—for example, the presence of paratose in antigen 2 versus abequose in antigen 4 versus tyvelose in antigen 9.

In addition to mutation as a source of antigenic variation, sexual conjugation, transduction, and lysogenic conversion have been found to produce new serotypes. Genes for certain O-antigenic determinants appear to be carried exclusively by lysogenic bacteriophages. Changes in serotype from 3, 10 to 3, 15, to 3, 15, 34 produced by lysogenic conversion in the E group of *Salmonella* are illustrated in Fig. 3—6. When O-serotype 3, 10 is infected with phage E^{15}, a new serotype soon appears which is either 3, 15 or 3, 15, 34, depending on whether the original strain carried E^{34} prophage prior to infection with E^{15}. If both phages are present the conversion is to 3, 15, 34. The change from 3, 10 to 3, 15 involves a switch from α to β linkage of the galactosyl to mannosyl, while the conversion from 3, 15, to 3, 15, 34 requires an addition of α-glucosyl to the repeating trisaccharide sequence. Both phage genomes cause chemical modification of the linkages of a galactose residue, most likely in the order predicted from the biochemical and serological findings. It is remarkable that most of the O-antigen phage conversions so far studied in *Salmonella* lead to the addition of an antigenic component. Changes of specificities have also been detected in *Shigella* after conversion by phage.

Genetic analysis of flagellar antigen systems has been accomplished by phage-mediated transduction and by sexual conjugation. Transduction between different diphasic serotypes, e.g., from *S. typhimurium i:1.2* to *S. abony b: enx* gave *i:enx* and *b:1.2* recombinants, but none of the *b:i* or *1.2:enx* types. This indicates that the specificities of the two alternative antigenic phases 1 and 2 are mediated by "independent" loci designated H_1 and H_2, respectively. In other words, these bacterial chromosomal loci are sufficiently separated so simultaneous transduction by a single phage does not occur. Additional transductional experiments in the opposite direction and between different serotypes have

Phage   Polysaccharide   O -antigen

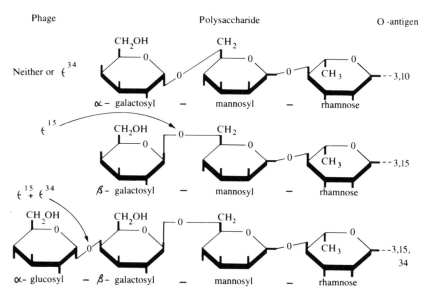

Figure 3–6. Schematic representation of structural changes in O-antigens of *Salmonella* group E brought about by lysogenic conversion with phages ϵ^{15} and ϵ^{34}. The phages provoke the appearance or derepression of bacterial enzymes which produce the new sugar linkages shown by the arrows. Phages may lead to replacement of one antigen by another or to the addition of one or more new antigenic specificities. (Modified from Robbins and Uchida, *Federation Proc.*, Vol. 21: 704, 1962.)

revealed two series of multiple alleles of H_1 and H_2. The H serotype of each phase includes multiple antigenic determinants. These determinants are presumed to reflect differences in the sequence of 15 to 17 amino acids comprising the homogeneous protein monomers of the flagellins that are primarily responsible for the characteristic antigen type. The difference in tryptic peptide maps is greater between phase-1 flagellins and phase-2 flagellins derived from different serotypes. This finding is analogous to the situation in ciliate protozoa mentioned earlier where allelic serotypes were found to be very similar in chemical structure to each other in contrast to nonallelic serotypes. The separate antigenic determinants manifested by a given flagellin are transferred as a unit in genetic recombination experiments, again supporting the working principle of "one gene locus → one complex macromolecule → multiple antibody specificities." However, it is evident that flagellar antigenic subunits may mutate independently of each other, suggesting a sequential arrangement of mutational sites or mutons comprising both the H_1 and H_2 locus. One may note that flagellins with unrelated antigens such as (b) and (g) differ by as many as thirty-nine amino acid substitutions whereas antigenically similar flagellins, e.g., (g,m), (g,m,s,), and (g,s,t,), differ by only a few amino acids from a total of nearly 380.

Several regulatory genes recently studied by Iino at the Japanese National Institutes of Health are involved in the production of flagellar antigens. One group designated *fla* includes numerous *fla⁻* mutant genes that cause impairment of the ability to produce flagella both in phase 1 and phase 2. The wild-type allele *fla⁺* is dominant over *fla⁻* alleles at all known *fla* loci. One group of *fla⁻* mutants produces a "flagellin-CRM" (cross-reacting material) which is immunologically indistinguishable from wild-type flagellin whereas another group, probably affecting the synthesis of flagellin from amino acids, produces no detectable flagellin-CRM. Transduction from *fla⁻*CRM⁺ mutants to any other *fla⁻* strain yields *fla⁺* recombinants. No difference between the *fla⁻*CRM⁺ mutant and its parental flagellated strains has been detected in other cell surface antigens. At the level of gene action, the *fla* gene may be responsible for the formation of flagella from their component flagellin molecules produced by the H_1 or H_2 loci. Other regulatory genes designated *ah* appear to function as operators of H_1 and H_2 gene activity. Phase-1 antigen is synthesized only when H_2 is in the inactive state in diphasic *Salmonella*. Otherwise active H_2 is epistatic to H_1. When the *ah* gene is active, the adjoining *H* is active. In the *ah* inactive state, the *H* gene is also inactive; thus *ah* inactive cells do not produce flagellin in the corresponding antigenic phase. The nature of the frequent *ah* state change in antigenic phase variation is unknown. The comparable serotype transformations of ciliary antigens pose similar developmental problems.

In addition to H and O antigens, some *Salmonella* strains possess a polysaccharide somatic antigen often associated with virulence known as Vi antigen. Although only one type of Vi antigen has been detected by agglutination, precipitation, and protection experiments, subtle differences in this antigen can be recognized via specific bacteriophages. Differing components of Vi antigen evidently serve as receptors to which specific phages are adsorbed. Nearly eighty distinctive Vi serotypes of the typhoid bacillus have now been identified on the basis of their susceptibility to lysis by specific phages. From a basic standpoint, it should be apparent that the number of antigenic or serotypic differences detectable in a species or genus is limited only by the resourcefulness and persistence of the investigator.

The virulence of pathogenic microorganisms for their natural hosts is, as previously indicated, often dependent upon the presence of certain antigens at the cell surface. Nevertheless, few genetic studies of characters determining virulence have been undertaken. Burrows has identified four properties essential for full virulence of *Pasteurella pestis*, the etiologic agent of plague. These properties are two virulence antigens (VW⁺), capsular antigen (Fl⁺), and genes that govern synthesis of purines (Pu⁺) and formation of pigmented colonies (P⁺) on synthetic medium. Two antigens V and W, demonstrable by agar immunodiffusion methods in VW$^+$ strains, are of major importance for virulence. The VW$^+$ state is associated with resistance to phagocytosis in mice, guinea pigs, and rabbits. Antiserums with demonstrable antibodies to V and W are more highly protective and opsonic than are those devoid of these antibodies. Although VW$^+$ bacteria are ingested by monocytes, they multiply and destroy these cells and are liberated in a state more resistant to phagocytosis by both granulocytes and monocytes.

Presence of the capsular (Fl) antigen appears to be necessary for full virulence in guinea pigs, but not in mice. Genotypically Fl$^+$ clones produce capsules only at temperatures about 37°C. Although Fl antigen does not appear as a surface specificity at 28°C, it is produced intracellularly as shown by agar-immunodiffusion tests and by the capacity of cells grown at this temperature to evoke Fl antibodies. Clones of Fl$^-$ genotype do not form Fl antigen either at 28°C or at 37°C and do not stimulate production of Fl antibodies. A third antigenic type designated Fl$^\pm$ shows intermediate properties in comparison to Fl$^+$ and Fl$^-$ types. The Fl$^\pm$ strains have intracellular Fl antigen when cultured at 28°C or 37°C, but fail to develop capsular antigen at 37°C. Such strains can elicit Fl antibody just as readily as Fl$^+$ strains. However, as pathogens they act like Fl$^-$ strains, showing high virulence for mice and reduced virulence for guinea pigs. Moreover, Fl antibody will not protect hosts against Fl$^\pm$ strains. The Fl$^+$ state appears to be controlled by at least two genetic loci—one mediating Fl antigen synthesis and the other its secretion as a surface capsule. On this basis, the latter locus would be inoperative in Fl$^\pm$ clones and the former or both loci would be nonfunctional in Fl$^-$ clones. Mutations from Fl$^+$ to either Fl$^-$ or Fl$^\pm$ have been detected, but the reverse mutations have not. Other recent evidence, beyond the scope of present considerations, suggests that episomes may confer additional characteristics upon *Pasteurella* species that substantially affect their virulence. Known genetic transfer systems such as conjugation, transduction, transformation, and lysogeny have yet to be demonstrated and exploited in *Pasteurella*.

Many strains of diverse species of bacteria are known to possess antigens which elicit antibodies cross-reactive with vertebrate tissue components, including blood-group active substances and histocompatibility antigens. Surprisingly, all Group A streptococci as well as *Staphylococcus aureus* and *albus* are capable of inducing allograft immunity in guinea pigs. The streptococcal antigens have also been shown to evoke skin allograft immunity in mice, rats, and rabbits. A bacterial cell membrane component, quite possibly *N*-acetylglucosamine of the Group A streptococcal carbohydrate, is responsible. Chemically, the blood-group specific structures of bacteria are similar to but not identical with the oligosaccharide determinants of the human blood group ABH glycoproteins. However, there is no convincing evidence incriminating the blood groups as selective forces in diseases caused by enteric or other bacteria.

Oncogenic Viruses and Tumor-Specific Antigens

The newest area in which immunogenetic characterization of microorganisms has provided substantial insights involves the many viruses capable of inducing cancer in vertebrate hosts. One may begin with the solid generalization that viruses, like other microorganisms, can be nicely identified serologically on the basis of group-, species-, and strain-specific antigens. Almost all virus-induced tumors show perpetuation of viral genes as a heritable factor in the tumor cells. These genes usually elaborate virus-specific antigens even when no infectious virus is produced. With oncogenic viruses, a central issue is whether the induced tumors acquire new antigenic characteristics distinct from viral antigens. It can now be stated unequivocally that new cellular alloantigens have been found in all classes of virus-induced solid tumors and leukemias that have been adequately studied. These antigens are demonstrable by both transplantation and serological tests. Many of the critical experiments in this field have been performed in the laboratories of Habel and of Heubner at the U. S. National Institute of Health, in Klein's laboratories at the Karolinska Institut in Stockholm, and by Old and Boyse at the Sloan-Kettering Institute in New York. Let us inquire then to what extent the process of malignant transformation and of immunity to tumor cells is associated with the viral genome and viral antigens.

The solid tumors induced in newborn rodents following inoculation of oncogenic DNA viruses (i.e., polyoma, SV_{40}, and adenovirus types 3, 7, 12, 18, and 31) may be conveniently considered together because these different viruses have quite similar effects. Early antigens appearing in tumor cells are mainly virus-specific protein found in the nucleus. These so-called "T antigens" are not essential for tumorigenesis since adenoviruses which are non-oncogenic can still induce T antibodies in hamsters. New transplantation or histocompatibility antigens additionally found in DNA virus-induced tumors are detectable by the resistance of adult, isogenic animals to challenge with viable tumor cells consequent upon previous infection with the homologous virus. This acquired immunity following infection is attributable to the appearance of transformed antigenic cells. Consequently, the host becomes resistant to subsequent inoculation of tumor cells induced by the same virus. That such immunity is referable to a common virus-specific alloantigen is revealed by the finding that a given virus will induce identical immunity to homologous tumor cells in diverse host strains and species. In other words, the antigens induced by a given virus are very similar or identical. This "one virus genome → one transplantation antigen" relationship appears to be remarkably specific in that different strains of polyoma virus produce different transplantation antigens. By contrast, the antigens of solid tumors induced by a given chemical carcinogen are generally distinct for each tumor. The apparent diversity of tumor antigens associated with a given chemical carcinogen, like methyl cholanthrene in inbred strains of mice, is usually taken as a strong argument against a viral etiology of these tumors. However, the number of distinctive antigens demonstrable in chemically induced tumors, as studied especially by Prehn, may well be limited (for example, 20–30) in a given host genotype. Activation of latent viruses or direct mutation of histocompatibility genes, or both, could be involved. Alternatively, Prehn supposes these antigens may arise through some type of derepression of normal cellular genes, especially genes active only during early embryonic development. The rationale here is that tumors and embryos may share antigenic properties not present in the normal adult; the "tumor-specific" antigens of chemically induced tumors could represent derepressed early fetal antigens.

Although induction of immunological tolerance (Chapter Seven) might be invoked to account for the susceptibility of perinatal animals to oncogenesis by DNA viruses in contrast with the resistance of adults, there is evidence against this possibility. Newborn mice inoculated with polyoma virus not only develop viral antibody in conjunction with tumors, but may become resistant to later transplants of polyoma tumor cells from isogenic animals. Moreover, a markedly diminished incidence of tumors consequent upon neonatal administration of SV_{40} virus or adenovirus type 12 can be achieved by subsequent inoculation of more virus or of irradiated tumor cells during the period preceding oncogenesis. These experiments also indicate that appropriate immunization can prevent the progressive proliferation of incipient tumor cells. Apparently the immunogenicity of the initial tumor cells is insufficient to cause their rejection.

These oncogenic DNA viruses also induce an additional class of antigen, the so-called "CF tumor antigen," detectable by complement-fixation (CF) tests. Thus, antiserums from Syrian hamsters bearing tumors produced by one of these viruses regularly show CF activity for the homologous tumor antigen. Because the CF tumor antigens appearing in cells from different species infected with a particular virus are quite similar, these antigens may well be products of the viral genome rather than the genome of transformed cells. However, these antigens are not found in the intact virus. The CF tumor antigens are distinguished from those known to be present in the virus on the basis of heat stability, molecular size, and absence of antibody cross-reactions. Lines of tumor cells induced by each of these DNA viruses retain their transplantation antigens and CF antigens long after infective virus is no longer recoverable. Moreover, transplanted polyoma and SV_{40} tumors do not evoke production of viral antibody. On the other hand, type-specific viral antigen persists in hamster tumors produced by adenovirus 12 while neutralizing and CF viral antibody are also present in host serums. Persistent viral antigen has been found only in tumors induced by this one type of DNA virus. Virus-specific tumor transplantation immunity may be elicted without the concomitant appearance of viral of CF tumor antibody. The timing and strength of the immunological response against the transplantation antigens probably determines whether a cluster of transformed cells continues to develop into a tumor. All the evidence taken together supports the assumption that the virus-mediated transplantation antigens, the soluble CF tumor antigens, and viral antigens are quite distinct. The nature of the specific interactions between virus and host cell nucleic acids responsible for the synthesis of new antigenic macromolecules is unknown.

A variety of oncogenic RNA viruses are now also known to evoke production of both transplantation antigens and soluble heat-labile antigens distinct from those of intact virus in tumor cells. These viruses include the different leukemogenic agents named Gross, Friend, Maloney, and Rauscher after their discoverers as well as the Rous sarcoma (RSV) and mammary tumor (MTV) viruses. As with tumors mediated by the DNA viruses, resistance to transplants of RNA virus-leukemias can be obtained in adult mice by preimmunization. Injection of virus, small numbers of histocompatible leukemia cells, irradiated leukemia cells, or allogeneic leukemia cells have all led to specific tumor transplantation immunity. In contrast to tumor cells caused by DNA oncogenic viruses, continued production of virus in leukemia cells has increased the difficulty of detecting transplantation antigens independent of viral antigens. Most RNA virus tumors continue to release infective virus indefinitely. Continued production of the RNA viruses and their apparent lack of effective antigenicity in their natural hosts is generally attributable to immunological tolerance consequent upon virus infection before birth or during neonatal life. Thus, the mammary tumor virus which infects newborn mice via the milk may continue to replicate thereafter under conditions of complete immunological tolerance. Reciprocal crosses between MTV+ and MTV- inbred mouse strains yield MTV- hybrids resistant to transplants of mammary tumors whereas MTV+ hybrids are entirely susceptible. However, mammary tumors may show immunogenicity in certain strains of MTV+ mice, which suggests either incomplete tolerance or the presence of additional nonviral antigens in these tumors. Mammary tumor transplants will grow more rapidly in mice previously infected with MTV than in uninfected isogenic mice.

Among the several distinct systems of antigens associated with leukemic cells, soluble antigens occur in the plasma of animals with primary or transplanted leukemias induced by leukemogenic viruses. These heat-labile antigens, which are not found in infective virus, appear to have the same specificity as the cellular antigen responsible for the sensitivity of leukemia cells to specific cytotoxic antiserum. This is shown by the finding that negative indicator cells to which soluble antigen is readily adsorbed then become sensitive to cytotoxic tumor antibodies. The acquisition of specific cellular antigens by normal cells as a consequence of virus infection has been termed *antigenic conversion*. A further example of such conversion is the appearance of a new cellular antigen in an established transplantable leukemia following infection by an unrelated leukemogenic virus. Also, viruses can infect and impart new antigenicity to nonviral tumors. The phenomenon of antigenic conversion may not be equivalent to malignant transformation since tumor antigens may be detectable in the normal cells and plasma of infected mice that have not yet developed tumors. Moreover, viral tumor-specific antigens appear in cells inoculated in vitro soon after infection and long before morphologic transformation of the cell cultures. Despite difficulties in determining the origin and nature of the diverse antigens of virus-induced tumors, it is clear that the antigens of tumors produced by any one virus are quite similar or identical in their serological reactivity. In this situation, one faces the complex problem of characterizing viruses in relation to transformed host cell specificities. Since part or all of the genome of the RNA-containing tumor viruses is present in the malignant cells, it may be argued that continued functioning of the viral genome is necessary to maintain the malignant change. With the DNA tumor viruses, it appears likely that the viral genome is important only in the initiation of the malignant change and not in its perpetuation. It remains to be determined whether the transplantation antigens induced by DNA viruses are specific virus-coded proteins or enzymatically altered host-cell surface components. The chemical nature of virus-specific transplantation antigens is unknown. Among both virally and chemically induced neoplasms, either relatively strong or weak antigenicity may be found. More provocatively, stronger antigenicity is associated with shorter latent periods for oncogenesis. The identification and characterization of cellular alloantigens in general are considered in the next chapter.

We have emphasized the essential principles and methods employed in the typing and immunogenetic dissection of protozoans, bacteria, and viruses. Many other examples could be cited from the extensive literature of microbiology. It seems appropriate to leave the reader with the thought that the apparent lack of antigenic polymorphism in some species almost certainly reflects inadequate study to date.

KEY REFERENCES

1. BEALE, G. H. *The Genetics of* Paramecium aurelia. Cambridge Univ. Press, London, 1954; and "The Antigen System of *Paramecium aurelia." Internatl. Rev. Cytol.,* Vol. 6: 1—23, 1957. These two reviews cover essentially all of the earlier work on ciliary antigens, their expression and detection.
2. BRAUN, W. *Bacterial Genetics,* 2nd ed. W. B. Saunders Co., Phila. and London, 1965. A well-written coverage of the general genetics of bacteria.
3. BURROWS, T. W. "Genetics of Virulence in Bacteria." *Brit. Med. Bull.,* Vol. 18: 69—73, 1962. Deals especially with strain differences in virulence antigens and capsular antigens of *Pasteurella pestis.*
4. HAYES, W. *The Genetics of Bacteria and Their Viruses.* John Wiley & Sons, Inc., New York, 1964. An excellent and advanced treatise.

5. HIWATASHI, K. "Serotype Inheritance and Serotypic Alleles in *Paramecium caudatum.*" *Genetics*, Vol. 57: 711–717, 1967. Differences among homologous serotypes from crosses of various stocks shown to be governed by alleles whereas crosses involving nonallelic serotypes show cytoplasmic control of gene expression.

6. IINO, T. "Genetics of Flagellar Antigen in *Salmonella.*" *Proc. XI Internatl. Congr. Genet.*, Vol. 3: 731–740, Pergamon Press, New York, 1965. A nice summary of genetic determination of flagellar antigen types and of gene regulation of antigenic expression.

7. JOHNSON, E. M. "Somatic Antigen 2 Inheritance in *Salmonella* Groups B and D." *J. Bact.*, Vol. 94: 2018–2021, 1967. One of the more recent and continuing transduction studies of serotype genetics in relation to defined antigenic specificities.

8. JONES, I. G. "Studies on the Characterization and Structure of the Immobilization Antigens of *Paramecium aurelia.*" *Biochem. J.*, Vol. 96: 17–23, 1965. Amino acid content of two allelic protein antigens and one controlled by a separate genetic locus were determined and numerous differences observed. Peptide maps of allelic types were more similar than those of nonallelic types.

9. LÜDERITZ, O., A. M. STAUB, and O. WESTPHAL, "Immunochemistry of O and R antigens of *Salmonella* and Related Enterobacteriaceae." *Bact. Rev.*, Vol. 30: 192–255, 1966. This is a thorough review of the chemical and biological properties of polysaccharide antigens of much studied enteric bacteria. See also LÜDERITZ, O., K. JANN, and R. WHEAT, "Somatic and Capsular Antigens of Gram-Negative Bacteria," in *Comprehensive Biochem.*, Vol. 26A: 105–228, Elsevier Publishing Co., Amsterdam, 1968, for a quite recent review of this field.

10. NANNEY, D. L., and J. M. DUBERT. "The Genetics of the H Serotype System in Variety 1 of *Tetrahymena pyriformis.*" *Genetics*, Vol. 45: 1335–1358, 1960; and NANNEY, D. L., S. J. REEVE, J. NAGEL, and S. DE PINTO. "H Serotype Differentiation in *Tetrahymena.*" *Genetics*, Vol. 48: 803–813, 1963. Multiple *H* alleles governing different immobilization antigens were investigated in terms of their expression, repression, and "differentiation" in inbred strains and in heterozygotes.

11. OLD, L. J., and E. A. BOYSE. "Antigens of Tumors and Leukemias Induced by Viruses." *Federation Proc.*, Vol. 24: 1009–1017, 1965. The complex relationships between various oncogenic viruses and tumor-specific antigens are thoughtfully evaluated

12. OSBORN, M. J., and I. M. WEINER. "Mechanism of Biosynthesis of the Lipopolysaccharide of *Salmonella.*" *Federation Proc.*, Vol. 26: 70–76, 1967. The detailed biosynthesis of O-antigens in *Salmonella* species is considered, especially in relation to the structural organization of the lipopolysaccharide.

13. PHILLIPS, R. B. "Inheritance of T Serotypes in *Tetrahymena.*" *Genetics*, Vol. 56: 667–681, 1967; and "T Serotype Differentiation in *Tetrahymena.*" *Genetics*, Vol. 56: 683–692, 1967. In addition to quite new work, these two papers summarize and interrelate immunogenetic studies of *Tetrahymena* and *Paramecium*.

14. PREER, J. R. "Genetics of Protozoa," in *Research in Protozoology*. Ed. T. T. Chen, Vol. 3, 1969, Pergamon Press, New York. A current and thorough review of protozoan genetics especially appropriate for advanced students in this field.

15. PREHN, R. T. "The Significance of Tumor-Distinctive Histocompatibility Antigens," in *Cross-Reacting Antigens and Neoantigens*, Williams and Wilkins Co., Baltimore, pp. 105–117, 1967. A provocative evaluation of immunogenetic aspects of tumor antigenicity.

16. ROBBINS, P. W., and T. UCHIDA. "Determinants of Specificity in *Salmonella*: Changes in Antigenic Structure Mediated by Bacteriophage." *Federation Proc.*, Vol. 21: 702–710, 1962. Phage conversion of O-antigens in *Salmonella* is described in relations to particular structural changes in bacterial polysaccharides.

17. ROWE, W. P. "Virus-Specific Antigens in Viral Tumors," in *Cross-Reacting Antigens and Neoantigens*. Williams and Wilkins Co., Baltimore, pp. 74–84, 1967. A recent summary and discussion of this complex field.

FOUR

CELLULAR ALLOANTIGENS

In the introductory chapter, standard serological approaches for the identification of different antigenic determinants, especially by cross-absorption analysis and progeny testing, were considered. Serum antibody reagents from immunized animals and, to a lesser extent, serums from normal individuals have been very successfully employed in revealing inherited individual differences in erythrocyte and leukocyte antigens. Even seed extracts from diverse plants are a source of lectins or antibody-like molecules which may exhibit a high degree of serological specificity. Thus, *Dolichos biflorus* not only provides strong agglutinins for the human blood group substance A, but reacts so much more strongly with subtype A_1 than with A_2 that it is nearly specific for A_1. Although the specificity of serological reactions is usually quite sharp, it is rarely absolute. Antigens of very similar chemical structure, as noted with certain serotypes in *Salmonella,* may cross-react to a large extent with the same antibodies. Under these circumstances, appropriate absorption of a high titer antiserum may still yield a subpopulation of antibody molecules with precise specificity. It should be remembered then that every antiserum, even though produced via immunization with a highly purified antigen, will contain a heterogeneous population of antibodies in terms of combining site specificities as well as other molecular properties. The late Karl Landsteiner of the Rockefeller Institute contributed much to our present understanding of serological specificity by detailed studies of chemically defined antigenic determinants. In assigning letter symbols (cf. Chapter One) to different antigens revealed by particular antiserums, one should bear in mind that additional differentiation or subgroup distinctions may be achieved with other antibody reagents.

Since cells from a given vertebrate individual contain a multiplicity of potential alloantigens which may function as "strong" or "weak" immunogens depending on the genotype of a given recipient, extensive investigation is usually required to define the antigenic products even of a single gene locus. The term *phenogroup* is often used in reference to one or usually more antigenic factors transmitted genetically as the product of a single allele. For our present purposes, the term *gene* will continue to be used in reference to a *functional unit* or *locus* or *cistron*. The word *system* will be used synonymously with locus in reference to a unit of closely linked genetic information which cannot readily be separated into subunits at the level of resolution permitted by formal mammalian or vertebrate genetics. The term *allele*(s) will denote alternative functional states of a given gene or locus. In association with the more than 300 alleles or phenogroups of the complex *B* blood-group locus identified in cattle, some fifty blood factors or distinct antigens have been found in diverse combinations with such designations as $BO_1 Y_2 D'$ and $BGIO_1 T_2 A'$. In other words, given alleles as discerned by breeding tests usually determine the expression of multiple antigenic factors, many of which may be common to different alleles. Although each allele may be a structural gene for only part of a single macromolecule, the stereo-chemical consequence of such polymorphic substitutions may lead to several different antigenic determinants. The problems of relating antigenic symbols to details of molecular structure are still largely unresolved. This is a challenging area to which we shall return again.

Much of our present knowledge of cellular alloantigens derives from studies of erythrocyte antigens or blood groups of man and other mammals. Our immediate aim will be an incisive examination of principles and analytic techniques rather than a comprehensive survey of blood-group systems.

Erythrocyte Antigens

The human *ABO* blood-group system was discovered with naturally occurring alloantibodies as a result of Landsteiner's attempts to determine whether specific serological differences existed among individuals of the same species. The importance of the ABO groups in blood transfusions was gradually recognized. Subsequently, the *MN* and *P* systems, inherited independently of the ABO series, were found through absorptions of serums from rabbits immunized with human red cells. These antigens are weak in man in the sense that the corresponding antibodies are infrequently induced and rarely lead to deleterious transfusion reactions. More recently the *MN* locus has been found to be more complex—and this is typical of ongoing studies of blood groups in general—with the existence of an additional pair of alternative factors S and s. With antiserums available for all four antigens, and disregarding additional rare alleles encountered, it is now possible to identify nine phenogroups for this locus alone. The alleles in question, which have not been shown by crossing over to represent separable genetic units, are usually designated L^{MS}, L^{Ms}, L^{NS}, L^{Ns} or simply, *MS, Ms, NS,* and *Ns* to indicate the codominant expression of all four factors involved. *N* appears to be a base substance variably converted by *M* genes. Since each allele is responsible for the appearance of the two antigens noted in its formula, several alternative gene-antigen-antibody relationships may be postulated as indicated in Fig. 4–1. Although model (A) is the most straightforward generalization in

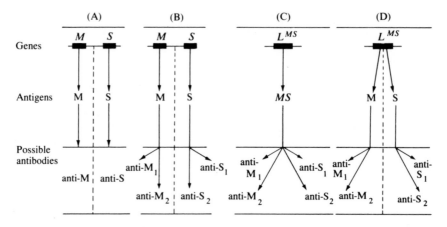

Figure 4–1.   Four models of possible relations among genes, antigens, and antibodies. (A) Two contiguously linked genes *M* and *S* produce two distinct antigens (determinants) M and S, each of which may cause, in a recipient lacking these antigens, the productions of antibodies of a single specificity, anti-M and anti-S. (B) Gene-antigen relation as in (A) but each antigen may evoke antibodies with different specificities, anti-M_1 and M_2 and anti-S_2. (C) A single gene produces a single, but chemically complex antigen MS which may evoke antibodies with multiple specificities. (D) A single gene produces two antigens, each of which may induce antibodies of more than one specificity. (Modified from Stern, *Principles of Human Genetics,* 2nd ed., W. H. Freeman & Co., San Francisco, p. 192, 1960.)

terms of interpretive symbols, Landsteiner clearly demonstrated that even a hapten (i.e., an ion or small molecule conjugated to a carrier macromolecule) will elicit a multiplicity of antibodies rather than a single population of specific antibodies. Thus the other models are more realistic from an immunological standpoint.

Some fourteen independently inherited human systems determining blood groups, including a sex-linked system are now known. These include more than sixty-five different erythrocyte antigens. It is not unreasonable to predict that the known number of reliably detectable groups will continue to increase to the extent that almost any two persons other than identical twins can be distinguished on serological grounds alone.

In 1940 Landsteiner and Wiener reported the discovery of the *Rhesus* (Rh) system which has turned out to be an important cause of maternal-fetal incompatibility in man. They detected the Rh system in an unusual manner by injecting blood from a rhesus monkey into rabbits; after the induced antibodies for previously known human antigens had been absorbed, the immune rabbit serums still agglutinated the red cells of about 85 per cent of the people tested. Since these people possessed a cellular antigen in common with the rhesus monkey, the factor was named Rh. Although Rh positivity is inherited as a dominant Mendelian trait, use of many different Rh antiserums has revealed the existence of eight common or "standard" *Rh* alleles, each leading to the expression of multiple blood factors or antigenic specificities. Most of these antiserums have been obtained from humans who have been immunized by Rh antigens from other humans, either as a consequence of blood transfusions, the passage of cells from a fetus into the mother, or experimental inoculation of Rh-negative volunteers.

Two contrasting nomenclatures, reflecting fundamentally different conceptions of the interrelation between genes, antigens, and antibodies, have been used to designate the genotypes and phenotypes of the Rh blood groups. Wiener, Stormont, and Owen, among others, interpret the evidence on the classic assumption of a single locus with multiple alleles. In Wiener's terminology these are given the letters R and r with distinguishing superscripts like R^0 and r'. The individual antigenic determinants or blood factors are called Rh, rh, and hr with superscripts or subscripts while the antibodies are correspondingly designated anti-Rh, anti-rh, and anti-hr. According to this viewpoint, a distinction is made between a complex antigen or "agglutinogen" and a "blood factor." The blood group substance or molecule as such is regarded as the antigen or agglutinogen while the blood factors are the constituent serological properties by which agglutinogens are recognized. Blood factors then are individually defined in terms of reactions (e.g., agglutination) with known antiserums. By contrast, an agglutinogen is defined in terms of two or more blood factors*. The following diagram is intended to summarize the sequence of relationships invoked:

---

* To minimize semantic confusion, the author prefers the term "complex antigen" over "agglutinogen," and the term "antigenic determinant" or simply "antigen" in the singular sense over "blood factor." However, the molecular meaning of the letter symbols assigned to complementary antigens and antibodies is still a source of some controversy. We shall return to this issue in several connections.

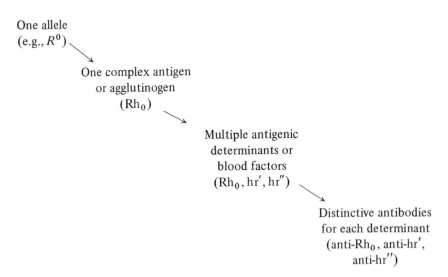

One allele
(e.g., R^0)

One complex antigen
or agglutinogen
(Rh_0)

Multiple antigenic
determinants or
blood factors
(Rh_0, hr′, hr″)

Distinctive antibodies
for each determinant
(anti-Rh_0, anti-hr′,
anti-hr″)

Fisher, Race, and Sanger, on the other hand, assume a complex *Rh* locus comprised of a series of very closely, if not absolutely, linked genes. Each of these genes is supposed to have two or more alleles, e.g., *C* and *c, D* and *d, E* and *e,* with correspondingly designated antigens and antibodies in a strictly one-to-one relationship (cf. Table 4–1).

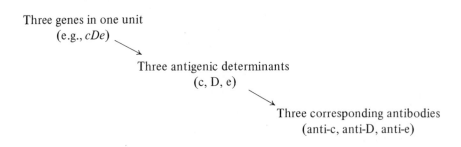

Three genes in one unit
(e.g., *cDe*)

Three antigenic determinants
(c, D, e)

Three corresponding antibodies
(anti-c, anti-D, anti-e)

One may note in Table 4–1 that the four "recessive" genes leading to Rh negativity (absence of Rh_0, D, or 1) nevertheless yield antigenic products which also occur in the presence of the dominant alleles. The existence of antigen *d* remains quite doubtful. More than twenty-five Rh antigens or factors are now known and many more variants will probably be identified, including partial amorphs (Table 4–2). A numerical system such as suggested by Rosenfield and already adopted for the analogous *H-2* locus in mice (see below) appears best able to cope with the increasing complexity.

Table 4–1. The Eight "Standard" Rh Alleles and Their Antigenic Products Compared by Three Nomenclatures

Major Grouping	Allele or Gene Frequency in Whites (%)	Wiener			Fisher-Race		Rosenfield et al.	
		Genes	Agglutinogens	Blood Factors (Antigenic Determinants)	Genes	Corresponding Antigens	Genes	Antigenic Structure of Products
Rh+ *	2.7	R^0	Rh_0	Rh_0, hr', and hr''	cDe	c, D, and e	$R^{1,4,5}$	Rh: 1,4,5
	41.0	R^1	Rh_1	Rh_0, rh', and hr''	CDe	C, D, and e	$R^{1,2,5}$	Rh: 1,2,5
	15.0	R^2	Rh_2	Rh_0, rh'', and hr'	cDE	c, D, and E	$R^{1,3,4}$	Rh: 1,3,4
	0.2	R^z	Rh_z	Rh_0, rh', and rh''	CDE	C, D, and E	$R^{1,2,3}$	Rh: 1,2,3
Rh–	38.0	r	rh	hr' and hr''	cde	c, d, and e	$R^{4,5}$	Rh: 4,5
	0.6	r'	rh'	rh' and hr''	Cde	C, d, and e	$R^{2,5}$	Rh: 2,5
	0.5	r''	rh''	rh'' and hr'	cdE	c, d, and E	$R^{3,4}$	Rh: 3,4
	0.01	r^y	rh_y	rh' and rh''	CdE	C, d, and E	$R^{2,3}$	Rh: 2,3

* Note the Rh positivity is determined by the presence of one or two genes (alleles) leading to the expression of the equivalent antigens or blood factors designated Rh_0, D, or Rh:1; over 90 per cent of the clinical cases of erythrobastosis are attributable to the production of antibodies against this antigen.

Table 4–2. Comparative Designations of Antigenic Products (Specificities) of Complex *Rh* Alleles According to Three Terminologies*

Wiener:												
Rh_0	rh$'$	rh$''$	hr$'$	hr$''$	hr	rh_1	rh^{wl}	rh^x	hr^v	rh^{w2}	rh^G	Rh^A
Fisher-Race:												
D	C	E	c	e	f (ce)	Ce	C^W	C^x	V	E^w	G	—
Rosenfield:												
1	2	3	4	5	6	7	8	9	10	11	12	13

Wiener:											
Rh^B	Rh^C	Rh^D	Hr	Hr	hr^s	—	—	—	—	—	—
Fisher-Race:											
—	—	—	—	—	—	VS (e^s)	C^G	CE	—	E^T	—
Rosenfield:											
14	15	16	17	18	19	20	21	22	23	24	25

* (−) indicates absence of alternative designation.

In view of the extensive evidence from microbial molecular genetics that most genetic loci are complex and comprised of distinctive informational units in multiple triplets of DNA base pairs, the long debate over the multiple allele versus linked-gene hypotheses now appears to be superfluous and largely semantic. Actually, it is now known that at least two genetically independent loci are needed for the normal manifestation of Rh antigens. A common precursor gene and product appears to underlie the *Rh* system. However, the opposing interpretations of the serological results remain a major issue. Is each discrete antigenic determinant detectable by a monospecific antiserum referable to a separate gene or codon? Or do single gene products confer upon a macromolecule multiple properties that evoke different subpopulations of antibody specificities? A final decision will have to await not only the immunochemical identification of the determinents of many alloantigens but the biochemical pathways involved in their assemblage.

There is at present no way to prove that any Rh antiserum contains antibodies elicited by only a single antigenic determinant. Attempts to determine the chemical nature of the antigens in the *Rh* system by the method of hemagglutination inhibition with low molecular weight inhibitors have involved so many diverse compounds that interpretation of the results is still doubtful. Specific inhibition of Rh_0 (D) antibody by compounds containing neuraminic acid has been repeatedly observed. Although a recent study suggests a human ganglioside composed of D-galactose, D-glucose, *N*-acetylgalactosamine, and N-acetylneuraminic acid as the serological determinant of Rh_0 (D), further confirmation is needed. Chemical distinctions among different Rh antigens will be of great interest since it is well established that single monosaccharides or even isomers may function as antigenic determinants. Indeed, changes in anomeric linkages may be all important in substitution of one specificity (as rh' or C or 1) for another (as hr' or c or 4).

The H-2 blood-group locus, also a major histocompatibility locus in mice, is similar to but apparently even more complex than the Rh blood-group locus in man. Various combinations of some thirty-three antigens or specificities have been detected in association with twenty H-2 alleles (Table 4–3). In mice, hemagglutination is the presence of polyvinylpyrollidone or certain dextrans has been most used for typing. It should be noted again that many of the same alloantigenic specificities are produced by different alleles. Thus H-2^a and H-2^b share antigenic determinants 5, 6, 14, 27, 28, and 29 in common. Antigen 5 is associated with thirteen of the twenty H-2 alleles whereas antigen 17 is a product only of H-2^q. The obvious objection to the old letter symbols for antigens in this and other complex systems is that there are many more known specificities than there are letters in the alphabet. Unlike the Rh locus, the H-2 complex has been subdivided by the observation of crossing over into at least three distinct regions tentatively designated D, C, and K in that order with a recombination frequency of about 0.4 per cent between D and K. The suggestion that H-2 substance may be essential to the viability of mouse cells is supported by failure to find any antigen-negative cells by immunofluorescence. The numerical designation of antigens associated with complex loci does not allow for direct indication of possible allelic relationships *within* the locus. If unequivocal evidence for the existence of mutually exclusive alleles within a locus such as Rh or H-2 is forthcoming, allelic symbolisms could readily be restored by using the same numbers with different small letter superscripts.

The blood group systems of cattle have been more extensively characterized than those of any other species. Alloimmune hemolysis in the presence of rabbit complement has proved to be the most sensitive and reliable technique for cattle blood typing. In contrast with most other species, cattle erythrocytes are not prone to agglutinate even when coated with antibodies in excess. Among the eleven systems or genetic loci known (Table 4–4), all degrees of immunogenetic complexity have been revealed, ranging from simple two-allele—one-alloantigen systems like L and N to the amazingly polymorphic B system with at least 300 alleles determining different combinations of some fifty potentially antigenic products or specificities. The number of possible diploid combinations or phenotypes of 300 B phenogroups is 45,150. However, Stormont estimates that about 15,000 of these phenotypes would be serologically distinguishable with anti-B system serums currently available. The number of distinguishable phenotypes in other systems is also limited by the quality and quantity of

Table 4–3. The Known Alleles and Alloantigenic Specificities of the H-2 System of Mice and the Inbred Strains That Carry Them (Modified by G. D. Snell, 1968, from Snell and Stimpfling, in *Biology of the Laboratory Mouse*, 2nd ed., McGraw-Hill, New York, p. 473)

H-2 Alleles	Alloantigenic Specificities. Old Symbol (Letters) Shown at the Top†																									Inbred Strains
	A	D^b	C	D	E	F	G	H	I	J	K	M	N	P	Q	S	V	Y	A^1	B^1	C^1	D^1	E^d	D^k	K^b	
a	1	–	3	–	4	5	6	–	*	–	10	11	13	14	–	–	–	–	25	27	28	29	–	–	–	A, AKR.K B10.A
b	–	2	–	–	5	6	–	8	–	–	–	–	14	–	–	–	22	–	27	28	29	–	31	–	33	A.BY, C3H.SW, C57BL/6, C57BL/10, C57L, CC57BR, CC57W, DI.LP, LP/J, ST/a, 129
c	–	–	3	4	?	*	–	8	–	10	–	13	*	–	–	–	*	*	27	28	29	–	31	*	*	D1.C
d	–	–	3	4	–	6	–	8	–	10	–	13	14	–	17	–	*	–	27	28	29	–	31	–	–	BALB/c, C57BL/Ks, B10.D2, DBA/2, ST.T6, WH, YBL/Rr, YBR/Wi, NZB
e	–	–	3	–	5	6	7	8	9	–	–	13	*	*	*	–	*	25	27	28	29	30	*	*	*	STOLI
f	–	–	–	–	?	7	*	?	*	*	–	–	14	*	–	–	*	27	27	*	*	31	*	*	*	A.CA, B10.M, RFM/Un
g	1	2	–	–	5	6	*	8	*	*	11	–	14	*	–	22	22	27	*	*	*	*	31	*	–	HTG
h	1	2	–	–	5	6	*	8	*	*	11	13	–	*	–	22	22	*	*	*	*	*	31	*	*	HTH, B10.A(2R)
i	–	–	3	4	5	6	*	8	*	10	–	13	–	*	–	22	22	?	?	*	*	–	–	*	33	HTI, B10.A(5R)
j	–	–	–	–	?	6	?	?	*	–	11	–	–	*	–	22	22	?	?	–	*	*	–	*	*	JK/St
k	1	–	3	?	5	–	–	8	–	11	–	–	–	–	–	25	25	?	*	*	*	32	*	32	*	AKR, B10.BR, CBA, CE, CHI, C3H, C57BR/a, C57BR/cd, C58, D1.ST. MA/J, RF/J, ST/bJ, 101
l	1	–	–	–	–	6	?	*	*	10	–	*	*	–	–	22	22	?	*	*	*	*	*	*	*	I/St, N/St(?)
m	1	–	3?	–	5	6	8	8	*	*	11 13	13	–	–	–	*	*	*	27	28	29	30	–	*	*	AKR.M
n	1	–	–	–	5	6	8	8	*	10	–	14	*	–	–	–	?	?	*	*	*	–	31	*	*	F/St
o	1	3	3	–	5	*	*	8	*	*	–	–	–	16	–	*	*	*	*	*	*	31	–	*	*	HTO/Sf
p	1?	3?	–	–	5?	?	–	8	*	*	–	–	–	16	17	–	*	*	*	*	*	–	–	*	*	P/Sn, C3H.NB
q	–	–	3?	–	5	6	8	8	*	*	11	13	–	–	–	–	25	25	27	28	29	30	–	*	*	DBA/1, C/St, BUB
r	1?	–	3?	–	5	7	8	8	*	11	11	–	*	–	–	25	25	?	–	28	–	?	–	*	*	RIII/J, RIII/Wy, LP.RIII
s	1	–	–	–	6	7	–	–	*	–	–	*	*	19	*	–	28	28	–	–	–	–	–	*	–	A.SW, SJL
w	–	2	–	–	*	*	*	*	*	*	*	*	*	*	*	*	*	*	*	*	*	*	*	*	*	WB/Re, WC/Re

† An asterisk indicates that no definitive test has been made for this antigen; a negative (–) symbol denotes absence of the component; a question mark indicates that presence or absence of the antigen is uncertain.

Table 4—4.   Eleven Genetic Systems of Blood Groups in Cattle*

Genetic System	Number of Alleles or Phenogroups (Minimum)	Number of Blood Factors or Alloantigens	Number of Distinguishable Phenotypes
A	10	6	13
B	300+	50	∿15,000
C	35+	10	>200
F-V	4	5	9
J	9	2	9(?)
L	2	1	2
M	3	2	4
N	2	1	2
S	5+	6+	12+
Z	3	2	3
R'-S'	2	2	3

*Clyde Stormont, personal communication.

monospecific antiserums available. The lack of correspondence between the numbers of alleles and alloantigens in nearly all genetic systems reflects the fact that different alleles may determine the production of none, one, or several antigens. The ten A-system alleles, for example, are designated a^{A_1}, a^{D_1}, a^H, $a^{A_1D_1}$, $a^{A_2D_1}$, a^{A_1H}, a^{D_1H}, $a^{A_1D_1H}$, $a^{A_1D_2Z'}$, and $a^{A_2D_1H}$ with the superscripts indicating the six distinguishable antigenic components in various combinations (phenogroups). Note that the factors D_2 and Z' occur only together and in conjunction with A_1 in the allele $a^{A_1D_2Z'}$. The distinction between D_1 and D_2 (or A_1 and A_2) is based on slight differences in reactivity. Absorption of a rabbit anti-D_1 serum with D_2 cells removes most of the D antibodies, but leaves unabsorbed antibodies specific for D_1. An exactly analogous situation obtains with the several A subtypes in man.

In the B system of cattle, factor K is another example of an interaction antigen since it appears only in combination with both B and G. The five known phenogroups in this subsystem are BGK, BG, B, G, and "—" (or no-BGK). The number of phenogroups and alloantigens in a genetic system is usually less than the number of distinguishable phenotypes for the simple reason that the phenotypes reflect diploid combinations of codominant alleles. If the possible phenotypes shown for each of the eleven systems in Table 4—4 are combined, about 2×10^{15} different blood types could occur, which is possibly more than all the cattle that have ever lived!

The J blood group system of cattle is especially interesting because the J substance naturally occurs in solution in body fluids and is secondarily absorbed onto erythrocytes. An animal with J on its cells and no J in its serum has never been found. The J character is inherited as a dominant trait and was detected until recently only with naturally occurring antibodies found in serums of cattle lacking J. Curiously, J-negative $(j^a j^a)$ cattle may or may not possess naturally occurring J antibodies, apparently depending upon the season. Clyde Stormont and associates at the University of California, Davis, and W. H. Stone and co-workers at the University of Wisconsin have extensively investigated this system from both immunogenetic and immunochemical standpoints. Wide variations in amounts of cell-bound J in different animals are apparent from the disparate reactivities of cells with given anti-J serums. Two J-positive classes (J^{cs} and J^s) were distinguished, each with four probable alleles determining different concentrations of cellular and serum J. Serums from J^{cs} cattle contain much higher concentrations of J than those of J^s cattle. Moreover, red cells from J^s cattle possess low levels of J detectable only by their ability to absorb anti-J. About twenty times as many J^s cells as J^{cs} cells are required to absorb the antibodies from an anti-J serum. Progeny tests involving J^{cs} and J^s classes revealed significant, genetically determined differences in concentrations of J attributable to multiple alleles. The j^a allele, yielding no J substance, does not contribute in heterozygous individuals to the variation found among progenies in the expression of the J^{cs} and J^s phenotypes. In these studies, the amounts of cellular J were determined by titration of cells with a standard anti-J serum while levels of serum J were determined by inhibition tests. Although the presence and concentration of cellular J is largely governed by the level of J substance in the serum, additional unidentified genes may also be involved.

Coating experiments in vitro indicate that the concentration of serum J rather than the nature of the cells is decisive in determining whether the erythrocytes become J-positive. However, this simple relationship is partially negated by exceptional cattle that have high levels of serum J with little cellular J evident. The J activity in purified preparations obtained from serum is associated with carbohydrate and protein while that derived from gastric mucosa appears to be carbohydrate alone. The determinant group of J specificity could well be an oligosaccharide bound to different macromolecules in different tissues since the best studied human blood groups suggest such molecular relationships.

With the apparent exception of Syrian hamsters, every vertebrate species that has been extensively studied, ranging from teleost fishes to primates, has shown multiple blood-group systems with allelic diversity. Thus, eight independent autosomal loci, each with two to five alleles, are now implicated in the control of at least sixteen blood factors in horses. It should not be assumed that all blood-group loci are on separate chromosomes. Numerous instances of genetic linkage between blood-group loci are now known in species of birds and mammals. Among some twelve blood-group loci and four serum-group loci recently studied in pigs, for example, three autosomal linkages have been detected. Thus, the loci for the C and J blood groups are closely linked. Also, the K blood-group locus and the Hp locus for hematin-binding beta-globulins (hemopexin) are in the same linkage group. Lastly, close association between the I blood-group locus and the Am locus for serum amylase probably represents close linkage rather than the pleiotropic effect of genes at one locus. Simple systems (loci) on continuing investigation have almost always turned out to be complex. Insofar as detection of new alleles and antigens is concerned, the total number discernible in a species appears to be limited only by the resourcefulness and persistence of interested investigators (Table 4–5). The largely unanswered

Table 4–5. Cellular Alloantigen Systems Known in Man and Various
Domesticated Animals

Species	No. of Independent Systems (Loci) Described*	Minimum No. of Cellular Alloantigens Detectable	Total No. of Linkage Groups (Chromosome Pairs in Species	Maternal-Embryo Incompatibility Reactions Reported
Human	17	81	23	yes
Mouse	14	60	20	yes
Pig	13	27	20	yes
Cattle	11	98	30	no
Chicken	10	23	39	yes
Horse	8	20	33	yes
Sheep	7	34	27	no
Dog	6	8	39	yes
Rabbit	5	13	22	yes
Rat	4	12	21	yes
Turkey	3	17	39	—

*All of these loci are not necessarily on separate chromosomes; some may well be loosely linked. Additional closely linked systems have been detected in pigs, mice, and chickens. The number and complexity of the systems described reflect in general the extent of investigative effort; additional systems probably remain to be discovered in most of these species. The seventeen loci indicated for man include fourteen blood-group loci and at least three loci specifying leukocyte antigens.

questions regarding the molecular basis and physiological significance of the distinctions between related antigens may now be considered in turn.

Sequence and Products of Gene Action

Although chemical studies of cellular alloantigens have just begun to elucidate immunogenetic findings, a revealing pattern of relationships between gene action, chemical structure, and immunologic specificity has been determined for the *ABO* and closely related *Lewis* blood group systems in man. Attempts to determine antigenic structure by direct extraction of erythrocyte components have not proved fruitful until quite recently because the desired determinants constitute only a small portion of the erythrocyte and are bound to lipoproteins of the cell membrane in a manner which makes purification quite difficult. However, blood groups A, B, H, Le^a and Le^b are present not only on red cells, but they also occur in water-soluble form in tissue fluids and secretions. These water-soluble determinants are identified and assayed by their capacity to react specifically with given blood-group antibodies so that agglutination fails to occur upon subsequent addition of the corresponding erythrocytes. Because the activity of most enzymes is inhibited by their products, enzymatic inhibition methods have also been used to support and confirm the results of serological inhibition tests. Molecules that specifically inhibit hemagglutination also occur in various plants and bacteria. Such heterogenetic antigens common to different species have provided another source of blood-group substances for chemical studies. The most concentrated sources of blood-group alloantigens in normal secretions are gastric juice and saliva.

Purified A, B, H, and Lewis substances (Le^a and Le^b) from secretions are glycoproteins containing about 85 per cent carbohydrate and 15 per cent amino acids. Their average molecular weights from different individuals range from 3×10^5 to 1×10^6. There is apparently some molecular heterogeneity in purified preparations even from a single individual and a single type of secretion. Although the detailed structure of these macromolecules remains to be determined, their properties are consistent with the assumption of many short oligosaccharide chains covalently bound to a peptide backbone. Integrity of the entire macromolecule appears essential for maximal serological reactivity, even though inhibition methods indicate that specificity is associated with the oligosaccharide units.

Our earlier consideration of ABO blood classification was based simply on one locus with three alleles (*O* being inactive) and two antigens (Chapter One). Actually, three additional but genetically independent loci, each with two alleles, are now known to be functionally interrelated with the *ABO* locus. These loci and their alleles are *H* (*H* and *h*), *Lewis* (*Le* and *le*), and *Secretor* (*Se* and *se*). Although A and B antigens are usually found in the secretions as well as on the red cells, about 20 per cent of persons with A or B on their erythrocytes do not have these antigens in their secretions. This characterisitic was found to be controlled by a locus designated Secretor, such that a dominant allele *Se* results in secretion whereas the recessive *se* leads to nonsecretion. Unlike the *A* and *B* alleles, the *O* allele does not yield a specific product. Secretions from *OO*, *Se*-individuals will neutralize only those antibodies in anti-O reagents that are also neutralized by A, B, or AB secretions. Since AB individuals cannot have an *O* gene, the neutralizing antigen associated with type O was named H. With the finding of rare individuals who lack H as a recessive trait (*hh*), H reactivity was assignable to a separate gene locus. The Le^a antigen of the *Lewis* system was found to be a product of the *Le* gene while the absence of Lewis antigen accompanies the recessive *lele* genotype. The Lewis B specificity of this system is *not* dependent upon an additional allele but occurs as an interaction product of the *H* and *Le* genes. These gene-antigen relationships are summarized in Table 4–6. Individuals of the rare "Bombay" phenotypes (*hh*) in groups 5 and 6 lack A, B, and H antigens both on their cells and in their secretions. However, the Le^a antigen is still normally synthesized in the absence of both *H* and *Se* genes (group 5). A meaningful understanding of these genetic relationships hinges upon immunochemical identification of the antigenetic determinents involved.

The different serological properties of A, B, H, and Le^a substances are not attributable to qualitative differences in composition. Each is composed of the same fifteen amino acids and each contains five sugars: a methyl pentose, L-fucose; a hexose, D-galactose; two amino sugars, *N*-acetyl-D-glucosamine and *N*-acetyl-D-galactosamine; and *N*-acetylneuraminic acid (sialic acid). However, purified A preparations show higher *N*-acetylgalactosamine values, Le^a preparations usually contain less fucose, and removal of *N*-acetylneuraminic acid does not lead to loss of serological activity. After years of painstaking investigation, especially by Watkins and Morgan in Britain and by Kabat in the United States, these blood-group specificities have been identified with particular sugars and their linkages at the nonreducing ends of the carbohydrate chains. The determinant monosaccharide constituents of A, B, and H, and the oligosaccharide determinants of Le^a and Le^b are as follows:

Table 4–6. Six Human Phenotypic Groups Characterized on the Basis of A, B, H, Le^a, and Le^b Antigens Detectable on Erythrocytes and in Secretions*

Group	Probable Gene Combinations	Antigens Found on Erythrocytes			Antigens Found in Secretions		
		ABH	Le^a	Le^b	ABH	Le^a	Le^b
1	ABO, H-, Se-, Le-	+++	–	++	+++	+	++
2	ABO, H-, se se, Le-	+++	+++	–	–	+++	–
3	ABO, H-, Se-, le le	+++	–	–	+++	–	–
4	ABO, H-, se se, le le	+++	–	–	–	–	–
5	ABO, hh, Se-, or se se, Le-	–	+++	–	–	+++	–
6	ABO, hh, Se-, or se se, le le	–	–	–	–	–	–

* Each individual has any two of the *ABO* genes; *H*, *Se*, and *Le* indicate individuals either homozygous or heterozygous at these loci. Entries: +++, strong specific activity; +, weak specific activity; –, no activity. Note that H activity is much stronger on *OO* individuals than in those of other ABO genotypes. (After Watkins, *Science*, Vol. 152: 174, 1966. Copyright 1966 by the American Association for the Advancement of Science.)

The involvement of L-fucose in the H, Le^a and Le^b antigens indicated that the linkage of the terminal sugar to the second sugar, or both the structure of the sugars and the nature of their linkage, was responsible for the observed serological specificity. Only oligosaccharides containing two fucose residues attached to adjacent sugars as shown were active inhibitors of Le^b hemagglutination. Thus the Lewis antigens appear to derive their specificity from the branching as well as the nature and sequence of sugar units. The difference between A and B, on the other hand, is reflected only in the occurrence of an $-NHCOCH_3$ versus an $-OH$ group on carbon 2 of a terminal galactose residue. Precipitation experiments with monospecific antiserums reveal these several antigens to be present on the same macromolecule. When purified soluble antigen from an AB person is precipitated with anti-B serum, both A and B activities are precipitated. Similarly, both H and Le^a antigens are found in macromolecules with A, B, or AB activity. Moreover, enzymatic release of a single sugar unit may unmask a different determinant, indicating that the antigens were originally part of the same carbohydrate chain. The chains in H and Le^a substances are identical to those of A and B after removal of the terminal sugar. The sequence and products of gene action described are summarized in Fig. 4–2.

Since A, B, H, and Le^a substances cross-react with horse antibody to Type XIV pneumococcal polysaccharide even after enzymatic or acid degradation to the extent that specific activity is lost, the Type XIV or a similar specificity appears to be the "precursor" oligosaccharide upon which the blood group genes act. The combined immunogenetic and biochemical evidence points to the conclusion that the *A, B, H,* and *Le* genes control specific glycosyl transferase enzymes that add sugar units to the carbohydrate chains of a preformed glycoprotein molecule. The recessive alleles at these loci may be regarded as inactive genes in view of their failure to yield detectable products. The addition of L-fucose to the "precursor" to give H specificity may be essential to the function of the transferases controlled by the *A* and *B* genes. This appears to follow especially from the observed absence of A and B antigens in *hh* individuals. In the presence of both *H* and *Le* genes, the addition of two fucosyl units to adjacent sugars results in a new antigenic determinant, Le^b. Le^b is made from the β 1,3 whereas A and B come from the β 1,4 "precursor" as illustrated in Fig. 4–2. There are some problems, however, with this straightforward interpretation of the biosynthetic events.

It will be noted from Table 4–6 that the Le^b antigen occurs only in the presence of the *H, Le,* and *Se* genes (Group 1). Nonsecretors (*se se*) fail to show Le^b either on red cells or in secretions even when the *H* and *Le* genes are present (Group 2). The presence of two *se* genes must somehow interfere with the operation of the *H* gene since ABH antigens occur on erythrocytes but not in secretions (Groups 2 and 4). Either the *se se* genes suppress the *H* gene and

GENES   OLIGOSACCHARIDE PRODUCTS   SPECIFICITY

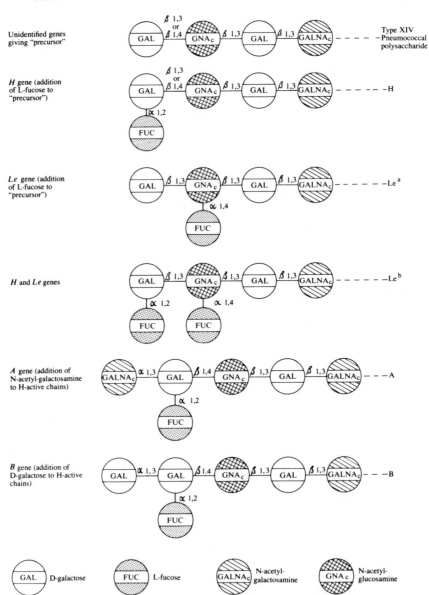

Figure 4–2.   Representation of the structures proposed for the carbohydrate chains in the precursor glycoprotein and the additions to these chains controlled by the *H*, *Le*, *A*, and *B* genes. (Modified from Watkins, *Science*, Vol. 152: 178, 1966.)

formation of sufficient H substance for Le^b production, or Le^b synthesis requires the combined interaction of *H, Le,* and *Se* gene products. According to recent work, secretor status is determined by the presence or absence of a GDP-L-fucose enzyme: B-D-galactosylsaccharide α-2-L-fucosyltransferase. This enzyme apparently attaches L-fucose in an α-$(1\rightarrow2)$ linkage to D-galactosyl residues, thereby converting "precursor" to H substance and Le^a to Le^b substance. The weak Le^a activity found only in the secretions of persons with Le^b activity (Group 1) obviously suggests that most potential Le^a substance is utilized in the formation of Le^b. Moreover, the strongest Le^a activity is found in nonsecretors with or without the *H* gene, indicating that the Le enzyme is not competing for substrate (Groups 2 and 5).

The existence of specific subgroups of A and B raises additional questions. If the major A_1 determinant, for example, is equated with N-acetylgalactosamine at the end of H-active chains, does the A_2 antigen represent a different linkage or some minor change in the availability of the molecule for reaction with antibody? Since anti-A_1 can be induced in A_2 individuals, it should follow that A_1 and A_2 are qualitatively different. A and B substances extracted directly from red cells are glycolipids, clearly of a different molecular species than the corresponding active glycoproteins obtained from secretions. On the assumption that both the glycoproteins and glycolipids have the same essential carbohydrate structure, the blood group genes (enzymes) may act only at the ends of the carbohydrate chains and thereby yield the same antigenic determinants in both types of molecules.

Considerable evidence now indicates that the M, N, P, and perhaps even Rh_0 (D) antigens are also associated with carbohydrate structures. M and N activity are found in the same macromolecule and terminal N-acetylneuraminic acid residues are involved in the antigenic specificity. The extent to which the pattern of genetic control and biosynthesis outlined for the *ABO* and *Lewis* systems applies to other blood group systems remains to be determined.

One can only speculate at present about the size and configurational nature of antibody combining sites in view of the variable structure, sequence, and linkage of the sugars conferring antigenic specificity. It is clear that an antigen such as H may be masked or unavailable for combination with antibody when single monosaccharides such as $GALNA_c$ (A) or GAL (B) are added to the ends of the chains. Similarly, the Le^a-like oligosaccharide within the A or B chains is not available to combine with Le^a antibodies. Yet A and B chains located on the same molecules in AB individuals lead to no apparent interaction or interference in terms of combination with their respective antibodies. The stereochemical questions raised may eventually be resolved when a series of very similar products of multiple alleles can be tested and compared.

Gene Interaction in Antigen Specification

We have already considered examples of blood group antigens in cattle such as K and Z' that appear to be interaction products dependent upon the presence of certain other alloantigens specified by the same allele. Thus, K occurs only in association with B and G as products of alleles of that order b^{BGK}; Z' in like manner has been found only in conjunction with the allele $a^{A_1D_2Z'}$. The molecular basis of the interaction between the independent H and Le genes yielding the Le^b antigen just considered was the addition of a single fucose (H-unit) to the Le^a trisaccharide. This is the only instance known at present where the chemical nature of the interaction product is defined. Even in this example, the role of the *Secretor* locus is still obscure and the Le^b oligosaccharide has yet to be identified directly from the degradation products of a blood group substance. Nevertheless, further consideration of examples of hybrid antigens, suppression of antigens, and epistatic action of genes is essential for a full grasp of known blood group systems.

An instance of apparent gene interaction resulting in a "hybrid" antigen was noted by Irwin in the hybrid progeny of two species of doves of the genus *Streptopelia*. Rabbit antiserum against hybrid cells after exhaustive absorption with cells of both parents or parental species was still strongly reactive with hybrid cells. This finding revealed a new antigen characteristic of the hybrids that was absent from the cells of either parent. This result may be symbolically diagrammed as follows:

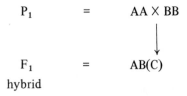

$$P_1 \quad = \quad AA \times BB$$

$$F_1 \quad = \quad AB(C)$$
hybrid

The new antigen (C) is dependent upon the concurrence of two or more genes (antigens) derived from the parents. As expected, hybrids between *Streptopelia chinensis* and *Steptopelia risoria* show both antigens that are common and those that are specific to the parental species. Backcross tests for allelism reveal that independent loci control nine different antigens specific to *S. chinensis*. *Inter se* matings of backcross birds demonstrate that progeny homozygous for *ch*-8 of *S. chinensis* lack the hybrid antigen whereas heterozygotes with the contrasting *ri*-8 of *S. risoria* possess it. The hybrid antigen then may be attributed to the interaction of the *ch*-8 and *ri*-8 alleles or their products. Actually, the backcross birds with ch-8/ri-8 antigens possess a minimum of five antigenic specificities of a hybrid substance not present in either parental species. Parallel instances of hybrid antigens have been identified in other interspecific hybrids among species of doves and ducks. However, hybrid antigens are not universal among species hybrids. Antibodies to hybrid antigens have been elicited by immunizing the actual parents with the hybrid cells, and mixtures of cells from the parental species fail to induce antibodies against the hybrid antigens in rabbits. Moreover, treatment of parental cells with trypsin or papain does not expose determinants reactive with hybrid antiserum. Thus no hybrid antigens are discernible in the parental species.

Comparable deviations from the one-gene—one-antigen relationship have been identified within species as well as in hybrids between species. In sheep, the appearance of the alloantigen R on red cells and in secretions requires the presence of two dominant genes, R and I, associated with different loci. Similarly in pigs, the A, O, and "—" (negative) phenotypes of the A-O blood-group system are controlled by genes at two loci. Here the independent genes designated S and A^A are necessary for the production of soluble A substance and its acquisition by red cells. Certain hybrid antigens in rabbits depend upon particular allelic combinations in heterozygotes rather than seperate loci. The hybrid specificity I has been found only on the cells of rabbits heterozygous for the Hg^A and Hg^{DJK} alleles of the Hg blood group system. The Hg^A and Hg^{FK} alleles of the same system likewise yield an antigen J in heterozygotes. However, rabbit J is also exceptional in that it occurs as a product of a single allele Hg^{DJK} as well as in Hg^A/Hg^{FK} heterozygotes. The Hg system and other blood group systems in rabbits are summarized in Table 4—7. The agglutinability of erythrocytes of different phenotypes, when compared by quantitative hemagglutination tests, suggests that interaction antigen I appears at the expense of A and D. No such competition of interference, however, is apparent with J.

Several examples of interaction or epistatic action of genes in the suppression of antigenic products have been discovered. Studies by Rendel in Sweden among others indicate that the R and O (or r) alloantigens controlled by alleles in sheep depend upon an independent dominant gene I for their expression. In the recessive (ii) genotype both antigens are suppressed. Erythrocytes from sheep of the ii group do not react with either anti-R or anti-O serums produced in cattle. The situation may be summarized as follows:

Group	R-Antigen on Erythrocytes and in Serum	O-Substance on Erythrocytes and in Serum	Naturally Occuring Anti-R in Serum
R	+	—	—
O	—	+	+ or —
i	—	—	+ or —

Table 4–7. Blood Group Systems and Antigens in Rabbits (Modified from Cohen and Tissot, *J. Immunol.,* Vol. 95: 152, 1965. Copyright The Williams and Wilkins Co.)

System	Genotype	Blood Type
Hg	Hg^A/Hg^A	A
	Hg^{DJK}/Hg^{DJK}	DJK
	Hg^{FK}/Hg^{FK}	FK
	Hg^A/Hg^{DJK}	ADI*JK
	Hg^A/Hg	AFJ*K
	Hg^{DJK}/Hg^{FK}	DFJK
Hb	Hb^B/Hb^B	B
	Hb^M/Hb^M	M
	Hb^B/Hb^M	BM
Hc	Hc^C/Hc^C	C
	Hc^L/Hc^L	L
	Hc^C/Hc^L	CL
He	He/He or He/he	E
	he/he	Lack of E
Hh	Hh/Hh or Hh/hh	H
	hh/hh	Lack of H

* I and J occur as interaction antigens in these heterozygous genotypes.

Although R is dominant to $O(r)$, recessive OO sheep nevertheless produce a distinctive antigen—an apparent exception to the rule that only dominant genes yield antigens. The O substance is completely absent from heterozygous R/O individuals. However, O-cells incubated in serum from R-individuals become positive for both R and O, and erythrocytes from group i may be similarly converted into R- or O-positive cells. Since R is present only in the serum at birth and later appears on the cells, it appears that R and O are acquired by the cells from the plasma, like the J antigen in cattle. A possible basis of the gene-product interactions in this sheep system is as follows:

Precursor
Substance $\xrightarrow{\textit{ii} \text{ genes (inactive)}}$ no O substance $\xrightarrow[\text{or } O \text{ gene}]{R \text{ gene} - R \text{ enzyme}}$ no R or O
substances

If this sequential relationship, so analogous to the ABO and H dependence in man, proves correct, the O antigen would have to be regarded as a product of the dominant *I* gene rather than the recessive *O* gene. It is noteworthy that one type of serum alkaline phosphatase activity is highly correlated with the presence of soluble O substance and is absent in groups R and i.

A parallel example of gene interaction in man resulting in suppression of blood group B is known. A woman who transmitted the *B* and *Se* genes to her offspring nevertheless possessed the cellular phenotype of a group O non-secretor. A recessive "suppressor" gene, like *i* in sheep, provides the simplest explanation for the lack of B in this mother. This supposition is in accord with the relevant phenotypes and genotypes for three generations of this family as determined by Philip Levine. Another very unusual family with eight members of three generations showed the *Rh* allele $R^{2,5}$ (*r'* or *Cde*) suppressing the expression of Rh 1 (D) on its partner chromosome, resulting in a variant Rh 1 designated D^u. This effect was demonstrated in two individuals of genotype $R^{1,2,5}/R^{2,5}$ (*CDe/Cde*) and a third of the uncommon genotype $R^{1,4,5}/R^{2,5}$ (*cDe/Cde*). Additional studies support this finding: whenever $R^{2,5}$ (*Cde*) is paired with the allele $R^{1,2,5}/R^{2,5}$ (*CDe*) or other alleles mediating Rh 1 (D), a weakly reactive Rh 1 or D^u specificity is produced. Strong reactions with anti-R 1 saline agglutinins can be demonstrated with Rh 1 positive cells, provided that Rh 2 (C) is not available to modify or surpress the reactivity of Rh 1. These and similar effects involving other *Rh* alleles have been attributed to cis-trans position effects on the assumption of closely linked genes, but the observed interactions are more probably at the final antigenic product or serological level.

The biosynthetic level of interactions resulting in hybrid antigens or apparent suppression of antigens may perhaps best be judged at present in the light of established evidence of gene action through DNA, RNA, and protein in general and through the *A, B, H,* and *Le* genes in particular. Hybrid blood group antigens probably do not result from any interaction of genes at the nucleic acid level, but from the specific enzymic attachment of saccharide units to macromolecules in linkages that lead to new stereochemical configurations. To the extent that this conception is generally valid, unusual antigens or masking of antigens primarily reflect complex properties of the final macromolecules. The concept of gene interaction may be limited to the involvement of sequential pathways, such that one gene and its functional enzyme require a precursor product of another gene(s)

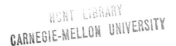

Conceptions of Gene-Antigen-Antibody Relationships

Earlier in this chapter we considered four models of possible relations among genes, antigens and antibodies, illustrated in Fig. 4–1. In the light of subsequent evidence concerning the sequence and products of gene action and gene interaction in antigen specification, additional relationships may be envisaged. First let us compare gene-product generalizations at different conceptual levels:

Microbial/Molecular Genetics	Immunogenetics
1. One gene → One enzyme	One gene → One complex or macromolecular antigen
2. One gene → One polypeptide	One gene → One micromolecular component or subunit of complex antigen
3. One operon → One polycistronic messenger	One complex locus → One multideterminant macromolecular antigen

The colinearity between the sequence of bases in DNA and amino acid sequences in their polypeptide products appears well established. From a mutational standpoint, one might suppose that because only four alternative DNA nucleotide pairs can occupy a single site, only four different products could result from a locus. However, loci in terms of functional genes or cistrons are composed of numerous nucleotide pairs, so there is no serious genetic fine structure problem in accounting for the multiple antigenic specificities associated with various alleles. Although the numbers of messenger RNA base triplets or codons (specifying given amino acids) referable to individual cistrons are not amenable to generalization, the one functional gene → one enzyme or polypeptide relationship still appears meaningful and tenable. In this connection, one may consider the sickle-cell gene in man which determines the substitution of a valine residue for a glutamic acid in the globin portion of hemoglobin. With the monosaccharide or oligosaccharide antigens characteristic of blood groups, each functional gene may be supposed to specify a transferase (enzyme) which in turn conjugates a particular saccharide unit to a precursor macromolecule. The operon-polycistronic messenger concept may be applicable in the immunogenetic context to such complex loci as *Rh* in man and *H-2* in the mouse. Since each allele or functional gene in these systems governs the specification of multiple antigenic determinants on the same macromolecular product, sequential biosynthetic pathways may be involved. This of course remains to be determined.

At the inescapable level of antigen-antibody relationships, the concept of a unique antibody specificity for each antigenic determinant is less tenable in the light of evidence given earlier. At least several possible relationships may be constructed for heuristic purposes.

Simple:	One gene	→	One antigenic determinant	→	One or more closely similar antibodies per antigenic determinant
Complex:	One complex locus	→	One complex antigen with multiple determinant groups	→	One or more antibodies per antigenic determinant ↑
More Complex	One structural gene (or complex locus)	→	One micro- or macro-molecule (precursor substance)	→	One complex antigen with multiple determinant groups

↑

One or more structural *or* regulatory genes

The two-allele-one-alloantigen *L* system in cattle might be an example of a simple system where only one antigenic determinant is directly associated with a given gene. The interactions of the *ABH, Lewis,* and *Secretor* systems in man appear to be an example of the "more complex" relationship indicated. The problem of multiple antibodies of similar specificity for each antigenic determinant is more likely to arise with the chemically related products of alleles than with the antigenic products of separate loci. One should remember that the quality and quantity of antibodies evoked by an antigen is also under genetic control. The degree of heterogeneity of antibodies produced by an individual, especially against a complex antigen, is almost certain dependent upon the genotype of the immunized individual (see Chapter Two).

Leukocyte Antigens

The identification of leukocyte alloantigens in man is one of the most rapidly developing areas of immunogenetics at present. Leukocyte alloantigens are shared by other nucleated cells but are not generally found in red cells. Although most blood-group antigens are present on leukocytes, mammalian erythrocytes in the course of their maturation generally retain a few of the antigens characteristic of leukocytes. However, it has been observed in chickens (with nucleated red cells) that antigens of the *A, D,* and *L* blood-group systems are erythrocyte specific whereas antigens of the *B* and *C* systems are common to lymphocytes and erythrocytes. Absorbed human anti-leukocyte serums have been obtained which react with antigens shared by lymphocytes, granulocytes, and platelets, but not by erythrocytes. Histocompatibility or transplantation antigens are also shared by nucleated cells of diverse tissues, including leukocytes, skin, and kidneys. Since leukocytes may confer tolerance in newborn animals toward subsequent skin grafts from the same donor (Chapter Seven), for example, it follows that leukocytes and cutaneous cells share all important transplantation antigens in common. Some, but not necessarily all, leukocyte alloantigens must also be general histocompatibility antigens. The principal focus of interest in leukocyte typing then is to facilitate histo-compatibility typing (Chapter Eight) so as to be able to match prospective donors and recipients of tissue and organ allografts.

Diverse techniques for leukocyte grouping have been used by different workers. The two methods most often employed are leukoagglutination and cytotoxicity. Cytotoxicity tests are generally performed with purified suspensions of lymphocytes whereas for agglutination tests one does not remove the granulocytes, as they are essential for the reaction.. Human leukocytes are usually harvested from blood made unclottable by EDTA in saline; the leukocyte yield may be increased by sedimenting the red cells with dextran. Defibrinated blood is more suitable than EDTA blood for detection of certain antigens in the agglutination test. Granulocytes, which tend to clump spontaneously, may be removed by defibrinated or heparinized blood by passage of leukocytes through columns of glass wool or beads to which granulocytes adhere. The test cells then consist primarily of lymphocytes with some red cell contamination. Red cells may be removed by lysis with hypotonic solutions or by selective agglutination. Human immune serums generally containing multispecific antibodies are obtained from persons immunized by multiple pregnancies, transfusions of whole blood, or multiple skin grafts. Doubling dilutions of immune serums in saline are used for titrations of leukoagglutinins against counted suspensions of leukocytes standardized to give maximal reactivity without false-positive or false-negative results. In the cytotoxic test, rabbit complement (preabsorbed in the cold to remove naturally occurring antibodies for human antigens) is added to the leukocyte-antiserum mixture and cell killing is scored on the basis of trypan blue dye uptake or on the basis of nuclear visibility (the nucleus of a dead lymphocyte can be readily distinguished) by phase contrast microscopy. The cytotoxic method is now generally preferred because of its superior sensitivity and reproducibility.

Other methods of leukocyte typing are complement fixation, mixed agglutination and inhibition of mixed agglutination. In the complement-fixation test, the supernatant from ultrasonically disrupted leukocytes is used as a source of specific antigens in conjunction with guinea pig complement and the standard indicator system of sheep red cells coated with rabbit antibodies. Cell monolayer cultures (e.g., human kidney cells) are the target cells of leukocyte antibodies in the mixed agglutination technique. The indicator system usually consists of human group O (Rh_0) cells coated with "incomplete" anti-Rh_0 serum and then with goat antihuman serum. If specific human antibodies are bound to the nucleated monolayer cells, the double antibody-coated erythrocytes will adhere to the culture cells in mixed agglutinates. Preabsorption of specific antibodies by leukocyte suspensions provides the basis for inhibition of mixed agglutination reactions. Details of leukocyte typing techniques may be found in the references cited at the end of this chapter. Analyses of patterns of positive and negative reactions of sets of mainly multispecific serums with random panels of donor cells has until recently been the basis of identifying alloantigens on human leukocytes. The difficulty of obtaining sufficient leukocytes from given individuals to facilitate absorption analyses of multispecific serums has also meant that monospecific reagents have not been available in needed quantity. Dausset, who discovered the first distinctive human leukocyte antigen in 1958, later identified ten such antigens in a panel of 133 persons with fifty antiserums by cytotoxicity or leukoagglutination tests or both. These ten antigens were associated with seventy-nine different phenotypes. Many important leukocyte antigens were initially discovered by Payne, working in California, and by van Rood in Holland. A total of twelve to fourteen antigenic specificities are now detectable as products of multiple alleles of one major H locus in man (see Chapter Eight). As in blood-group systems, some of these antigens are separately inherited while others always occur together in phenogroups of multiple specificities. Other investigators have also independently detected numerous leukocyte antigens given separate designations, many of which now turn out to represent the same antigens. Cross-comparisons of 158 antiserums from seven laboratories by Terasaki and co-workers revealed five or more major groups of similar or shared antigens. Whether such groups are equivalent to the products of separate leukocyte systems or genetic loci cannot, of course, be ascertained from serological evidence alone, especially with multispecific serums. The most recent and extensive family studies with increasing numbers of monospecific antiserums point to one major complex locus (HL-A) with forty or more alleles yielding diverse combinations of at least twelve to fourteen distinctive antigens. Whether such a large number of alleles represents a balanced polymorphism maintained by selection cannot be decided on available evidence.

A combination of population and family studies involving both multispecific and monospecific antiserums has led to the identification of at least three independent genetic systems beside the familiar ABO locus controlling leukocyte antigens. In addition to the major HL-A locus cited above, there is the independent HL-B locus with two known alleles and the tentatively designated TO 1(NA 1) and 9a systems. Since HL-B does not appear to be a histocompatibility locus, it is apparent that not all leukocyte antigens are necessarily transplantation antigens. The HL-A system appears to account for most of the antibodies produced as a consequence of fetal → maternal stimulation. The multiplicity of antigenic components associated with the numerous alleles of the *HL-A* locus is potentially analogous to the complex *Rh* locus in man or the *H-2* locus in the mouse. Other tactics of direct immunization may well prove fruitful for obtaining parent antiserums of new specificities. Indeed, Roy Walford has obtained serums from paired humans following reciprocal fourth-set skin allografts, or after a prolonged series of reciprocal intradermal injections of leukocytes, which showed potent cytotoxic activity against lymphocytes of certain individuals, but lacked reactivity with lymphocytes of other persons. Such serums are proving to be an excellent source of monospecific reagents, requiring a minimum of absorptions for family studies. It may be noted that early adoption of a suitable nomenclature for all human leukocyte antigen systems—with letter symbols for loci (alleles) and numbers for individual antigenic specificities—has now become highly desirable. The broader ramifications of histocompatibility typing are considered in Chapters Six and Eight.

A Model Study of Absorption Analyses

In the introductory chapter a simple absorption analysis leading to the recognition of two antigens was considered. At this juncture it will have become apparent that multiple and often complex individual differences in cellular alloantigens are commonly revealed when a panel of cells is tested against a battery of immune serums. The analytic procedures involved in resolving complex patterns may be illustrated in relation to actual data on leukocyte antigens in a family of five persons. In this instance, Lalezari and Spaet tested the cells by standard leukoagglutination technique against twenty-nine alloimmune serums known to contain leukocyte antibodies. The results are shown in Table 4–8. Arbitrary letter symbols are used to designate the antigens detected. Positive reactions are indicated by a plus sign and no reaction or absence of an antigen by a minus sign.

Table 4–8. Twenty-Nine Alloimmune Serums

Test Cells	1	2	3	4	5	6	7	8	9	10	11	12	13	14	15
1. I.C. (O⁺)	−	−	+	+	−	+	+	−	+	+	−	−	+	−	+
2. C.C. Jr. (O⁺)	+	+	+	+	+	+	+	+	+	+	−	+	+	−	+
3. A.M. (O⁺)	+	+	+	+	+	+	+	+	+	+	+	+	+	+	+
4. Mother (O⁺)	+	+	+	+	+	+	+	+	+	+	−	−	+	+	+
5. Father (O⁺)	+	+	+	+	+	+	+	+	+	+	+	+	+	+	+

Table 4–8. (*continued*)

Test Cells	16	17	18	19	20	21	22	23	24	25	26	27	28	29
1. I.C. (♂)	+	–	+	+	+	+	–	–	–	–	–	+	+	–
2. C.C. Jr. (♂)	+	+	+	+	+	+	+	+	–	+	+	–	+	+
3. A.M. (♂)	+	+	+	+	+	+	+	+	–	–	+	+	+	+
4. Mother (♂)	–	+	+	+	+	–	–	–	–	–	+	+	+	–
5. Father (♂)	+	+	+	+	+	+	+	+	–	+	–	+	+	+

All members of this family were of blood group O and Rh positive (♂). Each member of the family showed a different spectrum of leukoagglutination reactions. The twenty-nine alloimmune serums gave ten different patterns of reactions in this family, including no reaction (24) indicating an alloantigen lacking in all members of the family. Nine leukocyte alloantigens are required to account for the results above as follows:

Antigens	Serums Revealing Particular Differences	Total
C	1,2,5,8,17	5
D	3,4,6,7,9,10,13,15,18,19,20,28	12
E	11	1
F	12,22,23,29	4
G	14	1
H	16,21	2
I	25	1
J	26	1
K	27	1

Persons	Antigen Symbols Assigned								
I.C.	–	D	–	–	–	H	–	–	K
C.C.	C	D	–	F	–	H	I	J	–
A.M.	C	D	E	F	G	H	–	J	K
Mother	C	D	–	–	G	–	–	J	K
Father	C	D	E	F	G	H	I	–	K

Check for yourself that the factors arbitrarily assigned above account for the observed reactions. If it were assumed that these alloantigens represented all that were segregating in this family, then one would expect that A.M. and the father should accept skin grafts from I.C., and A.M. should also accept a graft from the mother. Since such acceptance is unlikely on empirical grounds, it follows that additional antigens are present but not detected. Alloantibodies for other antigens are probably present in the twelve serums that contain anti-D; such antibody reactivities would of course be inapparent since the leukocytes of all individuals were agglutinated by virtue of possessing the D factor. An absorption analysis of any one of these twelve serums might reveal additional individual differences as indicated below:

Absorption Analysis of Immune Serum 3

WBC	Unabs. Serum	Serum Absorbed by WBC of Persons:					Saline Control
		F	M	A.M.	C.C.	I.C.	
F	+	−	+	+	+	+	−
M	+	−	−	−	−	−	−
A.M.	+	−	+	−	+	+	−
C.C.	+	−	+	−	−	+	−
I.C.	+	−	+	+	+	−	−

Note that the negative reactions on the diagonal are essential controls showing that all antibodies for the respective cells were removed during the absorptions: thus absorption of the serum (3) by the mother's white blood cells removed all antibodies capable of reacting with the mother's cells but left behind antibodies for antigens on the cells of other members of the family. Reading down the column under F, one observes that his leukocytes removed all antibodies for all antigens present on the cells of members of this family. Thus, no member of the family has an antigen detected by this alloimmune serum that the father does not also have. (Note, however, that the father does lack a factor J occurring in other members of the family revealed by serum 26.) Conversely, reading down the column under M, one determines that every other member of the family has at least one antigen absent from the mother's cells. In this manner, one may assign symbols to the individual antigens detected as follows:

Initially read down the columns of positive and negative reactions to account for the observed result. Begin with the unabsorbed serum and previously identified D factor. No letter symbol is necessary relative to the column under F since no positive reactions were obtained. The letter L is assigned as shown below to indicate an antigen lacking on the mother's cells, but present in the remainder of the family, etc.

Persons	Initial Assignment of Antigen Symbols
F	D L M N O
M	D – – – –
A.M.	D L – N O
C.C.	D L – – O
I.C.	D L M N –

Unnecessary symbols can be deleted by reading across the columns of reactions:

Persons	Final Assignment of Antigen Symbols
F	D M N O
M	D – – –
A.M.	D – N O
C.C.	D – – O
I.C.	D M – –

Note that the L column is deleted in the final assignment of factors since all members of the family have at least one antigen not occurring in the mother on the basis of M, N, or O. Similarly, the N factor initially attributed to I.C. may be deleted since the M factor already accounts for an antigen lacking in the mother, A.M., and C.C. To check your understanding of the procedure, assign symbols of your own by reading across the columns of the absorption analysis; avoid unnecessary symbols as you proceed. This is really a direct, shortcut approach to the procedure given above. However, the longer procedure is generally preferable to avoid errors.

On the basis of this hypothetical analysis, one could proceed to prepare monospecific reagents for particular alloantigens. Thus, serum 3 absorbed by A.M. cells would give an anti-M reagent while absorption with C.C. *and* I.C. cells would give an anti-N reagent. This analysis would probably be just a first step in a thorough study. Leukocytes from other persons might reveal additional subpopulations of antibodies, even in what appeared to be monospecific serums in early tests. Absorption analyses of other immune serums would probably reveal further antigens in this family. The concept of monospecificity has an essentially operational meaning since all serums probably contain antibodies directed against separable determinants.

Maternal-Fetal Incompatibility and Natural Selection

The observed differences in frequencies of alleles (and phenotypes) for various blood groups suggest that natural selection plays an important role in the establishment and maintenance of alleles in populations. The ABO and Rh blood groups in man reveal several levels at which selection may operate. The Rh antigens are the most important cause of maternal-fetal incompatibility. Rh+ cells derived from the fetus often induce antibodies, mostly of IgG type, in Rh— women. These antibodies, particularly in second or later pregnancies, readily cross the placenta in sufficient concentration to produce severe hemolytic disease or embryonic death. Rh-negative women have the highest stillbirth rate. In North America, about one birth in every 200—300 shows disease attributable to Rh incompatibility. Incompatibility in the ABO system alone may have similar though less deleterious consequences in terms of injury to A, B, or AB newborns by the respective antibodies derived from the mother. Infants inheriting genes which determine weaker expressions of A or B do not usually show clinical evidence of disease. However, early embryonic deaths may also be caused by ABO incompatibility. Studies in European and Japanese populations indicate a smaller proportion of A children from marriages of O mothers and A fathers than in the reciprocal situation, suggesting that A antibodies from O mothers lead to the early death of A embryos. ABO erythroblastosis, in contrast with the Rh-associated form, is often observed in the first incompatible child and increasing severity of disease is not regularly seen in subsequent incompatible infants.

For a long time, the relative infrequency of hemolytic disease of the newborn from pregnancies involving Rh-negative mothers and Rh-positive fathers was unexplained. When such pregnant women, especially those who have already had an Rh-positive first child, are tested for Rh antibodies in their serum, fewer than half show evidence of sensitization. It turns out that ABO incompatibility of mother and child is strongly protective against Rh immunization. An O, Rh-negative mother is rarely sensitized by an A or B, Rh-positive fetus. Immunization to the relatively weak Rh antigen depends on substantial exposure to fetal red cells by "leakage" at the time of parturition; A, B, or AB cells entering an O mother are so quickly destroyed by the naturally occurring antibodies that the associated Rh antigens fail to reach the lymphoid centers in sufficient quantity. This same protective mechanism prevents sensitization to the Kell antigen—another potential source of hemolytic disease. However, if Rh antibodies have once been induced by pregnancy or blood transfusion, ABO incompatibility no longer protects. Thus, an *OO*, Rh-negative woman with a *BO*, Rh-positive husband might be immunized by her first child who happened to be *OO*. A second child, even if it were *BO*, would not be protected because even slight secondary Rh immunization leads to substantial, renewed antibody production. One may note that *AB*, Rh-negative women and O, Rh-positive men are most likely to have erythroblastotic children. The probable consequences of Rh maternal-fetal incompatibility in relation to ABO-compatible and ABO-incompatible marriages are illustrated in Fig. 4—3.

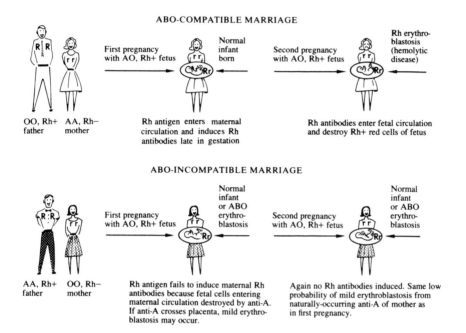

ABO-COMPATIBLE MARRIAGE

First pregnancy with AO, Rh+ fetus → Normal infant born

Second pregnancy with AO, Rh+ fetus → Rh erythroblastosis (hemolytic disease)

OO, Rh+ father   AA, Rh– mother

Rh antigen enters maternal circulation and induces Rh antibodies late in gestation

Rh antibodies enter fetal circulation and destroy Rh+ red cells of fetus

ABO-INCOMPATIBLE MARRIAGE

First pregnancy with AO, Rh+ fetus → Normal infant or ABO erythroblastosis

Second pregnancy with AO, Rh+ fetus → Normal infant or ABO erythroblastosis

AA, Rh+ father   OO, Rh– mother

Rh antigen fails to induce maternal Rh antibodies because fetal cells entering maternal circulation destroyed by anti-A. If anti-A crosses placenta, mild erythroblastosis may occur.

Again no Rh antibodies induced. Same low probability of mild erythroblastosis from naturally-occurring anti-A of mother as in first pregnancy.

Figure 4—3.   Second or later Rh-positive children of Rh-negative mothers may be severely anemic or die due to Rh antibodies induced by passage of fetal blood cells into maternal circulation in the absence of ABO incompatibility. Usually milder ABO erythroblastosis may occur in first or later pregnancies mainly in O type mothers with A- or B-positive fetuses, irrespective of presence or absence of Rh incompatibility.

A notable circumvention of Rh hemolytic disease has recently been achieved by passive administration of Rh antibodies (anti-Rh 1 or anti-D) which apparently blocks active immunization against this antigen. Thus, none of several hundred nonimmunized Rh-negative women given Rh antiserum at the time of delivery subsequently showed active immunization against Rh antigens. This fully effective protection, compared to about 80 per cent protection by natural ABO incompatibility, may depend upon sequestration of fetal Rh antigen or some form of feedback inhibition of active antibody production. Evidently the risk of primary Rh immunization prior to delivery is quite low or even nonexistent. The potential danger of hemolytic disease is of course much greater if the husband is homozygous, especially for Rh 1 or D; if he is heterozygous only half the children will be Rh positive. The actual incidence of hemolytic disease referable to particular systems is a function of gene frequencies—a point that may be illustrated with respect to the gene frequencies of *Rh* genes ($R(D) = 0.6$, $r(d) = 0.4$) and *Kell* genes ($K = 0.05$, $k = 0.95$) in Caucasian populations. The frequencies of the genotypes are:

	Rhesus		Kell
RR	0.36	*KK*	0.002
Rr	0.48	*Kk*	0.095
rr	0.16	*kk*	0.093

The proportions of marriages in which hemolytic disease may occur are:

♂ ♀		♂ ♀	
RR X *rr*	0.0576 X = 0.230	*KK* X *kk*	0.0018 X 4 = 0.007
Rr X *rr*	0.077	*Kk* X *kk*	0.086
	0.307		0.093

The homozygous mating frequencies above are multiplied by four since homozygous fathers are four times more likely than heterozygous fathers to have two Rh+ or K+ children in sequence. In other words, the chance of a heterozygous father having two successive Rh+ or K+ children is only $\frac{1}{2} \times \frac{1}{2} = \frac{1}{4}$ that of a homozygous father who must pass on the trait to all his children. Apart from consideration of the poorer antigenic efficacy of K, the summations of incompatible marriage frequencies indicate that about three times more Rh-related than Kell-related disease may be expected.

Some family studies indicate that ABO maternal-fetal incompatibility reduces fertility by about 6 per cent and causes loss of about 9 per cent of incompatible zygotes. ABO-incompatibility tends to manifest its deleterious effects mainly in early pregnancy, often so early that pregnancy is unrecognized. However, the data on this point are not conclusive. Although the existence of maternal-fetal incompatibility may lead to selection against heterozygotes in mothers incompatible for the *ABO* locus, heterozygotes appear to have an advantage in compatible mothers. It may be noted that human leukocyte antigens are also a source of maternal-fetal incompatibility. Because of preoccupation with well-known blood groups, the potential significance of leukocyte alloantigens in this connection is yet to be fully explored.

The ultimate goal of measuring the relative fitness of each genotype in each blood group system is complicated not only by poorly understood interactive effects of an immunological nature but by differential effects on reproductive performance at various stages of the life cycle. Reproductive performance in relation to blood groups has been measured as a function of number of pregnancies, probability of sterility, proportion of pregnancies terminating in spontaneous abortions, stillbirths or fetal deaths, and proportion of liveborn children dying nonaccidentally under five years of age. Blood-group phenotypes in six systems (*ABO, Rh, MN, Kell, Duffy, P*) and ABH secretor status were checked in one extensive study by a University of Michigan team for possible effects of husband's and wife's blood groups and types of matings. The highly significant correlations discerned are not amenable to simple explanation: Group O fathers and P_2-group mothers are associated independently with more deaths in liveborn children; Kell-negative women, independent of husband's group, have more pregnancies while group-N women are more sterile. ABO- and Rh-mating types also affect the numbers of pregnancies and spontaneous abortions, but the nature of the associations is still not clear because of conflicting evidence from different studies. Perhaps 20 per cent of ABO-incompatible zygotes are eliminated early in pregnancy, but superimposed on this effect is a probable 20 per cent differential in Rh selection pressure favoring ABO incompatible zygotes. Rh-negative daughters of Rh-positive women may possibly acquire some tolerance to the Rh antigen in utero, compared with Rh-negative daughters of Rh-negative women. The impact of ABO-Rh interactions on allele frequencies in future generations is not yet predictable. Infertility also appears to be related in part to occurrence of antibodies of the *ABO* system in uterine secretions and to the presence of sperm agglutinins in the serum of certain married women.

Among patients with duodenal ulcer there is a 17 per cent greater frequency of group O than in normal controls while among gastric carcinoma or pernicious anemia patients, group A is 10–13 per cent greater. However, these disease associations may have little selective value because of the relatively advanced age of the affected persons. On the other hand, the absence or extremely low frequency of Rh negatives in many regions where malaria is, or was, endemic strongly suggests effective natural selection. Natural selection should not be confused with genetic drift. The unusual blood group frequencies found in isolated Eskimo and aboriginal tribes are largely attributable to genetic drift—the random departure of gene frequencies from the norm caused by interbreeding in very small populations.

Hemolytic disease of the newborn occurs naturally or may be produced experimentally in diverse species of domestic animals (Table 4–5). Intrauterine selection caused by maternal-fetal incompatibility of blood types has also been found in whales. In horses, pigs, and dogs, the antibodies reach the newborn through the mother's milk rather than via the placenta. In the newly hatched chick, hemolytic disease may result from the passage of antibodies into the egg yolk before the shell is formed. The absence of hemolytic disease in cattle or sheep is probably attributable to digestion of antibodies during their passage through the gut after ingestion of the mother's milk. Why the antibody-containing colostrum ingested immediately after birth leads to hemolytic disease in some species and not others is puzzling. Antibodies protective against infectious agents passively derived in this manner are of obvious importance. Possibly only certain molecular species of antibodies may be passed to the young during a short period after birth via the digestive tract, and selective mechanisms may be involved.

Other Characteristics Associated with Blood Groups

Relationships between blood groups and production characters (butterfat yield, milk fat percentage, and heart girth) have been investigated in cattle in relation to linkage, pleiotropy, and heterotic effects. There is a significant relationship between the B locus and fat percentage of milk. Cows heterozygous at the B locus have higher fat percentages than homozygous cows, and animals possessing the allele $B^{BO_1V_2D'}$ also produce milk with more fat. In one extensive study involving progeny groups from sires heterozygous at the B locus, about 14 per cent of the variation in fat content was attributable to the particular B allele the offspring inherited from the sire. The J and M genes of the J and M systems led to increased milk fat whereas the L gene had the opposite effect. Total butterfat yield and heart girth measurements do not appear to be influenced by blood group genes.

Production traits have been similarly studied in sheep. Heterozygosity at one or more of seven loci ($A, C, D, M, R, I,$ or X) appears to be correlated with higher weaning weights and a more desirable meat-type lamb conformation. Different background genotypes show no consistent effect on associations between blood groups and production traits, and no genotype-environment interactions have been detected. Maternal-fetal blood-group differences evidently do not contribute to lamb mortality and no special survival advantage appears to be consequent upon heterozygous blood-group genotypes. In chickens, marked differences in the reproductive performance and viability of different B locus heterozygotes occur among progeny of crosses of inbred lines. Several heterozygous genotypes have an apparent advantage over homozygotes in egg production, hatchability of fertile eggs, and adult body weight. Just how heterozygosis for particular allelic combinations contributes to "hybrid vigor" is unknown. It is clear, however, that some blood group loci, such as the B loci in cattle and chickens, may influence morphologic or physiologic traits in addition to specifying cellular antigens.

KEY REFERENCES

1. "Blood Groups of Animals." *Proc. 9th European Blood Group Conf.*, Czech. Acad. Sci. Publ. House, Prague, 1965. A recent summarization of diverse work in this field.

2. COHEN, C., and R. G. TISSOT. "Blood Groups in the Rabbit." *J. Immunol.*, Vol. 95: 148–155, 1965. The five known rabbit blood group loci and the antigens they control are summarized. The I and J antigens of the *Hg* system occur as interaction products in certain heterozygous genotypes.

3. *Histocompatibility Testing*. Munksgaard, Copenhagen, 1967. This monograph contains a comprehensive and current summarization of ongoing investigations of the genetics and serology of leukocyte antigens.

4. LEVINE, P. "The Influence of the ABO System on Rh Hemolytic Disease." *Human Biology*, Vol. 30: 14–28, 1958. A classic study revealing the protective role of ABO incompatibility in reducing the incidence of Rh hemolytic disease.

5. MUSCHEL, L. H. "Blood Groups, Disease, and Selection." *Bact. Rev.*, Vol. 30: 427–441, 1966. The antigenic individuality of erythrocytes, other cells, and humoral factors is evaluated in relation to diverse diseases.

6. RASMUSEN, B. A. "Gene Interaction and the A-O Blood Group System in Pigs." *Genetics*, Vol. 50: 191–198, 1964. The phenotypes in this system in pigs like the *R-O* system in sheep are found to be controlled by genes at two loci.

7. REED T. E., H. GERSHOWITZ, A. SONI and J. NAPIER. "A Search for Natural Selection in Six Blood Group Systems and ABH Secretion." *Amer. J. Hum. Genet.*, Vol 16: 161–179, 1964. Certain significant associations of blood-group phenotypes in six systems—*ABO, Rh, MN, Kell, Duffy, P*–or ABH secretor status, were found with several indicators of reproductive performance.

8. ROSENFIELD, R. E. "The Current Status of Some Blood Group Problems." *Seminars Hemat.*, Vol. 4: 133–155, 1967. The biological role of blood groups and aspects of blood-group serology and of erythroblastosis fetalis in man most affected by recent investigations are discussed.

9. ———, F. H. ALLEN, JR., S. N. SWISHER, and S. KOCHUA. "A Review of Rh Serology and Presentation of a New Terminology." *Transfusion.*, Vol 2: 287–312, 1962. Despite two systems of Rh terminology, a numbered code was designed to cope with the total serological complexity of Rh since the *Rh* system involves multiple and overlapping genetic relationships between antigens.

10. SNELL, G. D., G. HOECKER, D. B. AMOS, and J. H. STIMPFLING. "A Revised Nomenclature for the Histocompatibility-2 Locus of the Mouse."

Transplantation, Vol 2: 777–784, 1964. This now generally accepted nomenclature should be adequate to encompass any foreseeable developments in our knowledge of *H-2* and similarly complex loci.

11. STIMPFLING, J. H., and A. RICHARDSON. "Recombination Within the Histocompatibility-2 Locus of the Mouse." *Genetics,* Vol. 51: 831–846, 1965. Results of linkage analyses provide evidence for at least three distinct regions of *H-2,* i.e., D(4,13)–0.21 per cent–C(3,8)–0.05 per cent–K(11) with a recombination frequency between the D and K regions of 0.36 per cent.

12. STONE, W. H., and M. R. IRWIN. "Blood Groups in Animals Other than Man," in *Advances in Immunology,* Vol. 3: pp. 315–350, Academic Press, New York. 1963. Covers detection of blood groups, genetic associations of blood factors, cellular antigens and gene interaction, soluble blood-group substances, and association between blood groups and other characters.

13. STORMONT, C. "Current Status of Blood Groups in Cattle." *Ann. N. Y. Acad Sci.,* Vol. 97: 251–268, 1962. The entire monograph "Blood Groups in Infrahuman Species" in which this article is contained is an excellent source of information about many species ranging from fish to primates.

14. ———, and Y. SUZUKI. "Genetic Systems of Blood Groups in Horses." *Genetics,* Vol. 50: 915–929, 1964. Eight independent autosomal loci, each with two to five or more alleles, are now implicated in the control of blood groups in horses.

15. UNDERKOFLER, J. W., and M. R. IRWIN. "Further Studies of Interaction Products of Genes Effecting Cellular Antigens in Species Hybrids in Columbidae." *Genetics,* Vol. 51: 961–970, 1965. Backcross hybrid doves with allelic *ch-8/ri-8* antigens found to carry a minimum of five antigenic specificities of a hybrid substance not present in either parental species. See also *Proc. Nat. Acad. Sci.,* Vol 56: 93–98, 1966, for evidence of interaction of nonallelic genes on cellular antigens in species hybrids of Columbidae.

16. WATKINS, W. M. "Blood-Group Substances." *Science,* Vol. 152: 172–181, 1966. This is a nicely detailed analysis of ABO, Lewis, and Secretor genes and antigens in man.

17. WIENER, A. S. "Blood Groups of Chimpanzees and Other Nonhuman Primates: Their Implications for the Human Blood Groups." *Trans. N. Y. Acad. Sci.,* Vol. 27: 488–504, 1965. At least nine distinctive erythrocyte antigens have been identified in chimpanzees. With their aid plus human-type ABO groups, more than 500 blood types of chimpanzees can be recognized. Many antigens similar to those in man are found in nonhuman primates.

FIVE

SERUM ALLOTYPES

Intraspecific differences in various serum proteins have become increasingly evident in recent years with the use of newer techniques, including electrophoresis and immunodiffusion in agar or starch gels. We noted in the preceding chapter that individuals as well as separate breeding populations may be uniquely characterized on the basis of cellular antigens alone. This same possibility now exists for serum proteins which show extensive polymorphism detectable by both chemical and immunological methods. We can be reasonably sure that molecular heterogeneity at all levels has functional and selective consequences under different conditions. However, the identification of particular cause-and-effect relationships is far more difficult and challenging. Although there is much continuing interest in inherited variants of molecules ranging from hemoglobins to serum albumins, our major focus in this chapter will be on immunoglobulins. Understanding the genetic and structural interrelationships among different molecular classes of antibodies and their constituent polypeptide chains holds obvious promise in revealing how immune processes are initiated and regulated. Both the ontogeny and phylogeny of immune responsiveness appear to hinge upon the biosynthesis of immunoglobulins—the only known family of molecules associated with specific immunity. The amazing heterogeneity of antibodies in both biological and chemical properties is in itself a crucial problem centrally relevant to the whole field of immunogenetics.

Classes and Properties of Immunoglobulins

Immunoglobulins may be defined as proteins with known antibody activity found in tissues and serum as well as other body fluids. These molecules differ widely in physicochemical properties such as electrophoretic mobility, sedimentation coefficient, amino acid composition, and carbohydrate content. It is now established that immunoglobulins consist of several polypeptide chains, just as do insulin and hemoglobin. Two types of polypeptide chains, H (heavy) and L (light), have been found, and it is possible to isolate these chains with retention of biological activity. A total of five major classes of immunoglobulins characterized by distinctive H chains have been found in man and various mammals. An internationally acceptable nomenclature for immune globulins is now in general use as summarized in Table 5–1. Only the IgM class of macroglobulins, representing molecules with 10H and 10L chains, appears to occur universally in all vertebrates ranging from cyclostome fishes to man. The finding of IgM as the only immunoglobulin in sharks implies that this protein originated early in evolution, before the other immunoglobulin classes now present in mammals. However, both large (19S) and small (7S) subclasses of IgM have been reported in elasmobranch fishes. The IgG class and subclasses have been identified in species of amphibians and higher animals, but may not occur in teleost or more primitive fishes. Much less is known about the extent of occurrence of the remaining three classes. IgD has thus far been detected only in man. The predominant antibody classes show striking differences in carbohydrate content—about 12 per cent in IgM, 10 per cent in IgA, and 3 per cent in IgG in man.

The H and L chains are readily distinguishable on the basis of molecular weight, amino acid composition, and antigenicity. Mammalian IgG antibodies have been most thoroughly analyzed and have a four-chain structure ascertained by Edelman and others which may be diagrammed as follows:

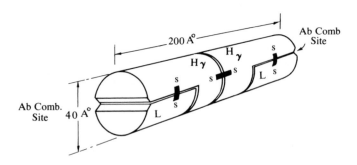

The two H and L chains are held together by multiple disulfide bonds and the two antibody-combining sites appear to involve both H and L chains. Half or less of the amino acids of each type of chain are constant or invariable whereas the remainder, involving at least thirty-two of the 107 residues including the antibody combining site, are notably variable. The same two types of L chains, kappa and lambda, are found in all immunoglobulins. Whether these L chains are actually part of the antibody combining sites, as the models above would suggest, or

Table 5–1. International Nomenclature for Immunoglobulins

Major Class			
Present Designation	Earlier Designation	Heavy Chain Type	Light Chain Type	Molecular Formula
γG or IgG	γ, 7Sγ, γ_2	γ*	K,λ	$\gamma_2 K_2$ or $\gamma_2 \lambda_2$
γM or IgM	$\gamma_1 M, \beta_2 M, 19S\gamma$	μ	K,λ	$(\mu_2 K_2)_5$ or $(\mu_2 \lambda_2)_5$
γA or IgA	$\beta_2 A, \gamma_1 A$	α	K,λ	$\alpha_2 K_2$ or $\alpha_2 \lambda_2$
γD or IgD	—	δ	K,λ	$\delta_2 K_2$ or $\delta_2 \lambda_2$
γE or IgE	—	ϵ	K,λ	$\epsilon_2 K_2$ or $\epsilon_2 \lambda_2$

* Four different γ chains give subclasses known in man as IgG1(We), IgG2(Ne), IgG3(Vi), and IgG4(Ge); these subclasses also differ in certain biological properties. In some publications, these four heavy chain subtypes are designated γ2a (=IgG2), γ2b (=IgG1), γ2c (=IgG3), and γ2d (=IgG4).

merely stabilize the reactive sites at the N-terminal ends of H chains is still not quite resolved. Most of the evidence favors the former assumption. Curiously, hybrid molecules with different types of L chains do not appear to occur naturally. It has been suggested that evolution of immunoglobulins initially occurred by duplication of primitive L-chain cistron(s) to produce the longer H chains. One might predict the existence of functional "antibodies" consisting only of L chains or half L chains in certain invertebrates on this assumption. However, L-chain formation may require many genes to code for the variable amino terminal halves of the molecules, even though a single gene is sufficient for the remaining invariable half. Kappa light chains of man and mouse actually show more amino acid sequences in common than do human kappa and lambda chains. This suggests a common evolutionary origin and early differentiation of L chains. Possibly genes for both light and heavy chains evolved from a common ancestral gene coding for some 110 amino acid residues. Knowledge of the detailed structure of various immunoglobulins is rapidly unfolding at this writing. Key references 1 and 15 are especially pertinent in this connection. The IgG antibody molecule may actually be V-shaped with the Fc piece (crystallizable fraction following enzymatic disruption) acting as the swivel and the two Fab pieces (identical fractions each with one of the two antibody-combining sites) functioning as the arms. The multivalent IgM antibodies may have starfish-like structures. A commensurate understanding of the biological properties and significance of the diverse subclasses of antibodies will certainly entail many more years of work. The nature of the genetic control of the structure and diversity of immunoglobulins, as revealed especially by distinctive antigenic determinants, represents the principal immunogenetic aspect of this subject.

Two types of immunoglobulin antigenicity may be distinguished at the outset: xenogeneic and allogeneic. Immunization of one species with globulins or other serum protein(s) of another, especially in adjuvant, regularly leads to rapid production of a multiplicity of antibody specificities, most of which are directed toward the predominant donor species-specific antigens (Fig. 5–1). The resulting antiserums provide useful antiglobulin reagents (e.g., goat antihuman globulin for Rh testing) which, however, are often unsuitable for the detection of individual or alloantigenic differences. Alloantigens or allotypes are best detected by production of alloimmune serums. In this situation, the host's response is restricted to the relatively minor structural differences among individuals. Failure to obtain alloantibodies in sufficient quantity for typing following xenogeneic immunization may be attributable to preemption of immunocompetent cells by "stronger" species-specific antigens or to antigenic competition on a similar basis. In other words, given a mixture of potential antigens, the more structurally foreign the molecule or portion thereof, the more likely it is to provoke an immune response. Even if alloantibodies are abundantly

Immunoelectrophoretic analysis
of human serum

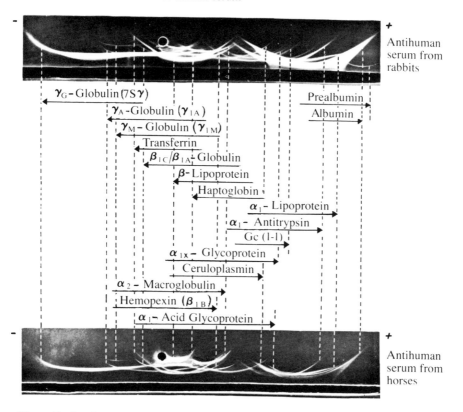

Figure 5—1.   Immunoelectrophoretic analysis of human serum. (Reproduced
by courtesy of Hoechst Pharmaceutical Co., Cincinnati, Ohio.)

present in xenogeneic serum, completely absorbing out the species-specific
antibodies can be a more difficult task than would be the case with cellular
antigens. Theoretically, such absorption can be readily accomplished by
conjugating the soluble species-specific antigens to a particulate carrier such as
latex spheres or sheep red cells. The less complicated approach of obtaining
reagents *within* the species has generally proved most fruitful thus far.

Serum allotypes (alloantigens) directly determined by known host genes have
been extensively characterized in the immunoglobulins of rabbits, humans, and
inbred strains of mice. Gamma globulin alloantigens have been distinguished in
pigs and their existence in most mammals appears highly probable. Both α_1-
and α_2-globulin as well as macroglobulin (IgM) allotypes have been found in

cattle. Though less thoroughly investigated, allotypic polymorphism has been discovered in certain amphibians, reptiles, and birds. Significant differences in gamma globulin allotypes among fourteen breeds of chickens showed some correlation with their geographic origins. Turkeys also possess immunoglobulin allotypes. It is probable that allotypic diversity is the rule among all vertebrates and even invertebrates. This remains an area inviting investigation. In mice and rabbits, allotypes are distinguishable with precipitating antibodies induced by injection of globulin fractions or an antigen-antibody precipitate derived from an allogeneic animal. Human allotypes, for unknown reasons, have not been detectable by direct precipitin reactions or by complement fixation but instead have been identified indirectly by inhibition of standard hemagglutination systems.

Allotypic Specificities in Man

In 1956, during experiments with nonagglutinating human Rh antibody bound to Rh-positive red cells, Grubb and co-workers observed agglutination of the coated cells by certain rheumatoid serums. This reaction was found to be inhibited by some normal serums but not by others. Moreover, the capacity to block this agglutination was shown by these investigators to reside in gamma globulin and to be genetically determined. Persons whose serums contained the inhibitor were designated as Gm positive and those lacking it as Gm negative. Numerous human allotypes have subsequently been identified by similar serological tests which measure the inhibition by the test globulin of the agglutination of erythrocytes precoated with nonagglutinating antibody. The indicator system of coated cells usually employed is anti-Rh:1 attached to 0,Rh:1-positive human erythrocytes. In this rather unusual methodology, the agglutinating antibodies are found in selected serums of normal subjects or of patients with rheumatoid arthritis. These agglutinating reagents are usually IgM macroglobulins, whereas the coating antibodies are IgG molecules. Because the specificity of antiserums from rheumatoid patients changes with time, these serums are not the first choice of workers in the field. An example of a test for Gm allotypes is given in Table 5-2 to illustrate the method. It should be noted that the Gm "antibodies" are naturally occurring in patients with rheumatoid arthritis and their origin is still obscure. However, anti-Gm globulins may be induced by direct immunization of Gm-negative individuals and by maternal-fetal incompatibility. Monospecific typing serums have recently been procured from rabbits following immunization with isolated human myeloma proteins or fragments thereof and subsequent absorption with normal human serum. Either whole serum, an isolated immunoglobulin, or a polypeptide subunit may be used as a source of blocking or inhibiting antigen in this test.

Table 5–2.   Hemagglutination-Inhibition Test for Gm1 Antigen in Globulins of
Two Unknown Human Serums

Test System	Agglutination Reaction
Agglutinating serum + coated cells (IgM containing anti-Gm 1) (0, Rh: 1 and γ G anti-Rh: 1)	
1. plus isotonic saline	+
2. plus normal serum 1	0
3. plus normal serum 2	+
Controls: Saline + coated cells	0
Agglutinating serum + uncoated cells	0
Conclusion: Normal serum 1 inhibits agglutination	=Gm(1)
Normal serum 2 fails to inhibit agglutination	=Gm(−1)

The reaction system employed should of course show essentially complete reproducibility. A significant difference between "inhibiting" and "noninhibiting" normal serums should be three or more doubling dilutions with the current hemagglutination-inhibition technique. When apparently new allotypes or reaction patterns are discovered, it becomes important to rule out the possibility that the results are attributable to antiserums containing a mixture of antibodies or previously known specificities. Tests with isolated immunoglobulin fractions from normal serums positive and negative for a new allotype should also be performed to establish the molecular localization of the new factor.

Some twenty-three different Gm allotypes determined by codominant alleles at a single autosomal locus have been identified. All are associated only with IgG globulins. The increasing complexity of factors governed by the *Gm* and other loci has recently led to the adoption of a new nomenclature with a numerical notation similar to that suggested for the *Salmonella* antigens, Rh blood groups, and histocompatibility antigens in the mouse (Table 5–3). This nomenclature has the decisive advantage of being noncommittal with respect to precise gene-antigen relationships that remain to be determined.

Family studies confirm the autosomal, allelic association of Gm types. Thus, heterozygous Gm^1/Gm^5 children invariably have parents who respectively possess Gm^1 and Gm^5 alleles. Likewise all children both of whose parents are homozygous Gm^1/Gm^1 test exclusively as Gm^1/Gm^1. Two methods are currently in use for recording the phenotype of an individual. For example, the notation Gm(1,−2,3,4,5) would indicate a person whose gamma G globulin tested positive with reagents for antigens 1,3,4,5 and negative with a reagent specific for antigen 2. Alternatively, only positive test results might be recorded, so this person would be Gm(1,3,4,5). In this instance, the alloantigens tested

Table 5–3.   Notations for Human Immunoglobulin Allotypes

Gm Allotypes				Inv Allotypes	
Original Designation	New Designation	Original Designation	New Designation	Original Designation	New Designation
a	1	b^3	13	ℓ	1
x	2	b^4	14	a	2
b^ω and b^2	3	s	15	b	3
f	4	t	16		
b and b^1	5	z	17		
c	6	R2	18		
r	7	R3	19		
e	8	20	20		
p	9	g	21		
b^α	10	y	22		
b^β	11	n	23		
b^γ	12				

cannot be ascertained from the recorded phenotype and reference must be made to a listing of the antibody reagents employed. The respective genes are indicated in italics with superscript digits according to established convention. A rare Gm^- null allele has also been identified. Although firm assignment of a genotype to a phenotype must depend upon analysis of family segregations, assignment of "the most probable" genotype in the absence of family data may sometimes be useful.

The gene symbols used in the following example do not imply that chromosomal subunits or codons corresponding to the *individual* numbers do or do not exist in the relevant genes.

Samples Tested for Gm(1), Gm(2), and Gm(5)

Phenotype	Population	Most Probable Genotype
Gm(1,5)	Caucasoid	Gm^1/Gm^5
Gm(1,5)	Negroid	$Gm^{1,5}/Gm^{1,5}$
Gm(1,2)	Caucasoid or Mongoloid	$Gm^{1,2}/Gm^{1,2}$ or $Gm^{1,2}/Gm^1$

It should be apparent to the reader that genetic symbols containing several numbers are especially appropriate to indicate phenogroups or individual alleles associated with multiple antigenic specificities. Note that Gm(1) and Gm(5) are usually determined in Caucasians by separate alleles versus a single allele

$(Gm^{1,5})$ in Negroes. Certain interdependent phenogroups, like those long known in various blood group systems (Chapter Four), have been recognized among the Gm allotypes. Thus, Gm(7) has been found only in association with Gm(1) while Gm(8) is apparently restricted to the phenotype Gm(2,5,8). The antigens Gm(3), Gm(5), Gm(13), and Gm(14) in Caucasian populations are almost always found to be inherited as a unit (cf. Table 5–4). Although interaction antigens appearing in the phenotype, but not found in the parental genotypes, have yet to be detected in human immunoglobulins, the new nomenclature (see key reference 13) may be readily used to record them.

In addition to the *Gm* system, another genetically independent system of allotypes designated *Inv* (Table 5–3) with four alleles, namely, Inv^1, $Inv^{1,2}$, Inv^3, and the rare Inv^- null allele, was discovered by Ropartz and colleagues working in France in 1961. The Inv antigens are detected by agglutination-inhibition techniques similar to those employed for the Gm antigens. All antibodies against Inv antigens have so far come from normal human donors and belong to the IgM class. They may be induced by deliberate immunization, by multiple transfusions, or possibly by maternal-fetal immunization. The Gm antigens are found on heavy polypeptide (γ) chains of IgG molecules whereas the Inv antigens are associated with light polypeptide chains which are common to all immunoglobulin molecules. In other words, Gm activity occurs on isolated H chains while Inv activity occurs on isolated L chains. However, Inv specificities appear to be found only on the kappa and not on the lambda type of L chains. Studies on the distribution of Gm and Inv antigens on fragments of IgG globulin produced by papain digestion indicate that Gm antigens are located mainly on the F(fast) or Fc fragments whereas Inv antigens are located only on the S (slow) or Fab fragments as determined by electrophoresis. Among the Gm allotypes, Gm(3) and Gm(4), which may be the same, have been found on Fab fragments. The position of the specificities in terms of known amino acid sequences has recently been determined as illustrated in Fig. 5–2. Inv(1) has been repeatedly correlated in isolated kappa L chains (Bence-Jones proteins) with the presence of leucine in position 191 of the 214 amino acids; Inv(3) appears to depend upon the presence of valine in this position. Whether the two products of the $Inv^{1,2}$ allele are simply referable to another amino acid at this position is apparently unknown. The near complete analysis of amino acid sequences in Bence-Jones proteins indicates that the COOH- terminal half (residues 108 to 214) is invariable except at position 191. Perhaps the *Inv* locus is responsible for coding this entire half of the molecule.

Comparable variation in lambda chains has recently been found at position 190 where lysine characterizes Oz (+) and arginine Oz (–) individuals. Other sequence differences in positions 144, 153, and 172 in the carboxyl half of certain lambda chains have been noted. Whether these amino acid interchanges are controlled by allelic genes is unknown.

IgG GLOBULIN CHAINS

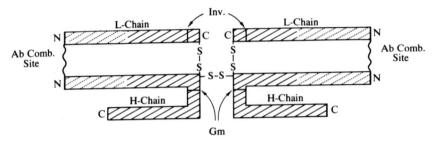

IgG GLOBULIN FRAGMENTS

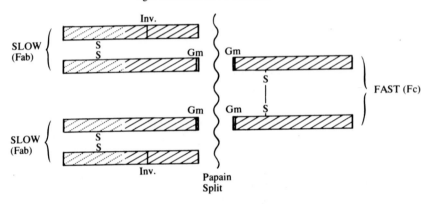

Figure 5—2. Association of polypeptide chains (above) indicating positions of Gm and Inv determinants in relation to N and C terminal amino acids. The relatively constant portions of the heavy and light chains are shaded in contrast with the remaining variable portions. Inv appears to be determined by a single amino acid at position 191 when the 214 amino acids of each kappa L chain are numbered from the N to C terminal ends. Papain splits the molecule (below) showing association of most Gm determinants with the Fc fragment of H chains; their exact position(s) is unknown. All Gm antigens except Gm 3, 4, and 17 are found on Fc fragments. Gm antigens are carried by three of the four immunologic subclasses of the gamma H chain (IgG1, IgG2, and IgG3), while Inv antigens occur only on the kappa subclass of L chains.

In the amino terminal portion of both kappa and lambda L chains, many amino acid interchanges are evident, suggesting that such structural variation may involve many genes. Each complete L chain almost certainly requires at least two and perhaps many more distinctive genes for its synthesis. The latter possibility would of course vitiate the "one gene → one polypeptide" concept.

Peptide mapping of tryptic hydrolysates of F fragments by Fudenberg and colleagues indicates that different Gm types differ in primary structure. A single peptide present in Gm(1) H chains and Fc fragments is missing from Gm(−1) subunits. Likewise, a single peptide distinguishes Gm(5) and Gm(−5) fractions. If these differences turn out to be consequent upon single amino acid substitutions, multiple genes may also be involved in the specification of complete H chains. Actually, the specification of H chains must be even more complicated. As noted in Table 5−1, at least four subclasses of γ heavy chains are known from different myeloma proteins on the basis of extensive antigenic as well as other differences. Gm(5) specificity has been found only in proteins of the minor IgG3 subclass while Gm(1) and Gm(4) activity is restricted to the major IgG1 subclass. Location of the Gm region near the site of papain cleavage, and perhaps involving several amino acids, follows from the finding that Gm(4) is localized on the Fab fragment whereas Gm(1) and Gm(5) are found only on Fc fragments. Furthermore, Gm(3) is also found on the Fab fragment but unlike other Gm types is not detectable on isolated H chains. Recombination of H and L chains restores Gm(3) reactivity as found in the intact IgG globulin. Occurrence of multiple antigenic specificities in *different* positions of the same heavy chains is the general rule. Whether each of these antigens results from independent amino acid substitutions at separate sites in the polypeptide chain is still conjectural. The above lines of evidence may be indicative of a series of closely linked genes or operon for H-chain synthesis as suggested by Kunkel and co-workers of the Rockefeller University. If Gm specificities are assumed to occur on essentially different H-chain molecules, (i.e., differentially on IgG1, IgG2 and IgG3 subclasses) a multigenic or polycistronic complex may well be involved. Litwin and Kunkel interpret family and population studies of Gm groups to indicate that heavy chains of each IgG subclass are products of genes at separate but closely linked loci. Three subclasses are very tentatively mapped in the order−IgG2−IgG3−IgG1−. It is clear that neither the Gm or Inv containing portions of IgG molecules are present in the region of the antibody-combining sites. The apparent absence of hybrid molecules with respect to Gm or Inv in heterozygous individuals raises the possibility that these molecular sites control the final coupling of the constituent polypeptide chains. In heterozygous Gm(1,5) individuals, fluorescent antibodies specific for Gm(1) and Gm(5), and conjugated with fluorescein isothiocyanate and tetraethylrhodamine isothiocynate, respectively, were found to localize in different plasma cells in the spleen and lymph nodes. However, in Gm(1,2,5) individuals, Gm(1) and Gm(2) were found in the same plasma cells. Here the genotype proved to be $Gm^{1,2}/Gm^{5}$. Evidently, only one *Gm* allele is functional in a given antibody producing cell. Similar studies reveal that individual spleen and lymph node cells may produce both H and L chains simultaneously, but they rarely if ever produce different types of L chains concurrently.

The Gm and Inv antigens not only occur with different frequencies in different populations within a race but are often specified by different alleles in different races. Hence, these allotypes are potentially useful for anthropologic and population studies. Many of the genetic studies in the field have been done by Arthur Steinberg and co-workers at Western Reserve University. The *Gm* alleles characteristic of diverse human races are set out in Table 5–4. Apart from

Table 5–4. *Gm* Alleles Commonly Present in Each of Several Races* (After Muir and Steinberg, *Seminars Hemat.*, Vol 4: 156–173, 1967. By permission)

Race	Alleles
Caucasoid	Gm^1, $Gm^{1,2}$, $Gm^{3,5,13,14}$
Negroid	$Gm^{1,5,13,14}$, $Gm^{1,5,14}$, $Gm^{1,5,6}$
Mongoloid	Gm^1, $Gm^{1,2}$, $Gm^{1,13}$, $Gm^{1,3,5,13\ 14}$
Ainu	Gm^1, $Gm^{1,2}$,‡ $Gm^{1,13}$, Gm^2
Bushmen	Gm^1, $Gm^{1,5}$, $Gm^{1,13}$, $Gm^{1,5,13\ 14}$
Pygmy	$Gm^{1,5\ 13,14}$, $Gm^{1,5,6}$ §
Micronesian	Gm^1, $Gm^{1,3,5,13,14}$
Melanesian	Gm^1, $Gm^{1,2}$, $Gm^{1,3,5,13,14}$, $Gm^{1,5,13,14}$

*Based on tests for Gm(1), Gm(2), Gm(3), Gm(5) Gm(6), Gm(13), and Gm(14).
‡This allele, which is relatively rare, may have been introduced by breeding with Japanese.
§This allele, which is relatively rare, may have been introduced by breeding with Negroids.

its remarkable dependence on combined H and L chains, the Gm(3) antigen is also notable for its association with Gm(5) of Caucasians but not with that of Negroes. Gm(6), on the other hand is practically confined to Negroes, who in turn do not show Gm(2). The Gm(1) specificity is universal in all races with a variable frequency only in Caucasians. There is presumably some important selective advantage connected with Gm(1). Although the $Gm^{1,5}$ allele is frequent among Chinese and Micronesians, it is curiously rare among the Japanese. Gm(2) is notably frequent in American Indians but uncommon or even missing entirely from many other populations. Among smaller population groups, the otherwise common Gm(5) factor is not found in Aborigines from the western desert of Australia. The finding of various Gm and Inv phenotypes has been reported in chimpanzees, gorillas, orangs, gibbons, baboons, and monkeys. Intraspecific differences have been repeatedly found in chimpanzees and baboons, which suggests that immunoglobulin allotype polymorphism in man is ancient and physiologically significant. Chimpanzee serums contain at least four of the human Gm antigens and two of the three known Inv antigens.

The disease states represented by various hypo-, hyper- and dys-gammaglobulinemias have revealed some interesting associations with allotypic markers although given allotypes as such are not known to lead to special deficiencies or disease susceptibility. Among many diseases checked for possible association with Gm(1), for example, only rheumatoid patients showed an increased frequency of Gm(1), and even this finding is made doubtful by contrary evidence. It has been suggested that mutation in allotype genes could result in suppression of the synthesis or of the combination of H and L chains. Certain familial immunoglobulin abnormalities and various forms of hypogamma-globulinemia or aggammaglobulinemia might have such a basis analogous to hemoglobinopathies like thalassemia. Congenital agammaglobulinemia of the sex-linked recessive type results in boys lacking both IgM and IgA globulins but having very low levels of IgG globulins. Such individuals rarely produce detectable circulating antibodies to any antigen. In congenital, autosomal agammaglobulinemia which affects both sexes, there is a more extreme general failure of immunoglobulin production associated with thymic aplasia and atrophy of all lymphoid tissues, as already considered in Chapter Two. Separate genetic control of different types of H chains is also suggested by normal or increased levels of IgM in certain hereditary hypogammaglobulinemias and by the absence of IgA molecules in relatives of some agammaglobulinemics. Primary acquired agammaglobulinemia, usually beginning later in life, may have several as yet unknown etiologies.

In patients with "H-chain disease," an unusual plasma cell dyscrasia, there is excessive synthesis of γ-type H chains leading to an abundance of an unusual protein in the serum and urine. Such patients have thus far proved to be Gm(5)—a type infrequently encountered in other myeloma proteins. Abnormal synthesis of L-chain monomers and dimers is revealed by the occurrence of so-called Bence-Jones proteins in large quantities in the urine (and less frequently in the serum) of individuals with multiple myeloma (plasma cell tumors). A myeloma IgG is homogeneous with only one type each of heavy and light chains in contrast to IgG from normal serum which contains more than eight combinations of heavy and light chains. The paraproteins of multiple myeloma and Waldenströms macroglobulinemia, unlike normal serum globulins, are also essentially homogeneous with respect to subclass antigenic determinants and allotypic determinants. Thus, myeloma protein isolated from an individual may contain antigens representing only one of the possible Gm and Inv alleles. Still other restrictions are evident: IgG1 myeloma proteins may be Gm(1), Gm(1,2), or Gm(3), or none of these; IgG3 heavy chains from whites may be Gm(5,13,14), from Negroes Gm(5,13,14), Gm(5,6), or Gm(5,6,14), and from Mongoloids Gm(13). No Gm or Inv antigens have been detected on IgG4 myeloma proteins.

Intensive studies by Kunkel's group reveal as yet poorly understood but regular associations between certain Gm types and subgroups of myeloma proteins. Four subgroups of γ-H chains, as indicated before, are readily distinguished on the basis of reactions with different H-chain specific antiserums. Some 60 to 70 per cent of all myeloma proteins are found in the γ H-chain subclass IgG1. This subclass contains Gm(1) and Gm(4) if the appropriate alleles are present while Gm(5) and Gm(21) characteristics are found only in IgG3 myeloma proteins. Also, Gm(5) individuals, whether homozygous or heterozygous, have shown higher concentrations of IgG3-type globulins than Gm(−5) individuals. The IgG4 subclass of myeloma proteins appears to lack allotype antigens, but this conclusion is not unequivocally established. One is currently left with the impression that certain functional aspects of antibody specificity, especially among IgG molecules, may well turn out to be allotype associated. Moreover, both IgM and IgA immunoglobulins can each be subdivided into at least two different subclasses based on antigenic or allotypic differences in their heavy polypeptide chains. The extent to which the detailed findings with myeloma and other abnormal proteins may be applied to normal immunoglobulin molecules remains to be seen. Although myeloma globulins have been called "antibodies in search of an antigen," certain of these globulins are now known to have specific antibody activity. However, it should also be noted that chromosomal abnormalities have been observed in all types of monoclonal gammopathies.

Maternal-fetal incompatibility for Gm antigens may lead to production of Gm antibodies in successive pregnancies analogous to the situation in Rh immunization. Why only some mother-fetus combinations of appropriate Gm phenotypes lead to production of Gm antibodies is unclear. Production of anti-Gm is presumably stimulated by entrance of fetal blood into the maternal circulation. One family study demonstrated that synthesis of Gm(1) globulin was occurring in a fetus by the seventh month of gestation in sufficient quantity to immunize a Gm(−1) mother. Gm-anti-Gm interactions may have deleterious consequences in vivo as seen under conditions of repeated experimental immunization. Maternal antibodies against fetal Gm determinants may be involved in the etiology of transient hypogammaglobulinemia of infancy. However, it is not established that allotype incompatibilities have led to fetal deaths or disease in newborns. The Gm and Inv phenotypes of mother and newborn child are initially identical because much of the IgG present in the infant is acquired from the mother via the placenta. Only after a few months, when the child has metabolized its mother's globulin and concurrently acquired its own, does the phenotype reflect the infant genotype. Under these conditions one might expect infants to become tolerant (Chapter Seven) of maternal serum alloantigens, at least of the IgG species, but on the contrary, alloimmunization appears to occur.

Allotypic Specificities in Rabbits

At about the same time that the existence of the human Gm groups was discerned, Oudin in France detected globulin allotypes in rabbits directly by injection of specific precipitates of rabbit antibodies in Freund's adjuvant into other rabbits. The alloantibodies so induced were revealed by precipitin reactions in agar gels and by passive cutaneous anaphylaxis in guinea pigs. Extensive studies, especially by Dray and co-workers in the United States and by Dubiski and co-workers in Canada and Poland, have shown nine or ten allotypic specificities associated with rabbit IgG globulins. Two closely linked and one independent autosomal loci, each with multiple alleles, appear to control these allotypes. Typical codominant inheritance of these alloantigens has been observed. Serums from individual rabbits generally show at least three allotypes while rabbits heterozygous at one or more loci may reveal four or more allotypes. The present nomenclature for these loci, alleles, and allotypes is still something of a geneticist's nightmare. The best studied, independent loci have been designated *a* and *b*, while the alloantigens are currently noted as al, a2, a3, b4, b5, b6, *or* A1, A2, A3, A4, A5, A6, etc. The alleles in turn have also been given alternative designations (Table 5–5), which are inconsistent with established immunogenetic usage. It may be hoped that the type of nomenclature for human immunoglobulin allotypes previously described will be generally applied to other species for reasons already given. The suggested nomenclature indicated in Table 5–5 would do nicely with minimal modification of current usages. The *A* and *B* loci respectively control H- and L-chain antigens present in serum IgG and IgM and in IgG and IgA of colostrum of a given rabbit. The *C* or third locus may determine H-chain antigens in an IgG2 subclass and appears to be closely linked to the *A* locus governing at least three allotypes in the IgG1 subclass. Whether the *C* locus also affects the heavy chains of other classes of immunoglobulins is not clear. Still another gene locus tentatively designated *Ms* yields two allotypes (Ms1 and Ms2) found on rabbit IgM, but not rabbit IgG. When the structural units controlled by these four loci are better known, the locus symbols may be appropriately revised to indicate special relationships to given immunoglobulin classes or polypeptide chains. Thus, the *A, B, C,* and *Ms* loci could be designated *IH-1, IL, IH-2,* and *IM,* respectively, if their supposed restriction to H or L chains or to a given class (IgM) turns out to be valid.

The most common method of typing normal rabbit serums for presence or absence of given allotypes is illustrated in Fig. 5–3. Tests for possible linkage of the *A* and *B* loci in various classes involving doubly heterozygous sires and homozygous dams yield four phenotypes with about equal frequencies, thereby excluding close linkage, but leaving open the possibility that the two loci are far apart on the same chromosome. Various progeny tests indicating allelism for genes at the *A* and *B* loci, respectively, are shown in Table 5–6. The rather surprising one-to-one relationships between alleles and alloantigens given for these systems already appears to be an oversimplification. Thus, dual precipitin bands indicating two allotypes invariably appear in association with the alleles *B1* and *B2*, respectively, strongly suggesting two distinctive antigenic determinants governed in each instance by single Mendelian genes. Moreover, the possibility exists that the *B* locus is complex and polycistronic in nature.

Table 5–5. Diverse Nomenclatures for Rabbit IgG Allotypes

Locus*	Suggested Nomenclature		Current Nomenclatures		
	Alleles	Alloantigens	Locus	Alleles	Alloantigens
A	A^1	A(1)	a	Aa^1 or a^1	Aa1, a1, or A1
	A^2	A(2)		Aa^2 or a^2	Aa2, a2, or A2
	A^3	A(3)		Aa^3 or a^3	Aa3, a3, or A3
B	B^1	B(1)	b	Ab^4 or b^4	Ab4, b4, or A4
	B^2	B(2)		Ab^5 or b^5	Ab5, b5, or A5
	B^3	B(3)		Ab^6 or b^6	Ab6, b6, or A6
	B^4	B(4)		Ab^9 or b^9	Ab9, b9, or A9
C	C^1	C(1)	"third	—	Ac7, P, As7, or A7
	C^2	C(2)	locus"	—	As8 or A8

*The A (or a) locus produces H-chain allotypes and the independent B (or b) locus produces L-chain allotypes. The C or third locus may govern H-chain antigens in an IgG2 subclass and appears to be closely linked to the A locus determining allotypes in an IgG1 subclass. The alleles designated at the C locus are not firmly characterized.

Table 5–6. Some Progeny Tests for Segregation at the *A* and *B* Allotype Loci in Rabbits (Modified from Dray *et al.*, *J. Immunol.*, Vol 91: 410–411, 1963. Copyright The Williams and Wilkins Co.)

Phenotypes of Parents	No. of Litters	No. of Progeny	Expected (E) and Observed (O) Segregations		Phenotypes of Offspring		Probability
A(1) × A(2)	11	46	E	0	A(2) 46	A(1,2) 0	A(1) 0
			O	0	46	0	A(1) 0
A(2) × A(1,2)	56	232	E	116	A(2) 116	A(1,2) 0	A(1) 0
			O	122	110	0	A(1) 0.3–0.5 0
A(1) × A(1,2)	28	140	E	0	A(2) 70	A(1,2) 70	A(1) 0
			O	0	66	74	A(1) 0.3–0.5 0
A(1,2) × A(1,2)	12	45	E	11.25	A(2) 22.5	A(1,2) 11.25	A(1) 0.02–0.05
			O	11	30	4	
B(1) × B(2)	39	164	E	0	B(2) 164	B(1,2) 0	B(1) 0
			O	0	164	0	B(1) 0
B(2) × B(1,2)	39	149	E	74.5	B(2) 74.5	B(1,2) 0	B(1) 0
			O	67	82	0	B(1) 0.2–0.3 0
B(1) × B(1,2)	57	253	E	0	B(2) 126.5	B(1,2) 126.5	B(1) 0
			O	0	127	126	B(1) 0.90–0.95
B(1,2) × B(1,2)	49	200	E	50	B(2) 100	B(1,2) 50	B(1) 0.3–0.5
			O	48	93	59	

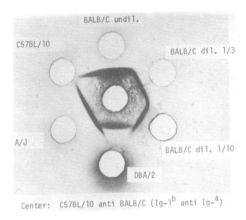

Center: C57BL/10 anti BALB/C (Ig-1^b anti Ig-^a)

Figure 5–3. Ouchterlony experiment showing the method of typing normal rabbit sera for presence or absence of Ab5 or B(2) γ globulins. Alternate holes of the center row were filled with an Ab5 reference normal serum (as shown) and with anti-Ab5 serum (unmarked). Twelve normal rabbit sera were placed in the numbered holes; sera 1, 2, 3, 6, 9, and 11 contain Ab5 globulins. (Modified from Dray *et al.*, *J. Immunol.*, Vol. 91: 408, 1963. Copyright the Williams and Wilkins Co.)

It may not be mere coincidence that the *A* locus produces H-chain allotypic specificities and the *B* locus L-chain allotypic specificities quite similar in effect to the *Gm* and *Inv* loci of man. However, the rabbit allotypes determined by these two loci appear to be included in all types of immunoglobulin, in contrast to the Gm specificities in man. Dray and co-workers identified a third (*C*) locus governing two additional alloantigens found on rabbit IgG molecules. Hamers and colleagues in Belgium have probably also detected the *C* locus in the same linkage group as *A*. The C2 (or A8) alloantigen yields a second precipitin line in immunodiffusion tests with certain anti-A(1) serums. The new specificity is not clearly attributable to a new allele of *A* or *B* since it is present in animals supposedly heterozygous for both loci. Because this new dominant trait may also be found in rabbits homozygous for known A and B allotypes, it probably is not an interaction antigen.

Although considerably less is known about the fine structure of rabbit IgG in comparison to human IgG, Dray and Nisonoff have recently established certain gene-rabbit IgG globulin relationships of fundamental interest. Quantitative analysis of allotypes was achieved by labeling purified gamma globulin or its papain-digested fragments with I^{131} or I^{125} and determining the amount of label precipitable by monospecific antiallotype serums. To ensure complete removal of a precipitable allotype, supernatants were tested for co-precipitation with unlabeled carrier gamma globulin together with additional antibody.

Soluble complexes remaining after the initial reaction were also precipitated through indirect (antiglobulin) reactions involving a second antiserum specific for an allotype present on the initial antibodies, but not present on the globulin serving as antigen.

The key findings were as follows: Most but not all whole IgG molecules have allotypic specificities controlled by both the A and B loci. At face value, this would imply that neither of these loci is absolutely essential for the synthesis of IgG molecules. Moreover, not all IgG molecules with B locus allotypes have A locus allotypes and vice versa. Whether other undetected allotypes, perhaps involving other genetic loci, are present on the unusual molecules remains to be seen. Although alloantigens of both loci are usually found on the same IgG molecules, specificities of different alleles are never present on the same molecules. Even though both alleles, contrary to the Gm situation in man, may function in a given antibody producing cell, hybrid allelic molecules for unknown reasons are not naturally occurring. In heterozygous B^1/B^2 rabbits, both B(1) and B(2) appear to be produced in the same cell as evidenced by fluorescent antibody tagging. Whether all four allotypes are produced in the same cell in double heterozygotes remains to be established. Curiously, the distribution of alloantigens governed by the two loci in the double heterozygote appears to be random. Thus, in an $A^1A^3B^1B^2$ double heterozygote, 68 per cent of the IgG precipitable with anti-A(1) are also precipitable with anti-B(1) while only 16 per cent of the IgG possessing A(1) also have B(2). Although the data indicate random assortment of A(1) with B(1), this may not be so for A(1) and B(2). In this instance, the A(1) and B(1) specificities came from different parents. Other studies indicate that the relative concentrations of A and B allotypes vary greatly in different populations of purified antibodies produced by the same rabbits. One can only speculate about the functional significance of such differences in terms of the assumption that the allotype region in some way influences the conformation of the antibody-combining site. Conceivably, antibodies of a given specificity are selectively formed from certain subclasses and allotypes. However, both IgG and IgM hapten antibodies in one study showed allelic light chain allotypes in the same relative proportions as found in the total IgG of the serum from which they were isolated.

Heavy chain antigenic determinants of rabbit IgG controlled by the A locus have been found on serum IgM and IgA from colostrum by immunodiffusion tests, as already noted. This occurrence of the same or similar heavy chain antigens in three different classes of immunoglobulins suggests certain common peptide sequences which presumably reflect evolution from a common precursor.

Papain digestion shows the allotypic regions controlled by both the A and B loci to be in both antigen-binding fragments (I and II or Fab) where the H and L chains are conjoined. The H-chain portion containing the carbohydrate (fragment III of Fc) is apparently lacking in alloantigens. Differences of A or B locus genotypes apparently do not restrict the recombination of half molecules of IgG globulin following reduction and alkylation. Indeed, hybrid IgG molecules with allelic allotypes B(1) and B(2) have been formed from half molecules of B(1) and B(2) specificity. Presumably, the absence of two different allelic specificities on the same natural molecules is central to the biosynthesis rather than the joining of the constituent heavy and light polypeptide chains. In the light of present knowledge, there is no reason why polypeptide chains of nonallelic allotypes should fail to pair in antibody synthesis. Quantitative differences in the amounts (and sequence) of seven amino acids have been found with respect to isolated L chains from rabbits homozygous for B(1) and B(2), respectively. In the absence of inbred lines or antibodies of similar specificity, the significance of such differences is open to question.

The remarkable phenomenon of *allotype suppression* in heterozygous rabbits is worthy of special mention. Heterozygous B^1/B^2 offspring of B^1/B^1 mothers immunized with paternal B(2) antigen show suppression of production of immunoglobulins with the B(2) allotype concurrent with a compensatory increase in immunoglobulins of B(1) allotype. Such offspring then have normal levels of IgG globulin. B(2) allotype suppression can also be specifically achieved, for example, by injection of newborn B^1/B^2 rabbits with anti-B(2) serum. Passive or trans-placental allotype suppression persists at least up to sixty weeks of age or throughout life whereas the antibodies causing the suppression remain detectable for only six weeks. Similarly, A^1A^3 offspring of A^1A^1 mothers producing anti-A(3), or offspring of the same genotype from A^3A^3 mothers producing anti-A(1), exhibit only low levels of the respective paternal allotypes. The phenotypic expression of the B^2 allele derived from the paternal genome was unaffected in these same $A^1A^3B^1B^2$ offspring. This alteration of A locus allotypes persisted for at least twenty-three months. Thus, allotype suppression may occur separately in relation to either heavy or light chains in doubly heterozygous rabbits, although normal total IgG levels are maintained. Presumably some central or feedback control of synthesis of IgG immunoglob-ulin is triggered by alloytpe-specific antibodies early in life, and continued suppression is not dependent upon indefinite persistence of the anti-allotype molecules. These findings provide some searching questions for future studies.

Allotypic Specificities in Mice

Genetically controlled differences in the allotypes of four of the five immunoglobulin classes of mice have been demonstrated during the last few years. Much of this work was undertaken by the Herzenbergs at Stanford University and by Dray and co-workers at the U. S. National Institute of Health. These immunoglobulin classes have been designated γM, γA, γG_1, γG_{2a} and

γG_{2b}. The most extensively studied locus designated *Ig-1* controls some eleven antigenic specificities found on H chains (F fragments) of γG_{2a} globulins. We shall follow the established usage in mice by designating the immunoglobulins with a γ(gamma) prefix and the allotype loci (genes) with an *Ig* prefix. These antigens are all cross-reactive as determined by precipitation of labeled gamma globulin of the immunizing strain-type with alloimmune serums. However, cross-reactions have been most sensitively detected by inhibition assays measuring quantitative inhibition of precipitation of I^{125}-labeled alloantigens. The Ig-1 antigens (phenogroups) indicated by numbers and their controlling alleles, as identified by tests of F_2 and backcross progenies of inbred strains, are given in Table 5–7. In contrast with the *A* and *B* allotype genes in rabbits, where single antigenic specificities are surprisingly limited to single alleles, each of the *mouse Ig-1* alleles determines multiple (3–7) antigenic specificities, and there are extensive overlaps. In general, mice heterozygous at the *Ig-1* locus show the antigens of the different alleles on different immunoglobulin molecules. Each mouse phenogroup is characterized by different combinations of antigenic determinants. Only the *Ig-1^b* and *Ig-1^f* alleles specify unique antigens (4 and 11) which are individually restricted to these phenogroups. This general pattern of complex gene-antigen relationships is of course common in blood group systems, so much so in fact that the ultimate reality of the simple one-to-one relationships tentatively ascribed to rabbit allotypes may be doubted. Although a minimum of eleven antigens has been related to the *Ig-1* locus, at least one antigenic unit is common to γG_{2a} and γG_{2b} molecules. The Ig nomenclature employed is consistent with and has all the advantages of the nomenclatures recently recommended for the analogous *Rh* and *H-2* blood-group systems. The distribution of *Ig-1* alleles in sixty-eight inbred mouse strains is summarized in Table 5–8. These assignments were deduced from the reactions and cross-reactions of normal serums with various antiserums. In the absence of any deliberate selection for these allotypes, the *Ig-1^a* allele appears most frequently and the *Ig-1^d* allele least frequently. This same system, independently investigated by Lieberman and Dray, led to the identification by double diffusion and immunoelectrophoresis in agar gel plates of five allotypes (Asa 1-Asa 5) on a one allele—one antigen specificity basis in thirty-eight inbred strains of mice. The two schemes of classification of alleles do not correspond: the Asa^1 group includes strains separately classified as *Ig-1^a* and *Ig-1^h*; the Asa^3 group includes strains listed as *Ig-1^c* and *Ig-1^g* (Table 5–8). Both groups of investigators made their allele-allotype correlations on the basis of F_2 and/or backcross progeny tests. Moreover, each inbred mouse strain tested exhibited as expected only one of the allotypes characteristic of a given allele. The conflict then hinges on accounting for cross-reactions in terms of the antigenic symbols (numbers) assigned. There is no doubt that the same or similar antigenic components may be represented in different allotypes (alleles) since some allotype antibodies cross-react with other

Table 5–7. Allotypic Specificities of Mouse γG_{2a} and γG_{2b} Immunoglobulins* (Modified from Warner and Herzenberg, J. Immunol., Vol. 99: 677. Copyright The Williams and Wilkins Co.)

Type-Strain	Allele	Ig-1 Locus (γG_2)	Ig-3 Locus (γG_{2b})	γG_2 Common Allotypic Specificities		
				1(1.9)†	2(3.5)†	3(3.6)†
BALB/c (or C3H)	a	1 2 – – – 6 7 8 10–	1 2 – – 4 7 8	1	2	3
C57BL/10	b	– – – 4 – – – 7 – –	– – – 4 7 8	1	–	–
DBA/2	c	– 2 3 – – – – 7 – –	1 2 – 4 7 8	1	2	–
AKR	d	1 2 – – 5 – 7 – – –	1 – 3 – 7 or 8	–	2	3
A/J	e	1 2 – – 5 6 7 8 – –	1 – 3 – 7 –	–	2	3
CE	f	1 2 – – – – – 8 – 11	1 2 – 4 – –	1	2	3
RIII	g	– 2 3 – – – – – – –	1 2 – 4 ? –	1	2	3
SEA	h	1 2 – – – 6 7 – 10–	1 2 – 4 7 8	1	2	3

*Number indicates presence of antigen while dash indicates its absence. The distinctive phenotype of an $Ig\text{-}1^a/Ig\text{-}1^b$ hybrid might, for example, be written Ig-1.1,2,4,6,7,8,10.
†Previous designated name of specificity.

Table 5–8. Distribution of *Ig-1* Alleles in Inbred Mouse Strains. (Modified from Herzenberg *et al.*, *J. Exp. Med.*, Vol. 121: 430, 1965.)

$Ig\text{-}1^a$			$Ig\text{-}1^b$		$Ig\text{-}1^c$	$Ig\text{-}1^d$	$Ig\text{-}1^e$	$Ig\text{-}1^f$	$Ig\text{-}1^g$	$Ig\text{-}1^h$
BALB/cJ*	C58/J	PL/J	C57BL/10J*	SM/J	DBA/2J*	AKR/J*	A/J*	CE/J*	RIII-J*	SEA/Gn*
C3H/HeJ	F/Ao	POLY1/Ao	B10.D2(new)/Hz	STA/Je	DBA/1J	AL/N	NZB/B1	DE/J	DA/Hu	BDP/J
BUB/Bn	H-2G/Go	POLY2/Ao	B10.D2(old)Hz	WB/Re	I/Ao		NZO/B1	N/Ao	FZ/Di	BSL/Di
CBA/J	JK/Bi	PRUNT/Ao	C57BL/H	WC/Re	JB/Di		NZW	NH/N	STB/Je	P/J
CHI/Ao	MA/J	ST/J	C57BL/Ka	WH/Re	RF/J					SEC/Gn
C3H/Hz	MA/MyJ	STR/N	C57BL/6J	WK/Re	SWR/J					
C3H.SW/Hz	NZY/B1	T6/H	H-2H/Go	58N/Sn						
C57BR/cdJ	PBR/Ao	129/RrGa	H-21/Go	101/R1						
C57L/J			LP/J							
			SJL/J							

* Asterisk indicates "type-strain" for each allele.

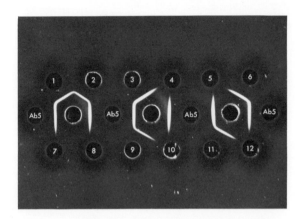

Figure 5—4. Cross-reaction of DBA/2 (*Ig-1ᵈ*) and A/J (*Ig-1ᵉ*) with BALB/c (*Ig-1ᵃ*). Center well contains C57BL (*Ig-1ᵇ*) anti BALB/c (*Ig-1ᵃ*). (Courtesy of L. A. Herzenberg).

allotypes. An example of such cross-reactivity is illustrated in Fig. 5—4. The shared specificities are almost certainly components of the same molecules. Absorptions of multispecific antiserums in Ouchterlony-type double diffusion tests may be conveniently achieved by prefilling the antibody wells with different allogeneic serums. This procedure permits the absorbing serum to permeate the surrounding agar and provide a zone of excess antigen.

The Asa notations in effect assume a unique specificity for each allotype whereas the *Ig-1* alleles mostly reflect different combinations of the same antigenic determinants. Overall, the available evidence is more in accord with the conception of *Ig* loci as given in Table 5—7. The general rules followed in the analysis of the Ig antigens are potentially appropriate to analogous studies. They may be cited as follows:

1. The immunizing strain should possess *all* the antigens to which the antiserum reacts, while the recipient strain should have *none* of the alloantigens corresponding to antibodies produced by it.

2. An antiserum produced in a given donor-recipient combination will not necessarily detect all of the antigens characteristic of the donor strain.

3. The antigens detected by an antiserum in a strain other than the immunizing strain may include all or only some of the antigens found in the immunizing strain.

4. Complete, partial, or no inhibition of an antiserum by an alloantigenic preparation means that the test preparation has all, only some, or none of the antigens, respectively, for which antibodies are present.

5. Two strains other than the immunizing strain, each of which partially inhibits an antiserum, do not necessarily share the same antigen(s), but each may share different antigens in common with the immunizing strain.

6. The number of antigens assigned to a locus (alleles) should be the minimum number compatible with the results—by application of Occam's razor.

The conflicting conceptions of one gene → one antigen *versus* one complex locus → one complex antigen with multiple determinant groups are once again raised (cf. Chapter Four) by investigations of the genetic control of immunoglobulin allotypes. The reader should not be confused by the various terms used by different authors to identify the same entities. The generic term *antigen* remains by essential definition a molecule or submolecule capable of eliciting and combining with specific antibodies. Although it is convenient to use such terms as antigenic specificity, antigenic determinant, antigenic factor, determinant group, or even hapten in relation to serological properties of antigens, these terms are still synonymous with antigen in the immunogenetic sense of molecular identification. The indication of *an* antigen as comprised of multiple specificities is no different from, though it is less precise than, referring to a phenogroup or complex antigen as comprised of multiple determinants or specificities. The term *antigen* in these descriptions is obviously being used in a plural sense. What is often not clear in reality is whether a *singular* antigen (= one serological specificity) or *plural* antigen is referable to a single structural gene acting alone.

Three additional genetic loci, *Ig-2*, *Ig-3*, and *Ig-4*, controlling immunoglobulin alloantigens found on different heavy chains have recently been defined. The *Ig-2* locus is closely linked to *Ig-1* but specifies heavy chain amino acids of γA globulins. The Ig-2 antigens, readily detectable by lines of alloprecipitation in Ouchterlony tests, have been localized in the fast fractions (from papain digestion) and in the class-specific polypeptide chains of γA globulins. Three or four alleles at this locus have been recognized, two of which, *Ig-2^a* and *Ig-2^c*, occur in the DBA/2 and C3H strains, respectively. The close linkage of *Ig-1* and *Ig-2* has been revealed by appropriate test crosses (Table 5–9). Among sixty-four strains, the *Ig-2^a* associated antigen was found solely in certain strains possessing the *Ig-1^a* allele while the *Ig-2^c* antigen was detected in all strains carrying *Ig-1^c*. No other combinations of these alleles or recombinants have been detected. The assumption of two separate loci rather than pleiotropic effects of the same complex locus hinges on the evidence that two substantially different polypeptide chains are involved. An arbitrary definition of a gene locus as the length of DNA which codes for one molecular species of polypeptide chain is implied in this connection.

The *Ig-3* locus has been associated with six alloantigens of the $\gamma^{\leftrightarrow}_2$ subclass and two antigens also found among the γG_2 subclass of immunoglobulins as

Table 5–9. Linkage of *Ig-1* and *Ig-2* (From Herzenberg, *Cold Spring Harb. Symp. Quant. Biol.*, Vol. 29: 460, 1964.)

Cross	Progeny	
(C3H × DBA/2)F$_1$, × C57BL	Parental Types	
	$\dfrac{Ig\text{-}1^a \ \ Ig\text{-}2^a}{Ig\text{-}1^b \ \ \ —}$	78
$\dfrac{Ig\text{-}1^a \ \ Ig\text{-}2^a}{Ig\text{-}1^c \ \ Ig\text{-}2^c} \times \dfrac{Ig\text{-}1^b \ \ —}{Ig\text{-}1^b \ \ —}$	$\dfrac{Ig\text{-}1^c \ \ Ig\text{-}2^c}{Ig\text{-}1^b \ \ \ —}$	71
	Recombinant Types	
	$\dfrac{Ig\text{-}1^a \ \ Ig\text{-}2^c}{Ig\text{-}1^b \ \ \ —}$	0
	$\dfrac{Ig\text{-}1^c \ \ Ig\text{-}2^a}{Ig\text{-}1^b \ \ \ —}$	0
	Total Tested	149

shown in Table 5–7. Note that three heavy chain allotypic specificities may occur in either γG_{2a} or γG_{2b} immunoglobulins. Because clean separation of γG_{2a} and γG_{2b} immunoglobulins from normal mouse serums has not been achieved, γG_{2b} antigens have thus far been analyzed by use of γG_{2b} myelomas. Inhibition tests with γG_{2b} myeloma proteins as labeled antigens have revealed the Ig-3 antigens whenever suitable antiserums have not been inhibited by γG_{2a} myeloma proteins. The Ig-3 antigens so detected appear to be generally independent of Ig-1 antigens found on γG_{2a} immunoglobulins. In other words, diverse combinations of allotype specificities occur on the different H chains of the type strains. Nevertheless, the *Ig-3* locus is closely linked genetically to *Ig-1*. About five *Ig-3* alleles are suggested by the different combinations of antigens evident.

Most recently, an *Ig-4* locus, closely linked to the other three H-chain gene loci, has been designated to account for phenotypic differences in the heavy polypeptide chains of γG_1 immunoglobulin. At least two alleles have been invoked for strain differences in electrophoretic mobility, but *not* antigenicity, of both whole γG_1 and γG_1 Fc fragments. Since no recombinants between *Ig-1* and *Ig-4* loci were found among 201 F$_2$ animals derived from several different heterozygous *Ig-1* intercrosses, these loci should be close together—probably less than one map unit apart. Although the chromosomal sequence of the four *Ig* loci and their homologies with respect to amino acid sequences are unknown, these structural genes may well have arisen by duplication during mammalian evolution. There is the attractive analogy with hemoglobin α, β, γ, and δ chain genes which yield homologies in amino acid sequences, suggesting derivation by gene duplication.

Each *Ig* locus also manifests multiple alleles coding for H-chain components comparable with those of the closely linked H-chain loci identified in rabbits and humans. A contemporary summary of mouse allotype relationships is given in Table 5—10. Note that neither light chain nor γM heavy chain polymorphism has

Table 5—10.   Summary of Mouse Immunoglobulin Allotype Relationships

Locus	Immunoglobulin (H-Chain) Class	Minimum No. of Alleles Recognized	Total No. of Antigens (Separate Specificities) Recognized
Ig-1	γG_{2a}	8	11
Ig-2	γA	4	4
Ig-3	γG_{2b}	5	8
Ig-4	γG_1	2	0

yet been discerned in mouse populations. Both the Ig-2 and Ig-3 loci have at least one allele that has not yet been correlated with the presence of an antigenic substitution. Most of the same alloantigens found in inbred strains have also been demonstrated in wild Mus musculus. Although it appears likely that the numerous allotypes in evidence depend on known differences in amino acid sequence, the possibility that these alloantigens reside in carbohydrate or other prosthetic groups attached to the polypeptide chains has not been ruled out.

Several loci affecting the production of serum proteins other than immunoglobulins in mice have been identified. The loci controlling production of a prealbumin, a transferrin, and several esterases have been discovered by non-immunological methods involving electrophoresis and selective staining of products. Separate loci independently controlling a β-migrating serum protein (Sas-1), a protein dependent upon a gene intimately associated with the H-2 locus (Ss), and a hemolytic complement component (Hc) have been revealed by immunodiffusion techniques. As indicated previously, there appears to be no limit to the potential number of variations in properties of macromolecules discernible by chemical and immunogenetic methods. Many such differences may be of interest only as genetic markers.

Serum complement of course has special interest because of its central role in host resistance and immunity to certain infectious agents. Hemolytic complement activity in certain mouse strains has been shown to be dependent on several genes involving product and linkage relationships not yet well understood. The Hc^1 allele leads to complement activity inherent in a protein that is alloantigenic on injection into complement-deficient strains homozygous for the Hc^0 allele. Strain and sex differences in hemolytic complement activity appear for the most part to reflect differences in the C'3 complex. The Hc^0 allele evidently yields no antigenic product recognizable by rabbits or mice. Another mouse complement component designated MuB1 is an alpha-globulin probably identical with $C'5$. As an antigen, MuB1 is determined by an autosomal dominant gene which is inherited independently of the immunoglobulin allotypes. Inherited deficiencies in MuB1 appear to be closely linked with or identical to the Hc^0 deficiency. MuB1 antigen is completely absent from certain inbred strains. In the MuB1-positive strains, it occurs in higher concentration in males than in females beyond three weeks of age. However, MuB1 concentration is nearly twice as high in homozygous as in heterozygous animals and is male-hormone dependent. The physiological significance of these genetically determined differences in mouse complement are still obscure. The deficient strains appear quite capable of coping with the usual pathogens and insults of the environment. These strains also reject tissue allografts with unimpaired vigor. The supposed deficiencies may well be misleading since they are mostly based on an artificial test system involving rabbit antibodies. The decisive and unanswered question is how effectively these different mouse complements function in the presence of known mouse antibodies. Substantial sex-associated differences in the serum concentrations of α-, β-, and γ-globulins, with females either higher or lower than males depending on the strain, also invite further study.

Allotype suppression by specific antibodies is obtainable in young mice as in young rabbits. Heterozygous mice of $Ig\text{-}1^a/Ig\text{-}1^b$ genotype prenatally and/or postnatally exposed to maternal anti-Ig-1b showed a lower rate of synthesis of Ig-1b antigens compared with control mice. This suppression persisted for only one to two months in the absence of continued anti-allotype treatment and was less severe than that observed in rabbits under similar conditions. This species difference may hinge on the presence of the suppressed antigens on rabbit IgM, IgA, and IgG whereas the Ig-1 antigens are nearly all restricted to the γG_{2a} subclass comprising less than half the total immunoglobulins of mice. In contrast to the seemingly slight effects of Gm maternal-fetal incompatibility in man, both maternal and fetal deaths have been observed in pregnant mice with allo-antibodies against paternal gamma globulin allotypes. Thus, when BALB/c females were immunized with C57BL/6 gamma globulin and then mated to C57BL/6 males, the number of progeny surviving per pregnant mouse was 30 per cent of the control value, and nearly half of the BALB/c females succumbed at term. In the reverse situation, immunized, pregnant C57BL/6 mice all survived, but no live progeny were delivered. These mouse data have been seriously questioned and this work still lacks independent confirmation. It would be surprising if maternal-fetal allotype incompatibility should lead to infant deaths only under certain circumstances. Perhaps viral rather than immunologic disease is responsible. From a human standpoint, it seems entirely possible that whole blood transfusion of a woman could by chance lead to immunization against certain paternal allotypes with serious consequences during a later pregnancy. Compelling evidence in this connection is not available.

Applications of Allotypes as Genetic Markers

The potential usefulness of serum allotypes as genetic markers should be at least as great as erythrocyte or leukocyte antigens. Indeed, serum has the advantage over viable cells of being more readily and safely stored for indefinite periods. Several applications have already been cited in this connection. For family and population studies, globulin allotypes are already in the mainstream of genetic research. Because of their distinctive distributions, the Gm antigens of man are much more useful than the Inv antigens for distinguishing populations. Ever-increasing interest in mechanisms of antibody production and amino acid sequences of heavy and light chains make allotypic markers especially valuable. In rabbits, for example, RNA from peritoneal macrophages can apparently elicit synthesis by lymph node cells of IgM globulin which exhibits the light chain allotype of the RNA donor rather than that of the recipient. In other words, IgM antibody produced by lymph node fragments from homozygous B^1/B^1 rabbits in response to RNA extracted from antigen-stimulated macrophages of B^2/B^2 genotype was of B(2) allotype. However, IgG antibody formed under the same circumstances was of B(1) allotype. Presumably, from this evidence which needs further confirmation, either macrophages are directly capable of IgM production or their two or more classes of RNA differentially stimulate or program lymphocytes for specific antibody synthesis.

Other areas of relevance are apparent. Hybrid progeny from turtledove-ringdove, pigeon-ringdove, and bison-cattle crosses, respectively, show serum antigens characteristic of each parental serum as well as additional components present only in the hybrid serum. Interaction specificities then may be nicely studied on molecules naturally occurring in serum as well as on cells. However, intraspecific diversity needs to be ruled out in such studies by testing the actual parents involved before the existence of hybrid or interaction specificities may be firmly established.

Finally, rabbit gamma globulin allotypes have been used as genetic markers for the source of antibody produced in adoptive immunity experiments. Rabbits homozygous for the $B1$ and $B2$ alleles were used as donors and recipients of lymph node cells from animals previously immunized with Shigella. In each instance, cells from donors of one allotype were transferred to recipients of the other. The allotype of agglutinins to Shigella appearing in the recipients was determined, following adsorption to Shigella, with fluorescein-conjugated rabbit anti-B(1)- and anti-B(2)-gamma globulin serums. The results showed that only donor-type antibodies appeared in the serums of moderately X-irradiated recipients. These same recipients subsequently produced Shigella agglutinins of their own allotype after active immunization. Analogous approaches to ascertain lymphoid cell chimerism, existence of immunological tolerance or immunity, and effectiveness of immunosuppression may have decisive merit.

KEY REFERENCES

1. *Antibodies.* Cold Spring Harb. Symp. Quant. Biol., Vol. 32, 619 pp., 1968. The articles in the sections on structure of antibodies and on evolution and genetics of antibodies are especially pertinent.

2. CINADER, B., S. DUBISKI, and A. C. WARDLAW, "Genetics of MuB1 and of a Complement Defect in Inbred Strains of Mice." *Genet. Res.,* Vol. 7: 32–43, 1966. Genetically determined differences in mouse complement are of obscure physiological significance since individual variations do not affect immune responsiveness or other known homeostatic factors.

3. DRAY, S., and A. NISONOFF. "Relationship of Genetic Control of Allotypic Specificities to the Structure and Biosynthesis of Rabbit γ-Globulin," in *Molecular and Cellular Basis of Antibody Formation,* Academic Press, New York, pp. 175–191, 1965. Immunochemical analyses of allotypes in homozygotes and heterozygotes clarifies structural control by *A* and *B* loci and reveals that not all 7S gamma globulin molecules exhibit allotypes determined by these loci.

4. ———, G. O. YOUNG, and L. GERALD. "Immunochemical Identification and Genetics of Rabbit γ-Globulin Allotypes." *J. Immunol.,* Vol. 91: 403–415, 1963. Agar gel methods for identification of ten allotypic specificities associated with three gene loci governing IgG are presented. See also *Nature,* Vol 214: 696–697, 1967, for more recent work in this connection.

5. ERICKSON, R. P., D. K. TACHIBANA, L. A. HERZENBERG, and L. T. ROSENBERG, "A Single Gene Controlling Hemolytic Complement and a Serum Antigen in the Mouse." *J. Immunol.,* Vol. 92: 611–615, 1964. The same *Hc* locus determines a serum antigen and the presence of complement activity in various strains of mice. Deficient strains appear to carry a null allele which yields no recognizable product.

6. HAMERS, R., C. HAMERS-CASTERMAN, and S. LAGNAUX. "A New Allotype in the Rabbit Linked with As1 Which May Characterize a New Class of IgG." *Immunology,* Vol. 10: 399–408, 1966. A new locus and allotype is apparent for H chains in an IgG2 subclass; this locus appears to be closely linked to the *A* locus determining allotypes in the IgG1 subclass.

7. LIEBERMAN, R., and S. DRAY. "Five Allelic Genes at the Asa Locus Which Control γ-Globulin Allotypic Specificities in Mice." *J. Immunol.,* Vol. 93: 584–594, 1964. Thirty-eight inbred strains of mice were grouped into five allotypes based on alloprecipitin reactions in double diffusion and immuno-electrophoresis in agar gel plates.

8. ——— and ———. "Maternal-Fetal Mortality in Mice with Iso-Antibodies to Paternal γ-Globulin Allotypes." *Proc. Soc. Exp. Biol. Med.,* Vol. 116: 1069–1074, 1964. A high incidence of maternal and fetal deaths was observed in pregnant mice with antibodies against paternal gamma globulin allotypes.

9. LITWIN, S. D., and H. G. KUNKEL, "The Genetic Control of γ-Globulin Heavy Chains. Studies of the Major Heavy Chain Subgroup Utilizing Multiple Genetic Markers." *J. Exp. Med.*, Vol. 125: 847–862, 1967. Different areas of human heavy chains appear to be under control of the same gene although heavy chains of each IgG subclass may be products of genes at separate but closely linked loci. See also *J. Immunol.*, Vol. 99: 603–609, 1967, for comparable study of *Inv* genes and antigens by these investigators.

10. MAGE, R. G., G. O. YOUNG, and S. DRAY, "An Effect upon the Regulation of Gene Expression: Allotype Suppression at the *a* Locus in Heterozygous Offspring of Immunized Rabbits." *J. Immunol.*, Vol. 98: 502–509, 1967. Allotype suppression may occur separately in relation to either heavy or light chains in doubly heterozygous rabbits although normal total IgG levels are maintained.

11. MINNA, J. D., G. M. IVERSON, and L. A. HERZENBERG. "Identification of a Gene Locus for γG_1 Immunoglobulin H Chains and Its Linkage to the H-Chain Chromosome Region in the Mouse." *Proc. Nat. Acad. Sci.*, Vol. 58: 188–194, 1967. An *Ig-4* locus, closely linked to the other three H-chain gene loci in mice, is designated to account for phenotypic differences in heavy polypeptide chains of γG_1 immunoglobulin.

12. MUIR, W. A., and A. G. STEINBERG. "On the Genetics of the Human Allotypes, Gm and Inv." *Seminars Hemat.*, Vol. 4: 156–173, 1967. An excellent and concise review of the independent *Gm* and *Inv* systems in man.

13. *Notation for Genetic Factors of Human Immunoglobulins.* Bull. World Health Org., Vol. 33, No. 5, 1965. Explains and justifies notations for genes, for new antigens, and for new systems. Criteria for recognition of new antigens are also given.

14. OUDIN, J. "Genetic Regulation of Immunoglobulin Synthesis." *J. Cell. Physiol.*, Vol. 67: Suppl. 1, 77–108, 1966. Compares the control and diversity of antigenic specificities characteristic of mice, rabbits, and humans.

15. PUTMAN, F. W. "Immunoglobulin Structure: Variability and Homology." *Science*, Vol. 163: 633–644, 1969. Neither the multiple germ line theory nor the somatic hypermutation theory of antibody variability successfully explains the genetic and evolutionary stability of the constant portion of the chains including the allotypic variations.

16. RAPACZ, J., N. KORDA, and W. H. STONE, "Serum Antigens of Cattle. I. Immunogenetics of a Macroglobulin Allotype." *Genetics*, Vol. 58: 387–398, 1968. An allotype controlled by an autosomal dominant gene which occurs with variable frequencies in different cattle breeds is described. Earlier work on other allotype systems in cattle is reviewed.

17. WARNER, N. L., and L. A. HERZENBERG. "Immunoglobulin Isoantigens (Allotypes) in the Mouse. IV. Allotypic Specificities Common to Two Distinct Immunoglobulin Classes." *J. Immunol.*, Vol. 99: 675–678, 1967. Allotypic specificities of mouse γG_{2a} and γG_{2b} immunoglobulins are further defined and compared. See also *J. Immunol.*, Vol. 97: 525–531, 1966.

SIX

HISTOCOMPATIBILITY GENETICS OF TISSUE TRANSPLANTATION

Successful transplantation of solid tissues, especially of intact organs in attempted replacement of diseased or atrophic organs, has long been a major lifesaving goal. Unfortunately, from an immediate medical standpoint, rejection of grafts between unrelated individuals has been the rule. Such rejection, as we shall see in this chapter, is a prime manifestation of the "uniqueness of the individual"—a fundamental biological attribute. This uniqueness entails much more than mere chemical polymorphisms associated with the mutation-selection process. The uniqueness manifested by tissue or cellular incompatibility has the immediate significance of enabling the individual to cope with a multitude of pathogens, potentially malignant cells, and foreign substances. Indeed, the very integrity of the whole animal must depend on recognition of foreignness and reaction to it.

Immunogenetic Basis of Tissue Allotransplantation

The now generally accepted genetic basis of transplantation incompatibility was first demonstrated in 1916 by C. C. Little, a geneticist, and E. E. Tyzzer, a pathologist, as a result of tumor transplantation experiments with closely inbred lines of mice. In succeeding years, Little and co-workers showed that the same principles applied to transplants of normal tissue in mice. Thus, parents (closely inbred waltzers and albinos) failed uniformly to support implants of the splenic tissue of their hybrid progeny whereas F_1 progeny (waltzer $\times$ albino) grew regularly the splenic tissue of either parent strain. Many subsequent studies have confirmed this unidirectional compatibility between the F_1 and inbred parent strains of mammals. The full interpretation of these results, however, requires additional test-graftings and correlations between the genetic constitutions, sexes, and ages of donors and recipients. The type and quantity of tissue grafted may also be important. One should understand the most basic relationships and terms at the outset.

Transplants of skin and organs can be made successfully from one part of the body to another (autografts), and from one identical twin or equivalent highly inbred animal to another (isogenic grafts or isografts), but *not* normally between other individuals (allografts or homografts), with very few exceptions. Other pertinent terms are defined in Table 1–4.

The rules or "laws" of transplantation, as established with different inbred strains of diverse species of experimental animals may be set out as follows:

Donor	Adult Recipient	Accept/Reject
Inbred strain	Same strain	Accept
Inbred strain	Another strain	Reject
Inbred strain	F_1 hybrid between donor strain and another inbred strain	Accept
F_1 hybrid	Inbred strain	Reject
F_2 hybrid	F_1 hybrid	Accept
Inbred parent strain or F_1 hybrid	F_2 hybrid	Reject (proportion depending on number of different H genes segregating)

Note that F_1 hybrids in such a pedigree should behave as "universal recipients" when the parent strains have been sufficiently inbred to be isohistogenic. In other words, all members of the F_1 between two inbred lines of mammals appear to possess all the antigens of the parent lines and no more. The very high frequency of rejection of parent or F_1 hybrid grafts by F_2 hybrids indicates the existence of a large number of dominant histocompatibility genes. In general, the relationship "one dominant allele → one antigen specificity" is consistent with the evidence. A recipient will accept a graft only if the donor tissue has no genes for histocompatibility or transplantation antigens not also possessed by the recipient. This point brings us back to the inverse principle that a normal recipient will react only against antigens not present in his own cells. A summary diagram of the genetic rules of transplantation is given in Fig. 6–1 on the assumption that each histocompatibility antigen is determined by a single, autosomal, dominant gene (allele). These rules have been confirmed in xiphophoran (teleost) fishes, chickens, mice, rats, Syrian hamsters, and guinea pigs, at least in relation to female donors and recipients. We shall return to a consideration of some qualifications and exceptions to these classic rules.

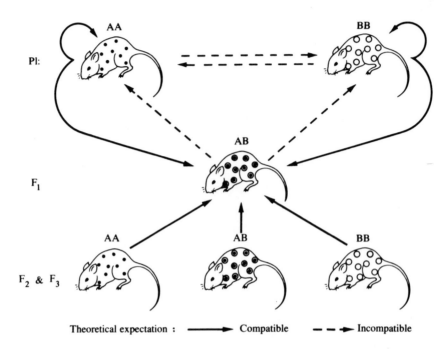

Figure 6–1. Diagram of genetic rules of transplantation on the assumption that each histocompatiblity antigen is determined by a single, autosomal, dominant gene (allele). Given separate inbred strains in the parental generation, A and B represent different alleles at each histocompatibility locus in diploid adults. Note that F_1 hybrids should accept grafts from each other, from either parent strain, and from progeny of subsequent generations. (Modified from Hildemann, in *Advance in Transplantation,* Munksgaard, Copenhagen, p. 19, 1968.)

Although graft rejection may be highly variable in its time course and severity as a manifestation of the strength of the histocompatibility barrier involved, an immunological rather than a mere biochemical incompatibility is evident. The primary immunological causation of allograft rejection is revealed by test grafting hosts previously exposed to donor cells or their lipoprotein constituents. Second-set or repeat test-grafts (skin grafts in most studies) made between an incompatible donor and recipient regularly show accelerated rejection in comparison with the first-set or initial graft. Thus, anamnesis or immunological memory is a constant feature of allograft reactions. Lymphoid cells transferred from graft rejectors to normal adults of the same inbred strain enable these animals to reject skin grafts from the original donor strain in an accelerated or immune fashion. The *adoptive immunity* is specific and referable to living, immunocompetent cells. Although specific serum antibodies are also regularly induced in conjunction with allograft and xenograft (interspecies) destruction as a further manifestation of immunity, the functional role(s) of such antibodies remain controversial. For present purposes, it will suffice to realize that the immunological events surrounding allograft rejection remain to be fully elucidated. Apart from special cases involving nonviable hard tissue such as bone or immunologically privileged sites as the brain or anterior eye chamber, allograft rejection is universal among random-breeding populations of adult vertebrates, including man. Transplantation reactions have been extensively studied in diverse species of fishes, amphibians, reptiles, birds, and mammals. Strong rather than weak incompatibility appears to be more common. However, chronic rejection of skin allografts reflecting "weak" histoincompatibility appears to be characteristic of Caecilian and Urodele amphibians, turtles, and certain mammals such as pigs and Syrian hamsters. Notwithstanding such differences in degree, the "uniqueness of the individual" and the "uniqueness of separate breeding populations" in terms of alloantigenic constitution have emerged as fundamental immunogenetic concepts.

In *Xenopus* toads derived by nuclear transplantation, reciprocal skin grafts between members of the same clone survive like autografts, regardless whether the recipient egg cytoplasm comes from the same or different (outbred) females. Since reciprocal grafts between toads from separate clones are rejected, compatibility between toads derived by nuclear transplantation must depend on their genetic identity at the nuclear level. Preexisting cytoplasmic or episomal differences in the egg or zygote evidently do not affect later allograft compatibility in immunologically mature recipients. Incidentally, clonal histo-compatibility is naturally occurring in certain species of Poeciliid fishes and confirms their gynogenetic origins. In these all-female species, inheritance is entirely matroclinous. Sperm from males of closely related, sympatric species merely serve to stimulate embryogenesis. With this background, let us now take a closer look at the genetic aspects of tissue transplantation.

The indefinite acceptance of grafts from either inbred parent strain by F_1 hybrids tends to rule out the possibility of alloantigens determined by recessive genes. If any antigen "a" present in one parent strain were determined by recessively functional alleles *aa*, this antigen should fail to appear in F_1 hybrids which would be heterozygous *Aa* whenever the other parent strain contributed a dominant allele. This situation should of course lead to rejection of grafts from one of the two parent strains by the F_1; this result has not been observed when sex-associated incompatibilities have been avoided. Thus, we are tentatively led to the conclusion that transplantation antigens are determined only by dominant or, more precisely, codominant genes. In other words, histocompatibility alleles express themselves even in heterozygous individuals. That alloantigens must be foreign to the recipient to evoke an immune response accounts for the *acceptance* of grafts which carry no histocompatibility alleles alien to the host and the *rejection* of grafts which do carry alien alleles. How many such genes must then be invoked to account for the low frequency of successful allografts from parent strain to F_2 or backcross progeny? The theoretical expectations are set out below with the simplifying assumption that the H genes are segregating independently from a Mendelian standpoint.

Expectation of Successful Allografts on F_2 Progeny from Either Parental Strain:

$$F_1: \quad AB \times AB$$
$$\downarrow$$
$$F_2: \quad \tfrac{1}{4}AA : \tfrac{1}{2}AB : \tfrac{1}{4}BB$$

3/4 of progeny accept grafts from either AA or BB donors if only *two* alleles or one locus are involved—the proportion of successful grafts (S) = $(3/4)^n$, where n is the number of independent H loci involved.

Expectation of Successful Allografts on Backcross (BC) Progeny from Opposite Parental or F_1 Donors:

$$BC: \quad AB \times AA$$
$$\downarrow$$
$$\tfrac{1}{2}AB : \tfrac{1}{2}AA$$

AB half of progeny accept grafts from either BB or AB donors if only two allelic genes involved—the proportion of successful grafts (S) = $(1/2)^n$, where n is the number of independent H loci involved.

In one extensive series of mouse skin grafting experiments done at the University of Birmingham in England, Barnes and Krohn found that two of 120 A-strain and one of 154 CBA-strain grafts survived transplantation to F_2 generation mice for at least one hundred days. On the now well-supported assumption that each separate antigen is capable of causing graft breakdown, at least fifteen independent loci must be invoked to account for the results. Since late rejections after one hundred days often occur in response to weak antigens, even the minimum number of loci estimated is probably too low. Similar experiments by others involving many hundreds of F_2 backcross recipients derived from other strains of mice and rats yield estimates ranging from nine to twenty genetic loci influencing histoincompatibility. Many of these experiments involved 200-day observation periods. More recent studies done by Donald Bailey at the University of California Medical School, San Francisco, lead to a higher estimate of a minimum of twenty-nine to thirty three loci distinguishing the BALB/c and C57BL/6 strains of mice. In one ingenious experiment, more than forty lines were derived by backcrossing (BALB/c ♀ × C57BL/6 ♂) F_1 females and their derivatives to C57BL/6 males through five successive generations. Tail-skin grafts from twenty sibs of each line in the fifth backcross generation were placed on C57BL/6 hosts of the same sex. The number (n) of histocompatibility loci still showing segregation of BALB/c alleles was estimated by the proportion (S) of grafts surviving through eleven weeks such that $S = (½)^n$ or $n = \log S/\log 0.5$. With a calculated mean of 1.8 loci per line, the original two strains should have differed by sixteen times this value or twenty-nine loci. This procedure is diagrammed in Fig. 6–2. Even the latter estimate must be considered too low as a potential total for the following reasons: (a) numerous H loci, at least in mice, are linked and therefore do not segregate independently as assumed in the calculations; (b) since some alleles will

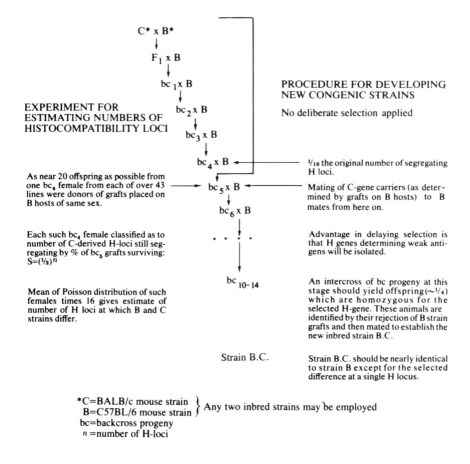

C* x B*

F$_1$ x B

bc$_1$ x B

bc$_2$ x B

bc$_3$ x B

bc$_4$ x B

bc$_5$ x B

bc$_6$ x B

. . . .

bc$_{10-14}$

Strain B.C.

EXPERIMENT FOR ESTIMATING NUMBERS OF HISTOCOMPATIBILITY LOCI

As near 20 offspring as possible from one bc$_4$ female from each of over 43 lines were donors of grafts placed on B hosts of same sex.

Each such bc$_4$ female classified as to number of C-derived H-loci still segregating by % of bc$_5$ grafts surviving: $S=(½)^n$

Mean of Poisson distribution of such females times 16 gives estimate of number of H loci at which B and C strains differ.

PROCEDURE FOR DEVELOPING NEW CONGENIC STRAINS

No deliberate selection applied

1/16 the original number of segregating H loci.

Mating of C-gene carriers (as determined by grafts on B hosts) to B mates from here on.

Advantage in delaying selection is that H genes determining weak antigens will be isolated.

An intercross of bc progeny at this stage should yield offspring (~1/4) which are homozygous for the selected H-gene. These animals are identified by their rejection of B strain grafts and then mated to establish the new inbred strain B.C.

Strain B.C. should be nearly identical to strain B except for the selected difference at a single H locus.

*C=BALB/c mouse strain ⎫ Any two inbred strains may be employed
B=C57BL/6 mouse strain ⎭
bc=backcross progeny
n =number of H-loci

Figure 6–2.   Bailey's procedure for estimating numbers of histocompatibility loci and for developing new congenic strains.

be held in common by any two strains under test, the loci involved will remain undetected; (c) H loci with weak antigenic products may remain undetected unless the graft observation period is at least 200 days.

Analogous studies involving tumor transplantation have used host death as the criterion of graft compatibility. Some representative data are summarized in Table 6–1. A transplantable mammary tumor indigenous to strain A grew in all animals of this strain but failed to grow progressively in strain DBA. Although it grew in all F_1 mice and all backcross progeny of the susceptible A-strain parent, the tumor grew in only 60 of 219 F_2 mice and 10 of 116 mice of the opposite backcross. When mice derived from crosses of BALB/c and C57BL were tested with a C57BL transplantable leukemia, most of the recipients succumbed. When, however, F_2 and backcross mice were preimmunized, all or nearly all became resistant (see Table 6–1). Even under the latter circumstances, a much lower minimum estimate of H loci could be assumed than was possible with Bailey's skin allograft data with the same or similar strains. Additional data also reveal that malignant tumors may often override weak transplantation barriers, even following preimmunization. Conversely, sensitive skin grafts are much more vulnerable to immune rejection and therefore more likely to yield meaningful estimates of H gene differences. Yet even skin grafts may show very prolonged survival in the face of weak immunity.

In a larger sense, use of inbred lines oversimplifies the genetic basis of allograft incompatibility with respect to outbred populations such as human beings because widespread multiple allelism is not taken into account. Indeed, the allelic diversity found at loci such as Rh and $HL-A$ in man, the B and C systems of bovine blood groups, and the $H-2$ system in mice points up the inevitable involvement of numerous alleles in the genetic control of normal tissue compatibility. Whereas the maximal number of alleles for each locus with any given parents is four, in view of the lack of restriction on the number of alleles which may be present in a random sample of a population, relatives and especially siblings should give better estimates of the nature of genetic diversity than unrelated individuals. Even goldfish (*Carassius*) exhibit complex transplantation genetics, such that numerous independent H loci must be invoked to account for the high frequency of incompatibility observed among siblings. Newth has calculated probabilities of allograft compatibility in various donor-recipient combinations as shown in Table 6–2 on the assumption that all alleles are antigenically effective and no immunosuppression is involved. Given the conservative assumption of some fifty effective antigens distributed in diverse phenogroups among twenty loci, the chance of complete compatibility is low even among relatives. As might be expected, successful grafts are generally more probable between relatives than between random pairs. Ceppellini and others have recently broadened the scope of the probability formulations of allograft compatibility. The probability of histocompatibility is of course different for

Table 6–1. Death Produced by Tumors Indigenous to Inbred Strains when Transplanted to F_1, F_2, and Backcross (BC) Mice (Modification from Snell and Stimpfling, in *Biology of the Laboratory Mouse*, 2nd ed., McGraw-Hill, New York, p. 459, 1966)

Cross	Tumor Donor	Recipients			Per Cent Mice Dying		
		Generation	Number	Number Dying	Observed	Expected	No. Loci Assumed
A × DBA	A	F_1	92	92	100	100	—
		F_2	219	60	27.4	31.6‡	4
		BC	116	10	8.6	6.2‡	4
C57BL × BALB/c*	C57BL	F_2	29	2	6.9	7.5‡	9
		BC	39	0	0	0.2‡	9

* The F_2 and BC mice in this experiment were preimmunized with 0.1 ml of strain C57BL blood 6 to 10 days prior to implantation of a c57BL leukemia.

‡ Calculated as $(\frac{3}{4})^n$ or $(\frac{1}{2})^n$ for F_2 and BC recipients, respectively, where n is the number of loci assumed.

Table 6–2. Probabilities of Compatibility of Allografts in Various Donor-Host Combinations, Expressed as Numbers of Successful Grafts per Thousand (Modified from Newth, *Transpl. Bull.*, Vol. 27: 454, 1961)

No. of Antigens	No. of Loci	No. of Alleles at Each Locus	Between Random Pairs*			Between Parents and Children*			Between Sibs*		
			A	B	C	D	E	F	G	H	I
10	1	10	37	513	18	190	526	111	354	860	38
10	2	5, 5	18	280	5.48	130	308	62	215	629	79
10	3	5, 3, 2	28	176	10	150	222	125	221	456	74
20	1	20	9.62	506	4.78	97	513	52	300	917	17
20	5	4, 4, 4, 4, 4	3.43	45	0.002	16	60	4	38	278.	0.0026
20	5	8, 4, 3, 3, 2	0.80	51	0.112	23	73	11.8	57	283	0.094
30	1	30	4.33	504	2.15	6.5	508	34	283	941	11
30	4	10, 10, 5, 5	0.025	73	0.002	4.6	85	0.77	26	465	0.012
30	5	6, 6, 6, 6, 6	0.009	39	0.0004	2.6	48	0.32	14	350	0.0018
30	8	8, 6, 4, 3, 3, 2, 2, 2	0.030	9.7	0.0025	4.0	17	2.36	15.0	133	0.0001
50	20	8, 4, 3, 3, 2, 2, 2, 2, 2, 2, 2, 2, 2, 2, 2, 2, 2, 2, 2, 2	0.0007	0.002	0.0003	0.307	0.161	11.8	1.4	4.6	0.0000003

* Columns A, D, G—unidirectional grafting between donor and recipient; B, E, H—reciprocal grafting from recipients to donors of accepted allografts; C, F, I—reciprocal grafting from recipients to donors of rejected allografts.

various genetic relationships between donor and recipient. In general, this probability is highest among siblings, intermediate between parents and children, and lowest between unrelated individuals. For each locus and any number of alleles, the lowest probability of compatibility is obtained when the alleles are equally frequent. Also, the chance of compatibility will decrease as the number of effective H loci increases. With unrelated combinations of donors and recipients, in particular, the chance of compatibility tends rapidly toward zero as the number of alleles per locus becomes larger. The calculated proportions of compatible grafts expected will of course differ as a function of the allelic differences and relative heterozygosity of donors and hosts. Now the prospects of prolonged or indefinite allograft survival in human patients are actually much better than most quantitative genetic considerations imply, but only through recourse to histocompatibility matching and immunosuppresion (Chapter Eight).

Strong and Weak Histocompatibility Barriers

The various combinations of some thirty-three antigens or specificities detected in association with twenty alleles at the major histocompatibility-2 locus in the ninth linkage group of mice were summarized in Chapter Four (Table 4–3). Additional alleles undoubtedly remain to be identified. This complex locus may be regarded as a "strong" H locus since any allelic difference at this locus, perhaps reflected in only a single alloantigenic specificity, regularly leads to acute graft rejection. The analogous B blood group locus in chickens and the Ag-B or H-1 locus in rats also appear to be especially strong and complex histocompatibility loci. The human counterpart now definitely appears to be the complex HL-A system of leukocyte antigens. Many other H antigens detected in these species are "weak" in various degrees as evidenced by relatively prolonged allograft survival times.

In addition to H-2, at least fourteen other loci generally determining weaker antigens have already been chromosomally identified in mice. The identified loci include thirteen autosomal loci, an X-linked locus, and a Y-linked locus. At least three of the autosomal loci are in the same fifth linkage group, sufficiently close together not to be inherited independently. The identification of separate H loci and their attributes has been a recent and major accomplishment of mouse immunogenetics. The key achievement has been the development of congenic strains in which the significant difference is at a single histocompatibility locus. Such strains can be produced by an appropriate series of crosses with continued selection on the basis of skin or tumor allograft rejection. An approach based on skin grafting is diagrammed in Fig. 6–2. Any two inbred strains (B and C) are crossed to give F_1 progeny which are then repeatedly backcrossed to one of the parental strains (B). If no deliberate selection is applied for four successive backcross generations, the bc_4 progeny should have only one sixteenth the original number of segregating H loci. The C-gene carriers among the bc_5 progeny may then be identified by rejection of their grafts on B hosts. The advantage in delaying selection is that H genes governing weak antigens are more likely to be isolated. To avoid sex-associated histoincompatibility and notably weaker male reactions which could confound this procedure, only female donors and hosts should be used. Such grafting is repeated in each subsequent backcross generation to select H genes of C-strain origin while otherwise increasing the background of B-strain genes. After ten to fourteen backcross generations, an intercross of bc progeny should yield offspring ($\sim$ ¼) which are homozygous for the selected H gene. These animals are identified by their rejection of female B-strain grafts and then mated to establish a new inbred strain B.C which is congenic with the original B strain. The number of backcross generations required may vary with the particular genes under selection. Compatibility represented by full viability of test grafts *within* the new B.C strain for at least 200 days may be taken as evidence that the new strain has become isohistogenic. Ideally, B and B.C should now be *coisogenic* strains defined as genetically identical strains except for a difference at a single genetic locus. This locus is always included in a transferred chromosome segment which contains certain "contaminant" genes. The length of the introduced chromosome segment and the number of contaminant genes will decrease as the number of backcross matings to the parent strain is increased. Since true coisogenicity is seldom attained because genes closely linked to the selected histocompatibility gene of C-origin are not readily eliminated by crossovers, the strains are called *congenic* to describe a useful approximation to the coisogenic state.

Congenic strains have also been produced by an appropriate series of crosses with tumor implantation used to select resistant animals every second or third generation. This method, first developed and widely applied by George Snell, is illustrated in Fig. 6–3. In this cross-intercross system, strain A is any inbred strain while B is some other strain, inbred or not. Strains A and B are crossed and an F_2 generation is raised. The F_2s and subsequent even numbered generations are inoculated with a transplantable tumor of A strain origin and specificity. The survivors or resistant animals, who have acquired a gene(s) for resistance from the B strain, are crossed to strain A in each odd numbered generation to progressively increase the background of A genes as in Bailey's procedure. In the fourteenth generation or later, two tumor graft survivors are mated to yield a new congenic resistant strain A.B. It must of course be demonstrated at this stage that grafts between A and A.B are rejected while grafts within either strain are accepted. Note that selection may only be applied every other generation in Snell's procedure. Selection for weak histocompatibility differences can be achieved in this procedure by preimmunization of tumor recipients with normal A-strain tissues. Then fast-growing tumor cells are less likely to override a weak histoincompatibility.

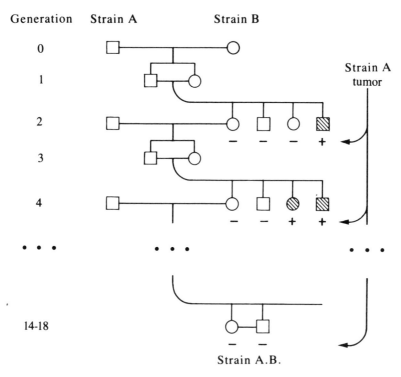

Generation   Strain A   Strain B

0

1   Strain A
                                                       tumor

2   − − − +

3

4   − − + +

• • •   • • •   • • •

14-18

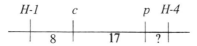

Strain A.B.

Figure 6–3. Diagram showing the cross-intercross method of producing congenic lines. Graft acceptance = +, graft rejection = −. Strain A.B should carry one histocompatibility gene derived from strain B which is different from the corresponding or allelic gene in strain A. Otherwise, strain A.B is essentially isogenic with A. (Modified from Snell, *J. Nat. Cancer Inst.*, Vol. 21: 844, 1958.)

Although development of congenic lines tends to select for an allelic difference at a single histocompatibility locus, the particular locus (or loci) involved will remain to be further identified or characterized. If a histocompatibility locus can be shown to be chromosomally linked to other genetic markers, this will serve to identify the locus in a unique and useful way. Thus, the *H-1* and *H-4* loci of mice are known to be in linkage group 1 in proximity to the genes for albinism (*c*) and pinkeye (*p*).

$$H\text{-}1 \qquad c \qquad\qquad p \quad H\text{-}4$$
$$\text{|}\underset{8}{\rule{0pt}{0pt}}\text{|}\underset{17}{\rule{0pt}{0pt}}\text{|}\underset{?}{\rule{0pt}{0pt}}\text{|}$$

The chromosome map distances or observed crossover frequencies are shown below the line. The close linkage between *H-1* and *c* as well as between *H-4* and

p became evident in the process of developing congenic strains. Indeed the C3H ($H\text{-}1^a$) and C3H$^{.}$K ($H\text{-}1^b$) pair of strains, though individually isohistogenic, conveniently have agouti and albino coat colors, respectively. The $H\text{-}4$ and p loci appear to be so closely linked that no crossover between them has ever been detected. One could even suppose that both traits are products of the same locus.

With the availability of spontaneous pinkeye mutants in the highly inbred CBA/J strain, it became possible to determine whether the *pinkeye* locus was also a histocompatibility locus. Skin grafts exchanged reciprocally between adult CBA/J and CBA/J-p were found to remain fully viable indefinitely whereas similar grafts across known $H\text{-}4$ barriers were rejected (Table 6—3). Moreover, reciprocal skin allografts between C3Hf/Ha (Pp) mice and otherwise isogenic pp animals were found by Hauschka to be permanently successful. It is highly probable then that p is not an H locus and that $H\text{-}4$ and p are separate loci. However, a mutation might conceivably have occurred at a single ($H\text{-}4\text{-}p$) locus to yield pinkeye without a concomitant effect on histocompatibility. Several other H loci in mice, including $H\text{-}2$ which is linked to Fu (fused-tail) on the ninth chromosome, have also been identified by their linkage relations. No H loci as such are known to determine any phenotypic traits in addition to histocompatibility. There is in fact considerable evidence to support the assumption that histocompatibility antigens serve as structural proteins of cell membranes in general. Nevertheless, very recent studies indicate that particular $H\text{-}1$ and $H\text{-}2$ alleles in congenic strains greatly affect the capacity to produce serum antibodies to certain haptens (see Chapter Two).

Because most congenic strains do not carry distinguishing marker genes, the alternative known as Snell's F_1 Test may be used to determine whether different loci or alleles distinguish strains having a common background. This test is diagrammed in Fig. 6—4. If two congenic lines on the same genetic background give an F_1 hybrid [A.B(1) $\times$ A.B(2)] resistant to an A-strain tumor, it may be concluded that the new strains differ from the A-strain at the same locus. In other words, these strains carry H alleles distinguishing them from the A-strain. If, however, the F_1 hybrid is susceptible to the test-transplant [A.B(2) $\times$ A.B(3)], a two-locus difference from the common partner strain is indicated. If three lines of common background give susceptible hybrids in all three possible F_1s, then three H loci are involved. The F_1 test may also be applied to the identification of alleles. If A.B(2) and A.B(3) in Fig. 6—4 were inbred strains unrelated to the other congenic strain pair and even to each other, their alleles could be determined at any locus for which A and A.B(1) are known to differ (e.g., R^a and R^b). Thus, if the F_1 hybrid between A.B(1) and A.B(2) is resistant, the unknown allele in A.B(2) differs from that in A. F_1 susceptibility, however, as following the cross A.B(1) $\times$ A.B(3), would indicate the same or similar alleles. In studies of allelic diversity, the main value of the F_1 test is in

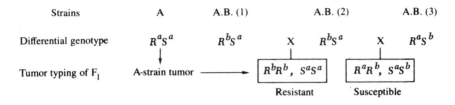

Strains	A	A.B. (1)	A.B. (2)	A.B. (3)
Differential genotype	$R^a S^a$	$R^b S^a$ X	$R^b S^a$ X	$R^a S^b$
Tumor typing of F_1	A-strain tumor ⟶	$R^b R^b,\ S^a S^a$	$R^a R^b,\ S^a S^b$	
		Resistant	Susceptible	

	Strain A (Tumor donor)	F_1 Hybrid	F_1 Response to transplant
One locus difference A.B. (1) x A.B. (2)	$H\text{-}R^a/H\text{-}R^a$	$H\text{-}R^b/H\text{-}R^b$	Resistant
Two locus difference A.B. (2) x A.B. (3)	$H\text{-}R^a H\text{-}S^a/$ $H\text{-}R^a H\text{-}S^a/$	$H\text{-}R^a H\text{-}S^a/$ $H\text{-}R^b H\text{-}S^b/$	Susceptible

Figure 6–4. F_1 test for different histocompatibility genes or loci in congenic strains.

typing various strains for already identified alleles. Numerous examples and extensions of this approach are given by Snell and Stimpfling in the reference cited at the end of this chapter. One should note that skin rather than tumor transplants might be just as well or better employed in the F_1 test. The common occurrence of tumor-specific antigens and of substantial variations in tumor virulence are at least theoretically objectionable in relation to "weak" transplantation barriers.

So-called weak histocompatibility barriers are found in all degrees as determined by allograft survival times under defined experimental conditions. Median survival times of reciprocal skin allografts between congenic strain pairs of mice are indicated in Table 6–4 in relation to host sex and ten autosomal non-*H-2* loci. The strengths of the barriers are quite variable, with median survival times for the various loci ranging from 15 to more than 300 days. The *H-1* difference represented by BL/10 → B10.BY gave an MST of 15 days in either sex—a survival time only slightly longer than the 10 to 14 days characteristic of strong *H-2* differences. Surprisingly, the reciprocal combination showed very prolonged graft survival in excess of 250 days, a markedly weak incompatibility. Note, however, that the B10.BY and other congenic strains listed were selected on the basis of resistance to a BL/10 tumor, not the other way round. The MSTs and ranges of allograft survival times found in other interallelic combinations reveal all degrees of transplantation immunity, including *H-9* differences so weak as to remain undetectable in either sex by skin grafting in the absence of preimmunization. Males often show prolonged or

Table 6–3. Reciprocal Skin Grafting Experiments with Cogenic Mouse Strains Strongly Suggesting That the *H-4* and *Pinkeye* Loci in the First Linage Group are Separate and That the *Pinkeye* Locus Is Not an *H* Locus (Snell and Hildemann, unpublished data)

Donor strain (Females)	*H* Allele	Host Strain (Females)	*H* Allele	No. Grafts Scored	Median Survival Time with 95 Per Cent Confidence Limits in Days	Range of Graft Survival Times in Days
BL/10	*H-4ᵃ*	B10:129(21M)-*p* -	*H-4ᵇ*	11	120 (46–309)	43 to > 309
B10.129(21M)-*p*	*H-4ᵇ*	BL/10	*H-4ᵃ*	13	27 (25–29)	25 to 34
CBA/J		CBA/J-*p*		12	No rejection	>300
CBA/J-p		CBA/J		14	No rejection	>300

Table 6–4. The Median Survival Time and 95 Per Cent Confidence Limits of Skin Grafts Between Congenic Strain Pairs (Modified from Graff, Hildemann, and Snell, *Transplantation*, Vol. 4: 429, 1966, Copyright The Williams and Wilkins Co.)

| | | Grafts from C57BL/10ScSn | | | | Grafts to C57BL/10ScSn | | | |
| | | Female | | Male | | Female | | Male | |
Locus	Congenic Strain	MST (Days)	95 Per Cent Conf. Limits	MST (Days)	95 Per Cent Conf. Limits	MST (Days)	95 Per Cent Conf. Limits	MST (Days)	95 Per Cent Conf. Limits
H-1	B10.BY	15	14–16	15	14–16	>250	—	>250	—
H-1	5M	25	23–27	26	24–28	>250	—	>250	—
H-3	B10.LP-*a*	21	20–23	30	27–33	52	24–110	46	25–84
H-4	21M	120	46–309	119	46–311	25	22–27	24	21–27
H-7	47N	23	21–25	25	23–26	33	28–40	47	34–65
H-8	57N	32	26–39	47	35–63	37	21–64	>200	—
H-9	45N	>400	—	>300	—	>300	—	>300	—
H-10	9M	91	67–122	>250	—	71	46–110	>300	—
H-11	10M	78	63–97	105	77–144	164	101–267	>300	—
H-11	55M	154	52–455	96	47–201	71	48–107	240	80–721
H-12	12M	259	132–510	>300	—	>300	—	>300	—
H-13	14M	38	33–45	67	60–75	73	22–239	116	40–330

indefinite allograft survival when females of the same strains show more vigorous immune responses reflected in curtailed survival times. This type of disparity cannot be simply sex-associated, however, since both sexes may show equally weak reactions toward certain antigens, as illustrated by the reciprocal *H-4* results in Table 6—4. Note that the "strength" of histoincompatibility between congenic lines of mice is a function of the interallelic combination rather than the genetic locus involved. This may be clearly seen in data gleaned from Table 6—4 for interallelic differences at four seperate loci as shown below

Interallelic Histoincompatibility

Stronger   Much Weaker

$H\text{-}1^c \rightarrow H\text{-}1^b$ $(15) \gg H\text{-}1^b \rightarrow H\text{-}1^c$ (> 250)
$H\text{-}3^a \rightarrow H\text{-}3^b$ $(21) \gg H\text{-}3^b \rightarrow H\text{-}3^a$ (52)
$H\text{-}4^b \rightarrow H\text{-}4^a$ $(25) \gg H\text{-}4^a \rightarrow H\text{-}4^b$ (120)
$H\text{-}11^a \rightarrow H\text{-}11^b$ $(78) \gg H\text{-}11^b \rightarrow H\text{-}11^a$ (164)

The numbers in parentheses are the MSTs in days of female to female allografts. The same relationships were found for males in these combinations. In certain weak congenic incompatibilities at least, heterozygous grafts survive longer than homozygous grafts, indicating that allelic dosage may also be a significant factor. Clearly, the quantity and distribution of cellular antigen as well as its quality may be important. The longer the median survival time, the greater was the range in survival times of individual grafts. The wide variation in survival times within supposedly homogeneous populations of grafts is only partly explicable in relation to slight differences in graft dosage. Variation in the time required for adequate host sensitization and a delicate balance between graft cell destruction and replacement may be involved. The latter assumption is supported by the repeated finding that second-set skin grafts may be destroyed during the vulnerable healing-in phase even though nearly fully viable first-set grafts continue to survive on the same hosts.

Multiple weak histocompatibility antigens may also have additive or augmentative effects leading to curtailed allograft survival. Double (and multiple H differences between strain pairs show a cumulative effect if the discrepancies between the MSTs of the constituent pairs are not large. This is reflected in a ratio between single difference MSTs of about 3:1 or less (Table 6—5). Conversely, no cumulative effect is shown if the discrepancies between the MSTs of the constituent pairs approach a ratio of 4:1 or higher. In this connection, this same prediction was fulfilled if the strain pairs differed at non-*H-2* loci or at a non-*H-2* locus and the *H-2* locus. Otherwise weak immunogens may become substantially stronger through their cumulative effect. However, once a recipient exhibits its maximum response to an allograft, the

Table 6–5. Comparison of the Rejection Intervals for Skin Grafted Across Double H-Locus Differences with Those for Skin Grafted Across the Constituent Single H-Locus Differences (Modified from Graff et al., *Transplantation*, Vol. 4: 610, 1966, Copyright The Williams and Wilkins Co.)

Double H-Locus Difference					H-Difference		Single H-Locus Difference					Ratio Between Single Diff. MSTs
Donor	Host*	No. of Mice	MST (Days)	95 Per Cent Conf. Limits	Host	Donor	Donor	Host*	No. of Mice	MST (Days)	95 Per Cent Conf. Limits	
5M ♀	B10.LP-a	17	26‡	24–29	H-1^c H-3^b	H-1^b H-3^a	5M ♀ C57BL/10 ♀	C57BL/10 B10.LP-a	10 23	>200 27	– 25–28	Infinity
21M ♀	10M	20	27‡	25–29	H-4^a H-11^b	H-4^b H-11^a	C57BL/10 ♀ 21M ♀	10M C57BL/10	19 18	102 25	89–116 24–27	4.1:1
B10.LP-a ♂	C57BL/10 ♀	15	16‡	15–17	H-3^a –	H-3^b H-Y	B10.LP-a ♀ C57BL/10 ♂	C57BL/10 ♀ C57BL/10 ♀	10 30	57 15	36–91 14.4–15.4	3.8:1
B10.LP-a ♀		10	18§	17–19	H-1^b H-3^a	H-1^c H-3	B10.LP-a ♀ C57BL/10 ♀	C57BL/10 ♀ 5M ♀	10 11	57 21	36–91 20–22	2.7:1
C57BL/10 ♂	B10.LP-a ♀	20	12§	11.2–12.4	H-3^b –	H-3^b H-Y	C57BL/10 ♀ C57BL/10 ♂	B10.LP-a ♀ C57BL/10 ♀	9 30	21 15	20–23 14.4–15.4	1.4:1
10M ♀	21M ♀	17	58§	49–69	H-4^b H-11^a	H-4^a H-11^b	10M ♀ C57BL/10 ♀	C57BL/10 ♀ 21M ♀	12 13	164 153	101–267 100–236	1.1:1

* All groups not otherwise designated were composed of nearly equal numbers of males and females.

‡ MST was not significantly shorter than the MST of the shorter of the two single-difference pairs.

§ MST was significantly shorter than the MSTs of both of the single-difference pairs.

addition of alloantigens may not further accelerate graft rejection. These considerations may be epitomized with respect to two reciprocal allelic combinations in congenic lines of mice as follows:

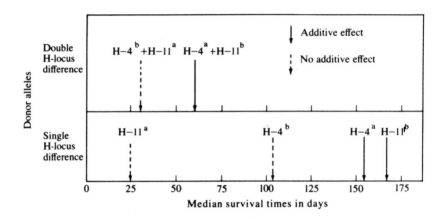

The nature of the cumulative effect is unknown. Absence of synergism could be attributed to interference or preemption by a strong antigen of an immune response otherwise available for a similar but weaker immunogen. The distinction between "strong" and "weak" immunogens at the molecular level is also unknown. Although the data cited refer only to skin allografts, the strengths and manifestations of rejection of skin and tumors across non-H-2 histocompatibility barriers parallel one another. Weak histoincompatibility barriers have also been investigated, though less extensively than in mice, in many other species including Syrian hamsters, rats, urodele amphibians, and even annelid worms. Certain rules and generalizations may now be stated in relation to weak histoincompatibility and associated chronic rejection, especially of skin transplants:

Rules

1. The later the time of onset of graft rejection, the greater is the interval between onset and complete rejection.
2. The longer the median or average survival time, the greater is the range or spread in survival times of individual grafts.
3. Multiple histocompatibility differences will exhibit additive or augmentative effects leading to curtailed allograft survival whenever the ratios between the constituent median survival times are not large (3:1 or less).
4. The "strength" of histoincompatibility (proven between many congenic strains of mice) is a function of the interallelic combination rather than the *H* locus involved.

Generalizations

5. Allograft survival times on females are usually shorter than on males of the same strain or genotype. (This is consistent with evidence—see Chapter Two—that females generally show more vigorous immune responses than males.)
6. Where only very weak histocompatibility differences exist, small grafts are usually rejected eventually while large grafts may survive indefinitely under the same conditions.

These six statements should continue to be useful operationally, although their bearing on clinical organ transplantation remains to be delineated. The less thoroughly studied generalizations invite further evaluation. Whether immunologic memory (anamnesis) is shorter-lived or longer-lived with weak histocompatibility antigens than with strong ones appears to depend on numerous factors, including the rules just cited. Results obtained are at least partly dependent upon the tactics of immunization and testing as well as probable intervention of enhancement (see page 187).

To a large extent, the immunogenetic findings made in relation to strong and weak skin graft reactions have been confirmed by tumor grafting (see page 187), transplantation disease induction (Chapter Seven), circumvention of alloimmune reactions (Chapter Eight), and parabiosis experiments. Parabiotic union of adult animals may be regarded as a severe test of relative incompatibility since a massive exchange of circulating immunocompetent cells is involved. Parabiosis between strains of mice or Syrian hamsters which show a high incidence of acute skin graft rejection also results in rapid parabiotic rejection. Despite physiological complexities, chronic parabiotic reactions are commonly induced by weak histocompatibility antigens (Fig. 6—5). In mice, but not in hamsters, persistent immunological tolerance may result from parabiosis across very weak histocompatibility barriers.

Present knowledge suggests that the *H-2* locus of mice is especially complex at both the genetic and end-product levels. This system was discovered with serological methods by Peter Gorer in the late 1930s in relation to potent cellular antigens found on erythrocytes as well as tumor cells. As noted earlier, each codominant *H-2* allele has been associated with multiple antigenic specificities. The linkage of *H-2* with *Fu* (fused-tail) and *T* (brachyury) on the ninth chromosome has facilitated detection of *H-2* alleles. The first accounts of crossing over *within* the *H-2* locus were published in 1955. Many instances of apparent crossing over within *H-2* support the view that the *H-2* region includes multiple determinant sites, some of which are separable by crossing over. Some five recons, designated in order as D, C, V, E, and K, have been identified as shown in Fig. 6—6. The recombination frequency within the *H-2* locus, i.e., between the D and K regions, though previously supposed to be as high as

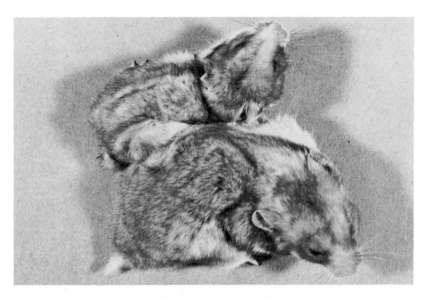

Figure 6–5.   Unilateral rejection well underway after eight weeks in parabiosis. Animals initially were of same size and weight. There is marked atrophy of one partner. (After Walford and Hildemann, *Transplantation*, Vol. 2: 101, 1964. Copyright The Williams and Wilkins Co.)

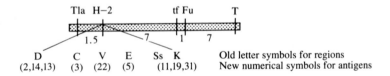

Figure 6–6.   The complex *H-2* locus and nearby loci in the ninth linkage group. Other locus designations are as follows: *Tla*, thymus leukemia antigen; *tf*, recessive hair loss; *Fu*, semidominant fused tail; *T*, brachyury abnormalities of the tail. The numbers between each pair of loci represent chromosome map distances.

1.0–1.4 per cent in relation to offspring from heterozygous females now appears to be only about 0.36 per cent for both sexes. The component percentages based on the extensive studies of Stimpfling and of Shreffler are about 0.55 per cent ± 0.22 in heterozygous females and only 0.19 per cent ± 0.14 in heterozygous males. Although observed crossovers have consistently revealed the same linear order of H-2 specificities, final evidence awaits test crosses involving independent markers at *both* ends of *H-2*. It already appears unlikely that each of the many serologically distinguishable components will be referable to separate gene sites within the locus. However, no mutually exclusive specificities determined by alternative or allelic subunits of *H-2* have yet been identified. Indeed, the thirty-three or more specificities determined by the *H-2* locus may be individually regarded at "nonallelic" or nonreciprocal in a fine structure sense until proven otherwise. A more exceptional aspect of *H-2* is the occurrence between the E and K regions of another locus *Ss* which controls a serum protein system phenotypically distinct from *H-2*. A pair of additively acting alleles (*Ss^h* and *Ss^l*) determining high and low protein levels has been characterized by Shreffler. *Ss* has no known effects on histocompatibility and is not antigenically related to any known H-2 specificities. The *Tl$_a$* locus about two crossover units from *H-2* determines three TL (thymus leukemia) antigens, TL.1, TL.2, and TL.3 present in the thymus and in leukemic cells of certain strains of mice. Unlike H-2, this antigen complex is absent from red cells, liver, spleen, and lymph nodes and is not a transplantation antigen. However, the TL antigen is detected by cytotoxic alloantibodies evoked by thymus or leukemic cells. Interestingly, phenotypic expression of TL antigens can be altered (antigenic modulation) by TL antibodies. Modulation of TL.1,3 components by corresponding antiserum also entails TL+ → TL− modulation of TL.2 in the absence of anti-TL.2. Thus, alterations in the expression of certain antigens may not be strictly dependent upon the presence of specific antibodies. Moreover, the content of H-2 antigens in thymus cells of TL− mice is greater than that of TL+ (TL.2 or TL.1,2,3) mice possessing the same *H-2* alleles.

A hybrid resistance factor has also been linked genetically to the D region of the *H-2* locus. When marrow cells of the genotype *H-2^b/H-2^b* are grafted to recipients heterozygous for *H-2^b* and some other *H-2* allele, the heterozygotes reject the transplant. Homozygous *H-2^b* hybrids are nonresistant, despite heterozygosity at one or several other *H* loci. The reaction of heterozygotes against *H-2^b* homozygotes appears to be an "F$_1$ hybrid effect" peculiar to lymphoid cell grafts and associated with the D region in tests of crossovers. This and other exceptions to the genetic rules of transplantation deserve special consideration.

Exceptions to the "One Autosomal, Dominant Gene → One Transplantation Antigen" Theory

The most straightforward exceptions are transplantation antigens associated with both X- and Y-linked genes in mice. Rejection of male skin grafts by adult female recipients is commonly found within many inbred strains, although comparable female to female, male to male, and female to male grafts are accepted. It is remarkable that this finding was not made until 1955 by the pathologist E. J. Eichwald, then working in Great Falls, Montana. Many earlier workers in their zeal to push on to new frontiers had simply not bothered to do these elementary experiments. The male-specific antigen(s) is moderately weak with MSTs of about twenty-five days (range $\simeq 14-100$ days) in mice of C57BL/6 background and considerably longer within many other inbred strains. This antigen appears to be present in all males and absent in all females although females of certain strains (e.g., A/J and BALB/c) have rejected only a fraction of skin grafts from males of their own strain. As noted earlier, minor differences may decisively modify responses to weak alloantigens. The male-specific antigen has been found in all tissues except testis and some tumors. The assumption that this H locus is nonautosomal and located on the unpaired segment of the Y chromosome is supported by consistent failure to detect the antigen in females, even under conditions of prolonged treatment with androgens. Indeed, testosterone treatment or castration of female hosts in one series of experiments failed to alter their capacity to reject male grafts. Nevertheless, the suspicion that autosomally determined but sex-limited antigens might be involved has persisted until quite recently. We now have rather compelling evidence for the existence of both X- and Y-linked antigens. Both A/J male skin grafts and BL/6 male skin grafts $\rightarrow$ (A/J ♀ × BL/6 ♂) F_1 male or reciprocal F_1 male hybrids regularly show chronic rejection at 21–180 days. Moreover, accelerated second-set rejection is demonstrable in both situations. Earlier rejections are usually found with smaller first-set grafts whereas large grafts promote prolonged or even indefinite survival. These results may be diagrammed as follows with the sex-chromosome sources of histoincompatibility italicized in each instance.

Parental Male Donor		F_1 Hybrid Male Recipients
C57BL/6	$(X_B Y_B)$	
		$\rightarrow X_A Y_B$ (A/J ♀ × BL/6 ♂)
A/J	$(X_A Y_A)$	
C57BL/6	$(X_B Y_B)$	
		$\rightarrow X_B Y_A$ (BL/6 ♀ × A/J ♂)
A/J	$(X_A Y_A)$	

Note that these sex-associated rejections are male to male, thus avoiding the intervention of possible hormonal or other physiological differences between males and females. Important controls in this type of experiment are to find female to female and male to male compatibility within each parental strain stock (preferably siblings) as well as female parental strain $\rightarrow$ female F_1 hybrid compatibility.

The Y-linked disparity between the A/J and BL/6 strains is novel because no alleles have heretofore been detected at this locus. Acceptance of CBA and C57BL male skin by their F_1 hybrid males and successful *interstrain* male → female tolerance induction experiments suggest that male mice of many strains have the same or similar Y antigens. The latter experiments involved injection of juvenile females of one strain with male cells of other strains (e.g., B ♂ → A ♀); when these females became adults, they were found to accept grafts from males of their own strain (A ♂ → A ♀) which would otherwise have been rejected. There are some peculiarities about the ease of induction, specificity, and persistence of tolerance in this situation that will be deferred to Chapter Seven. Studies of exceptional XO female and XXY male mice, involving continued immunologic function of transplanted spleen cells, demonstrate that the male-specific antigen is neither a result of the single-X condition normal to males nor is it suppressed by the double-X condition normal to females. In other words, XXY tissue can immunize against male-specific antigens whereas XO tissue apparently cannot.

X-linked histocompatibility genes were first discerned in 1963 in mice by the geneticist Donald Bailey, then working at the Cancer Research Institute of the University of California in San Francisco. Complete rejection of grafts of orthotopic, tail skin of (BL/6 ♀ × BALB/c ♂) F_1 hybrid males on reciprocal type F_1 hybrid males was observed, but only partial rejection of either reciprocal type F_1 hybrid female skin on the same type of male host. Slow or chronic rejection was the rule. Again, distinguishing the two parental sources of X-chromosomes as X_A and X_B,

$$X_A Y \ ♂ \leftrightarrows X_B Y \ ♂ \qquad \text{Complete rejection}$$
$$X_A X_B \ ♀ \to X_A Y \ ♂ \qquad \text{Partial rejection}$$
$$X_A X_B \ ♀ \to X_B Y \ ♂ \qquad \text{Partial rejection}$$

Partial rejection was scored in terms of a mosaic survival pattern of hair crops on female grafts, as opposed to obliteration of all hair in complete rejection. Although the partial rejections are consistent with the Lyon hypothesis of random X-chromosome inactivation, similar rejection patterns are also seen on grafts in relation to prolonged weak reactions associated with autosomal H genes. We have found the H-X disparity between the A/J and BL/6 strains to be demonstrable not only by skin allograft rejection but also by serum alloantibody production and graft-versus-host reactions. BL/6 adult females also mount a surprisingly early and vigorous antibody response to the H-Y antigen of their coisogenic males as demonstrated by the appearance of plaque-forming spleen cells. Both the H-X and H-Y loci clearly determine weak immunogens measured in terms of graft survival times. Although two or more H-X and H-Y alleles are apparent, it is not yet known whether one or more H loci occur on the sex chromosomes.

Our consideration of sex-associated antigens has been restricted to mice. Male-specific rejection has also been found in inbred strains of rats. This antigen(s) is species-specific to the extent that it does not sensitize female mice to H-Y mouse antigens. Since female-to-male skin grafts within highly inbred lines of chickens show slow rejection, one must invoke a histocompatibility antigen characteristic of the heterogametic female which is analogous to the H-Y antigen of mammals. Neither X-linked or Y-linked antigens have been detected in appropriate intrastrain and parent to F_1 hybrid tissue transplantation with inbred strains of platyfish (*Xiphophorus maculatus*) or of guinea pigs. Male-specific rejection also does not occur in inbred strains of Syrian hamsters examined so far. A sex-linked blood group system *Xg* was discovered in human beings in 1962, but it is not known whether the antigenic product plays any role in histocompatibility. Sex-associated histocompatibility antigens are apparently not universal, and their evolutionary significance is still conjectural.

New exceptions to the immunogenetic rules of transplantation were recently found in the rejection of skin grafts from F_2 and F_3 hybrid donors by F_1 hybrid mice. Although only 3.5 per cent first-set grafts from F_2 hybrid females to adult F_1 female mice derived from pedigreed A/J female × C57BL/6 male matings were rejected within six months, from 29 to 51 per cent of grafts from F_3 females to F_1 females in repeated experiments surprisingly showed variable, chronic rejection, reflecting weak histoincompatibility. Twice as many grafts (55 per cent) from F_3 males to F_1 males failed to persist as expected on the basis of known X-linked histoincompatibility. All other grafts from F_2 or F_3 donors to F_1 recipients remained fully viable indefinitely as expected on the basis of unmodified, codominant determination of histocompatibility antigens. Control skin isografts among parental females, F_1 females and parental strain female to F_1 female skin grafts also remained completely viable without exception. The above frequencies of rejection of F_2 and F_3 female grafts by F_1 females are probably due to gene-product interactions augmented by cumulative mutations among a large number of "weak" histocompatibility loci.

Spontaneous mutations of *H* alleles may first be considered in relation to the $F_2 \rightarrow F_1$ rejections cited. An apparent mutation rate of 3.5 per cent (4/113) per zygote is manifest if one ignores gain mutations that may have accumulated but remained undetected in the F_1 generation. This rate is halved to 1.75 per cent per zygote if one takes both hybrid generations into account. A comparable mutation rate of 1.35 per cent per zygote was estimated by Bailey and Kohn with regard to skin isograft rejections (9/667) among female (BALB/c × BL/6) F_1 mice. Since the total number of *H* loci is of course unknown, the average mutation rate per locus is conjectural. If a minimum of thirty loci is assumed, a high mutation frequency of 0.6×10^{-3} per locus per zygote is calculated from our $F_2 \rightarrow F_1$ data. However, on the not unreasonable assumption of a total of one hundred *H* loci, an average mutation frequency of 1.75×10^{-4} per locus per zygote or 0.88×10^{-4} per locus per gamete is found. The prevalence of apparent mutations leading to antigen gains in contrast to antigen losses in additional studies has suggested to Bailey that these histocompatibility changes resulted from incorporation of viral genomes into parental germinal cells analogous to lysogenic conversion in bacteria. Alternatively, the rarity of detectable mutations restricted to H antigen losses may usually be due to lethality early in development because these antigens may well be essential components of structural proteins of cell membranes in general.

Both the mutational and lysogenic conversion hypotheses run into difficulty in relation to the $F_3 \to F_1$ results cited. A gain mutation rate of about 17 per cent per zygote as an average over each of three generations (51/3) appears untenably high, especially by comparison to the $F_2 \to F_1$ results. Since the mice were raised in the same rooms under identical conditions, antigen gains via lysogenic conversion could hardly account for the large disparity between F_2 and F_3 generations. Numerous examples of gene or gene-product interactions leading to the production of new or hybrid antigens or to the suppression of parental antigens have recently been discerned, ranging from allotype suppression in heterozygous rabbits to the occurrence of red cell interaction antigens in rabbits, sheep, and human beings. Frequent "cosmetic crises" observed in female parental skin grafts placed on female F_1 hybrids in some strain combinations may represent a hybrid effect, perhaps reflecting one or more weak antigens not fully expressed in F_1 hybrids. However, recessive determination or possible suppression of antigens was not evident in the complete compatibility observed in parental female to $(A/J \, ♀ \times BL/6 \, ♂) \, F_1$ female transplants, nor would such suppression in F_2 or F_3 mice be expected to contribute to graft rejection by F_1 mice. Occurrence of new interaction antigens in F_2 and especially F_3 progeny should have a maximum potential probability because of many new combinations of segregating genes. Such grafts should of course not be rejected on the basis of a heterozygous allelic interaction antigen since that antigen would be present in the F_1. An interlocus interaction would presumably be required involving certain mixed homozygous-heterozygous genotypes in the F_2 or F_3. The new antigens need not necessarily represent new gene products, but could reflect new distributions or configurations of determinants on cell membranes. In other words, new antigens could result from new molecular arrangements in the cell membrane, analogous to the production of Le^b antigen through the interaction of the Le, H, and Se gene-products in man. However, production of new "hybrid" antigens alone does not readily account for the much higher frequency of rejection of F_3 as compared to F_2 grafts. All gene combinations possible in the F_3 are already possible, but not of course equi-probable in the F_2. In the absence of strong histoincompatibilities, the finding that otherwise weak and insignificant immunogens become manifest through their cumulative effect may partly account for the high frequency of ultimate rejection of $F_3 \to F_1$ grafts.

In some strain combinations, only a very low incidence of F_1 rejectors of F_2 or F_3 grafts has been found. Although questions of different skin grafting techniques, graft dosage, and scoring in different labs are not entirely resolved, apparent deviations from the "one dominant allele → one antigen" relation revealed by tissue transplantation are probably exceptional among hybrid progenies.

Some contribution to unexpected histoincompatibilities may conceivably derive from intracistronic recombination, unequal crossing over within complex loci, and cis-trans position effects. Given the protein nature of transplantation antigens, changes even in single codons could be sufficient to result in amino acid substitutions conferring new antigenic specificity on donor cells. An analogous example is the distinction between the allelic Inv[2] and Inv[3] alloantigens which depends only on the presence of leucine versus valine in position 191 of the 214 amino acids in isolated kappa L chains of Bence-Jones proteins. Possible effects of imperfect penetrance of H genes due to shifts in minor or obscure environmental factors may also be invoked: variables such as graft size, a weak level of host resistance, and a delicate balance between immunity and tolerance are known to influence disparities for weakly immunogenic loci.

Several classes of exceptions to the classic rules of transplantation are now evident. The existance of H loci on both sex chromosomes, cumulative effects of multiple, weak autosomal loci, and unexpected rejection of grafts from F_2 and F hybrid donors on F_1 hybrid recipients are established. These and other less well-defined exceptions invite further investigation. Taking the available evidence together, the "one dominant allele → one antigen" theory remains tenable as a unidirectional generalization in the limited sense that the presence of an antigen always requires the presence of a given allele. However, the reciprocal supposition that each alloantigen is referable only to the functioning of one allele now appears to be generally incorrect.

Immunogenetic Aspects of Tumor Transplantation

Our consideration of the principles of transplantation has included the assumption that normal and neoplastic tissues generally display the same reactivities. To the extent that tumor cells possess a full endowment of alloantigens characteristic of their strain of origin, they may be expected to elicit immune responses in foreign hosts just as readily as normal tissues. Nearly all of the congenic strains of mice developed by George Snell at the Jackson Laboratory in Bar Harbor, Maine, were selected on the basis of tumor transplantation. We have already noted, however, that malignant tumors may override the immune response of the host, especially when the histocompatibility barrier is weak. Also, residual heterozygosis within congenic lines is more likely to influence the fate of skin than of tumor grafts. Weak incompatibilities may nevertheless be made manifest by preimmunization and small tumor inoculums. The outcome of tumor transplantation experiments may be decisively influenced by a number of variables, some of which are still poorly understood.

Immunological *enhancement* is a frequently encountered failure to reject or promotion of the growth of a virulent tumor as a function of the host's immune response. This paradoxical phenomenon has been defined as the successful establishment of a tumor allograft and its progressive growth to death of the host or delayed rejection as a consequence of the tumor's contact with specific antiserum in the host (Fig. 6–7). Enhancement has been studied mainly in mice

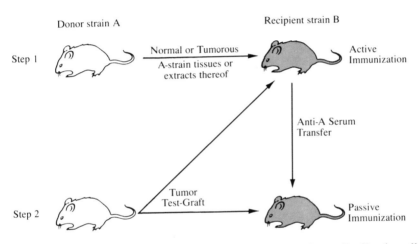

Figure 6–7.   Immunological enhancement requires specific antibodies (usually of the IgG class) in a recipient against the tumor-donor which may be achieved by either active or passive immunization.

with donor and host strains having different H-2 antigens. The demonstrated requirement for contact of the graft with specific serum antibody as the initiating factor in enhancement distinguishes this phenomenon from acquired tolerance (Chapter Seven) and various other forms of immune unresponsiveness. Enhancement following inoculation of allogeneic cells usually cannot be demonstrated until about two weeks after such immunization. The cellular immunity associated with allograft rejection comes into full force during the first five to ten days. Serum antibody production thereafter is accentuated, and enhancement, usually associated with IgG antibodies, may be obtained as the cellular immunity subsides. This sequence of events has been much studied with a strain-specific tumor designated Sarcoma I which is indigenous (originally methylcholanthrene-induced) to the A strain of mice. However, many other nonlymphoid tumors of diverse origins may be similarly enhanced. The provocative transition from heightened immunity to an enhanced state is illustrated in Fig. 6–8. Humoral antibody usually reaches peak production as

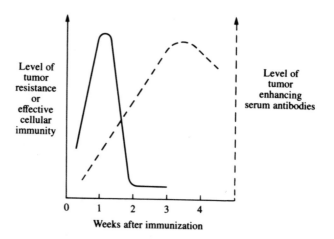

Figure 6–8. Early tumor immunity associated with immune lymphoid cells supplanted by tumor susceptibility associated with an increase in specific IgG serum antibodies.

cellular immunity disappears. The alternatives of effective resistance or enhancement are best demonstrated after immunization with living cells. Killed tissues or their extracts are less likely to promote tumor resistance. Enhancement by passive transfer of antiserum does not block, but does apparently delay the development of allograft (cellular) immunity. Such a delay can evidently be decisive in favor of a fast-growing tumor. Enhancement is more easily produced in males. A given tumor may be more readily enhanced in one strain of mice than in another, even though both strains yield enhancing antibody which is quite effective on passive transfer. Relative differences in histocompatibility barriers may be important, and serum antibodies against non-H-2 antigens have yet to be systematically studied in this connection. The IgG class of H-2 antibodies is much more effective than the IgM class in causing enhancement. This has led to the supposition that some form of feedback regulation governs the temporal shift in immune status. Whether the process of enhancement is mainly "central" at the immunocyte level or "peripheral" at the tumor target-cell level is not clear. The essential mechanism of tumor enhancement remains unknown.

Normal tissue allografts are not readily enhanced, at least in conjunction with strong histocompatibility barriers. However, enhanced or indefinite survival of test skin allografts has repeatedly been found in preimmunized hamsters and congenic strains of mice in association with weak histoincompatibility. In these instances, dependence on serum antibodies remains to be demonstrated. Slightly prolonged skin graft survival following passive transfer of alloantibodies has also been demonstrated in rabbits, guinea pigs, rats, and mice. Ovarian allografts in mice have proved more capable of being enhanced than skin.

Certain neoplasms, especially leukemias and lymphomas, are highly susceptible to the cytotoxic activity of serum antibodies in the presence of complement. The more vulnerable a tumor is to the cytotoxic effect of antibodies, the less likely it is to be enhanced. Vulnerability may depend on tumor cell antigen-antibody ratios as well as on the molecular species of antibodies involved. It is now widely appreciated that tumor immunity systems are delicately balanced. The type of tumor, antigenic changes in tumor cell populations and the dosages of cells frequently influence the outcome of experiments.

The widespread occurrence of tumor-specific antigens has been a major finding of the past decade. It has been repeatedly confirmed that many if not most tumor cells possess tumor-specific antigens. Such antigens, whether induced by chemical or physical agents or by viruses, are detectable by their induction of transplantation immunity in isogenic recipients. Obviously, progressive tumor growth, whether in a mouse or a human cancer patient, represents an ineffective host response to whatever tumor-specific antigens are present. Although these antigens are generally weak and often ineffective immunogens, they may play a critical role in tumorigenesis. Individual vertebrate animals may rid themselves of potentially malignant cells that have gained new antigens more often then we currently tend to suspect. Even tumors induced by DNA and RNA viruses possess both new transplantation antigens and soluble heat-labile antigens distinct from viral antigens. Indeed viral antigens often do not persist in tumors induced by DNA viruses although tumors mediated by RNA viruses may continue to release infective virus indefinitely. Oncogenic viruses were considered in more detail in Chapter Three.

Transplantable tumors of F_1 hybrid origin are usually rejected by either inbred parental strain. If strong antigens, such as H-2 in mice, of one parent disappear from the hybrid tumor, the tumor may then be able to grow progressively in the other parent strain. Variants lacking part or all of one parental H-2 complex have been identified and selected on this basis. Confirmation of H-2 association has been achieved by independent serological tests. Persistent loss of H-2 alloantigens has been demonstrated in a variety of carcinomas, sarcomas, and leukemias of F_1 hybrid origin. Prolonged serial passage through the F_1 hybrid in which the tumor originated has not led to reappearance of a missing antigenic phenotype. Complete loss of H-2 antigens is apparently unknown. Immunoselection following either mutation of somatic crossing over is a probable mechanism underlying antigenic simplification since loss or masking of immunogens should favor tumor cell survival. Now immunoselection may take diverse forms which still provide many challenging problems. Cytogenetic analysis of serially transplanted tumors has often shown loss of normal diploid status with the appearance of aneuploid or even polyploid clones having less specific histocompatibility requirements. Although antigenic variation and diminution of antigenicity within tumor cell populations is not uncommon, entirely nonantigenic variants appear to be rare. The generally accepted method for detecting tumor-specific immunity as distinct from alloimmunity is illustrated in Fig. 6—9. If strict specificity obtains, neither

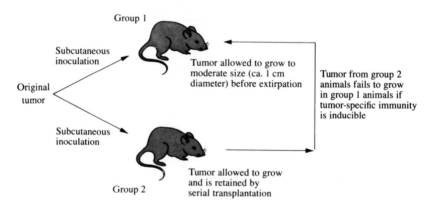

Figure 6—9. ,Experimental design to show active, tumor-specific immunity. Tumor and animals must come from the same highly inbred strain shown to be isohistogenic by persistent skin isograft survival between the same sexes.

normal tissues nor any other tumor substituted for the initial inoculum in group 1 should produce immunity against the original tumor being tested. Many tumors induced by chemical carcinogens such as 3-methylcholanthrene show strict immunospecificity under controlled conditions. However, some tumors, particularly after prolonged serial transplantation, become less specific in their histocompatibility requirements. A few, like the Ehrlich ascites tumor, become nonspecific and may even cross the host species barrier (e.g., by growing in rats as well as mice). Reduced antigenicity has been detected by absence of immunity in hosts challenged with a small piece of tumor or counted numbers of tumor cells after excision of a previous transplant. Effective immunogenicity is often a function of tumor cell dosage with larger challenge inoculums tending to override host immunity. Both quantitative and environmental factors tend to complicate evaluation of tumor transplantation studies.

So-called "F_1 hybrid effects" in tumor transplantation are especially interesting from an immunogenetic standpoint. Various sarcomas, carcinomas, and lymphomas originating in homozygous mice are found to yield a lower frequency of tumors with a longer latent period in F_1 hybrids than in isogenic mice. Snell originally observed that homozygous lymphoma cells of C57BL origin grew better in C57BL hosts than in various F_1 hybrids of C57BL with other strains. This growth differential, initially ascribed to nonhistocompatibility differences between isogenic hosts and their F_1 hybrids was later attributed to abortive graft-versus-host reactions by the lymphoid cells against foreign alloantigens of the hybrids. This unexpectedly deficient growth of parental tumors in F_1 hybrids, confirmed and substantially extended by the Hellströms at the Karolinska Institutit in Stockholm, has now been called syngeneic preference or allogeneic inhibition. Another provocative consequence of F_1 hybrid environments is the Barrett-Deringer transformation. Passage of various tumors indigenous to certain strains of mice through F_1 hybrids derived from crosses involving the tumor-carrying strain and unrelated strains rapidly leads to the appearance of tumors with less specific histocompatibility requirements. The new tumor cells do not appear to be rare mutant clones selected from a preexisting mixed population since only a very brief residence in F_1 hybrids is needed for the transformation to occur.

An important clue to the possible mechanism of tumor cell variant selection is inherent in the characteristics of allogeneic inhibition. It is not possible to strengthen or weaken it by pretreating F_1 hybrid recipients with either homozygous tumor cells or normal cells of the same strain. Similarly, allogeneic inhibition is not abolished by preirradiation of recipients with X-ray doses sufficient to inhibit immune responses in general. Proliferation of parental tumor cell cultures can also be inhibited by cell-free preparations of H-2 alloantigens from F_1 hybrids, but not by control isogenic preparations. Allogeneic inhibition then appears to be consequent upon exposure of grafted tumor cells to foreign alloantigens in heterozygous F_1 hybrids. It is not an immunological reaction in the usual sense. The Hellströms, Möllers, and Kleins, all working at the Karolinska Institutit, have suggested that allogeneic inhibition may function as a "surveillance mechanism" to eliminate cell variants with surface specificities different from normal, surrounding cells. Close contact between either immune or *normal* lymphoid cells and allogeneic target cells in vitro appears to be required for cytotoxicity in the absence of complement. Normal lymphoid cells become cytotoxic after agglutination to allogeneic target cells by phyto-hemagglutinin or by antiserum, although isogenic lymphoid cells appear to be ineffective under these circumstances. Moreover, lymphoid cells of F_1 hybrid origin may also kill parental tumor cells or fibroblasts after prolonged contact, even though hybrid cells should not be competent to react against parental cells.

How killing occurs when allogeneic cells make contact is unknown. The cytotoxic effect is not restricted to lymphocytes since liver cells and neoplastic cells may be equally effective. Cortisone is capable of abolishing allogeneic inhibition both in vivo and in vitro. Although cell-killing in vitro has been regularly demonstrable only with strong H-2 differences, cytotoxicity in vivo occurs in relation to weak transplantation antigens and tumor-specific antigens (also weak) as well. While immunological surveillance mechanisms are probably important in eliminating potentially neoplastic cells, other homeostatic mechanisms akin to allogeneic inhibition may be involved in maintaining the integrity of the body. However, recent experiments by Mintz and Silvers involving induction of persistent tolerance in allophenic mice (Chapter Seven) strongly suggest that allogeneic inhibition is operative only under certain conditions. An attempt by George Klein to summarize present understanding of tumor cell responses to immunoselection in relation to cellular concentration of strong and weak antigens is given in Table 6–6. The weaker the antigens and the lower their cell-surface concentration, the greater is the probability of their increased immunoresistance and effective enhancement by humoral antibodies. Complete antigen losses in response to immunoselection, as opposed to decreased antigen concentration with unchanged specificity, have thus far been demonstrated only in cells heterozygous for the H-2 complex. The various principles described in this section are known to obtain to a large extent in several species other than mice. However, much less definitive data are available than for mice.

Biochemical Properties of Histocompatibility Antigens

Many blood group alloantigens in mammals are known to have oligosaccharide or carbohydrate determinants. This point is clearly established for the classic A and B antigens of man (Chapter Four). Volunteers sensitized by multiple injections of purified ABO-incompatible erythrocytes regularly show accelerated rejection of skin grafts from other AB-incompatible donors compared with grafts from compatible (O) donors. Since the accelerated test-graft rejections occurred within a week or less, it is apparent that AB erythrocyte antigens can also act as strong transplantation antigens in man. This finding is consistent with the detection of AB antigens on nucleated cells and particularly in vascular endothelium and epithelium. The possible function of other human blood group antigens as transplantation antigens has yet to be directly demonstrated. Most erythrocyte alloantigens have long been considered to be nonhistocompatibility antigens or very weak ones because purified erythrocytes generally fail to immunize recipients against subsequent skin grafts from the same donors. Also, prematching of human donors and recipients for numerous blood groups has often failed to promote longer test-graft survival than that found with unmatched pairs. However, both the conditions and schedule of testing may be critical.

Table 6–6. Schematic Summary of Tumor Cell Responses to Host Defense Mechanisms (After Klein, in *Ciba Found. Symp. The Thymus: Experimental and Clinical Studies*, Little, Brown & Co., Boston, p. 354, 1966)

Surface Antigen Concentration	Probable Examples		Sensitivity to Humoral Antibody and Complement in Vitro	Likelihood of Enhancement by Humoral Antibody in Vivo	Sensitivity to Immune Lymphoid Cells	Demonstrated Response to Immunoselection
	Transplantation Antigens of the H-2 Type	Tumor Specific Transplantation Antigens (TSTA)				
High	Lymphocytes, bone-marrow cells, leukaemic cells, some carcinomas and sarcomas	Virus-induced leukemia	+	Low	+	Antigenic loss in H-2 heterozygotes only: decreased antigen concentration with increased immunoresistance in all categories
Low	Most carcinomas and sarcomas	Polyoma, SV4 0 MC-induced sarcomas	− or ±	High	+	Antigenic loss in H-2 heterozygotes only; none (in the case of mouse polyoma TSTA) or decreased antigen concentration with increased immunoresistance in all categories
Very low	Long transplanted nonspecific tumors	Tumors induced by films (?), some spontaneous tumors (?)	−	Very high	+ or ± (?)	Little likelihood of further change. No "zero" variants known in H-2

The protein or lipoprotein nature of mouse H-2 antigens has now been established and independently confirmed in several laboratories. These alloantigens, though found on erythrocytes, are more abundantly present in nucleated cells in particulate fractions derived from cell membranes. It may be quite significant that histocompatibility antigens are concentrated in cell membranes and endoplasmic reticulum. Purification of these antigens for identification of their immunological determinants has been hindered by their lability in many extraction procedures and by their association with insoluble fractions. A. A. Kandutsch at Bar Harbor, Maine, and D. A. L. Davies at High Wycombe, England, have concentrated their efforts especially on chemical characterization of histocompatibility antigens in genetically defined strains of mice. Assay procedures have been based on immunogenicity in relation to production of circulating antibodies and development of transplantation immunity. The serum antibodies have been measured as hemagglutinins, enhancing antibodies, and more recently as cytotoxins. Many preparations capable of eliciting specific antibodies have nevertheless failed to evoke transplantation immunity. Although these studies still have a long way to go, the latest work appears quite promising. Kandutsch has obtained at least four different lipoprotein preparations from the Sarcoma I indigenous to A-strain mice that are effectively immunogenic. These purified preparations include a detergent-soluble lipoprotein, a phospholipase A-treated lipoprotein, a succinylated lipoprotein, and a low-phosphorus protein. All four preparations not only elicited specific H-2 hemagglutinins, as had earlier extracts, but also sensitized mice for H-2 or non-H-2 antigens leading to rapid rejection of test-skin grafts as well. The effectiveness of the low-phosphorus protein containing only 1 to 2 per cent lipid suggests that the antigenic determinants are protein subunits and not necessarily dependent on the lipid components.

Purified H-2 alloantigens in soluble form have also been obtained by Davies, but from lipoproteins or glycoproteins derived from normal lymphoid cells. Several H-2 specificities have been found on the same molecules capable of inducing cytotoxic alloantibodies detectable against Cr^{51} labeled lymphoid target cells. Not surprisingly, F_1 hybrid mice have cells with "hybrid molecules" carrying specificities from both parental strains. Although these preparations with H-2 activity are mostly protein and give a single band of electrophoretic mobility, considerable carbohydrate and probably some lipid are also present. Additional studies suggest that non-H-2 antigens in mice are also protein or peptide in nature. Whether H-antigen determinants reside in the associated carbohydrate and lipid moities remains unknown.

Elucidation of the chemical properties of transplantation antigens is much to be desired. The various H gene-product relationships would then be much better understood. These antigens may be not only components of essential structural proteins but may also be critical to cellular "recognition" and homeostasis.

Evolutionary Aspects of Histoincompatibility

Except for identical twins and equivalent highly inbred lines, one can assert that allograft incompatibility is characteristic of *all* vertebrate species ranging from teleost fishes to man. This is perhaps the most impressive manifestation of the uniqueness of the individual. The situation among more primitive vertebrates and invertebrates is less well known and invites investigation. At this stage, far more questions than answers surround the phylogeny of immunological responsiveness. Earlier studies misleadingly indicated that skin allograft rejection and other manifestations of immunocompetence occurred in one cyclostome species (lamprey), but not in another (hagfish). Our own recent work clearly reveals that chronic skin allograft rejection is also characteristic of Pacific hagfish (*Eptatratus stouti*)—perhaps the most primitive vertebrate species amenable to such experimentation (Fig. 6–10). At a "higher" level, elasmobranchs and holostean fishes show general immunologic capacity and probably also reject tissue allografts. Until recently, histocompatibility and a lack of specific immunological competence were thought to be universal in all classes of invertebrates. Successful allotransplantation has been reported in protozoans, coelenterates, helminths, insects, and echinoderms. Although negative results in many early studies may be challenged on technical grounds and in relation to the short duration of the experiments, recent work on species such as crayfish (arthropod) and the octopus (mollusk) clearly reveal an absence of *acute* allograft rejection. However, weak histocompatibility reflected in chronic skin graft rejection has been unequivocally demonstrated by E. L. Cooper at the University of California, Los Angeles, for both xenografts and allografts in several species of annelid worms. Although immunological memory as reflected in accelerated repeat-graft destruction is specific in these annelids, it may be regarded as "primitive" because it is rather short-lived and not entirely predictable. At least some invertebrates then possess different histocompatibility antigens and are capable of reacting against them. Immunologic phylogenesis may be manifest in progressive differentiation and specialization of functions, especially in the transition from advanced invertebrates to primitive vertebrates. The extent to which immunological competence in general and transplantation immunity in particular exist in Eumetazoan invertebrates is problematical—a fascinating series of researches for the future. When one considers the profound differences in genetic and physiologic endowments among animal phyla, it should not be surprising if pathways of immune responsiveness substantially different from the familiar mammalian norms are found in invertebrates.

The essential uniqueness of separate breeding populations has long been known in terms of widely different frequencies of certain blood-group antigens. Similar distinctiveness has also been demonstrated in isolated wild populations

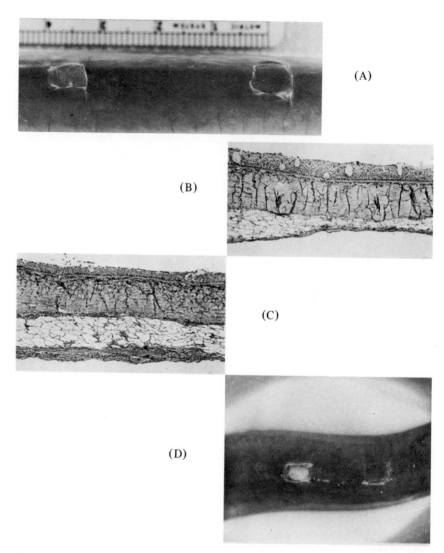

Figure 6—10. (A) Skin autograft (right) and allograft (left) on adult Pacific hagfish (*Eptatretus stoutii*) at sixty-five days after grafting at 19°C. Autograft is fully viable with normal pigmentation whereas allograft is edematous and pale with widespread pigment cell destruction indicating chronic rejection well underway. Biopsy sections of autograft (B) showing normal integument with abundant secretory cells (s.c.) in epidermis compared with allograft (C) showing atrophic epidermis and heavy lymphocyte infiltration (l.i.) in dermis. A similar hagfish with fully surviving autograft and completely rejected blanched allograft is shown in (D). (For further details, see Hildemann and Thoenes, *Transplantation*, in press, 1969.)

of bullfrog tadpoles and species of salamanders by skin allografting. Given the well-supported assumption that histocompatibility antigens are reliable genetic markers, populations may be characterized by allograft reactions without resorting to controlled breeding experiments. A test-grafting procedure employing two different donors and a common recipient will allow determination of both intrapopulation and interpopulation proportions of shared antigens (genes). An efficient design for such experiments involves reciprocal exchange of single skin allografts between randomly chosen animals in pairs. For the second test-grafting, pair combinations are changed as follows:

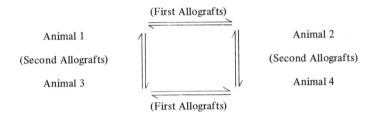

Each animal serves twice as a donor and concurrently becomes a recipient of two successive skin allografts from different donors. The second (test) allograft may or may not evoke accelerated rejection, depending on whether the two donors share one or more transplantation antigens. Note that weak antigens might not often be detected in the presence of strong ones since identification of antigen-sharing between successive donors requires accelerated test graft destruction. The percentage of antigen-sharing, which can vary from at least 10 (random tadpoles from large population) to 60 per cent (sibling tadpoles), may be taken as a measure of genetic diversity in population studies. Although it might be assumed that intrapopulation proportions of shared antigens (genes) would be higher than those found in interpopulation tests, both types of experiment should be done if quantitative, interpopulation comparisons are to be made. The "two successive donors → one recipient" design is also applicable to genetically defined populations, for example, inbred strains of mice. This method is limited to the extent that particular genes or antigens are not identified. Concurrent use of serological typing for cellular and/or serum alloantigens will of course augment the criteria available for population differentiations.

Estimates of the number of histocompatibility loci in many different species have been variable (3–30) and often unrealistically low, not only because of simplifying assumptions, but because very limited populations have been used. Given the abundance of newly discovered weak H loci in mice, it would not be surprising if one hundred or more loci affecting histocompatibility are eventually evident in various species. Furthermore, it is already apparent that most *H* loci show multiple alleles. Given the additional complication of gene-product interactions, naturally occurring allograft compatibility may be very rare between unrelated individuals.

The great precision of the immune response is necessary to enable the individual to cope with a multitude of pathogens and foreign substances from the external environment. Internal homeostasis with respect to disposal of self-products may be equally important. Potentially cancerous cells or any other mutant cells with aberrant properties including new antigenic determinants may be eliminated by the body in the same manner as infectious agents. From an immunogenetic standpoint, cancer and aging may be consequent upon prolonged histoincompatibility reactions among immunologically diversifying cells within an individual (cf. Chapter Seven). Immunogenetic homeostasis may have great survival value. Inborn antigenic diversity may be tied to adaptive flexibility, while rejection of foreignness is perhaps best understood as essential for preservation of the integrity of the individual.

KEY REFERENCES

1. BAILEY, D. W., and H. I. KOHN. "Inherited Histocompatibility Changes in Progeny of Irradiated and Unirradiated Inbred Mice." *Genet. Res.*, Vol. 6: 330–340, 1965. Mutants were classified according to gain, loss, or both a gain and loss in antigen specificity as determined by skin graft rejection among F_1 hybrid mice. Spontaneous and induced mutation rates are also calculated and compared.

2. BAUER, J. A., Jr. "Genetics of Skin Transplantation and an Estimate of the Number of Histocompatibility Genes in Inbred Guinea Pigs." *Ann. N. Y. Acad. Sci.*, Vol. 87: 78–92, 1960. Derives histocompatibility gene estimates based on proportion of parent-strain grafts surviving in F_2 and backcross animals and on the proportion of F_2 animals retaining both parent-strain grafts.

3. CEPPELLINI, R. "The Genetic Basis of Human Transplantation," in *Human Transplantation*, edited by F. T. Rapaport and J. Dausset, Grune & Stratton, New York and London, pp. 21–34, 1968. A recent evaluation of human histocompatibility systems with special attention to quantitative consequences of various genetic relationships.

4. DAVIES, D. A. L. "Soluble Mouse H-2 Isoantigens." *Transplantation* , Vol. 5: 31–42, 1967. Evidence is presented to show that several H-2 specificities are present on the same molecule and that in lipoprotein prepared from F_1 hybrid mice at least some hybrid molecules exist, carrying specificities derived from both parental strains.

5. GRAFF, R. J., W. H. HILDEMANN, and G. D. SNELL. "Histocompatibility Genes of Mice. VI. Allografts in Mice Congenic at Various Non-H-2

Histocompatibility Loci." *Transplantation*, Vol. 4: 425–437, 1966. Rejection characteristics of allografts were determined in congenic mice in many allelic combinations representing differences at ten autosomal, histocompatibility loci.

6. ———, W. K. SILVERS, R. E. BILLINGHAM, W. H. HILDEMANN, and G. D. SNELL. "The Cumulative Effect of Histocompatibility Antigens." *Transplantation*, Vol. 4: 605–617, 1966. Allografts exchanged between double, triple, quadruple, and multiple H-difference pairs of mouse strains showed a cumulative effect if the discrepancies between the median survival times of the constituent pairs of H differences were not large.

7. HELLSTRÖM, K. E., and G. MÖLLER. "Immunological and Immunogenetic Aspects of Tumor Transplantation." *Progr. Allergy*, Vol. 9: 158–245, 1965. A thoughtful review with major topics including immunological enhancement of tumor allografts, alloantigens as markers for cytogenetic studies, allogeneic inhibition, the Barrett-Deringer phenomenon, and tumor-specific antigens.

8. HILDEMANN, W. H., and N. COHEN. "Weak Histoincompatibilities: Emerging Immunogenetic Rules and Generalizations," in *Histocompatibility Testing*, Munksgaard, Copenhagen, pp. 13–20, 1967. Substantial immunogenetic evidence concerning weak histoincompatibility systems in various species is epitomized in six rules and additional tentative generalizations.

9. ———, and E. L. COOPER. "Transplantation Genetics: Unexpected Histoincompatibility Associated with Skin Grafts from F_2 and F_3 Hybrid Donors to F_1 Hybrid Recipients." *Transplantation*, Vol. 5: 707–720, 1967. Reviews and presents new exceptions to the "one autosomal, dominant gene → one transplantation antigen" theory.

10. ———, and R. HAAS. "Histocompatibility Genetics of Bullfrog Populations." *Evolution*, Vol. 15: 267–271, 1961. Results are consistent with the assumption that the percentage of antigen sharing shown by test grafting may be regarded as a measure of genetic diversity in population studies. See also N. COHEN and W. H. HILDEMANN. "Population Studies of Allograft Rejection in the Newt, *Diemictylus viridescens.*" *Transplantation*, Vol. 6: 208–217, 1968.

11. KALISS, N. "Immunological Enhancement: Conditions for Its Expression and Its Relevance for Grafts of Normal Tissues." *Ann. N. Y. Acad. Sci.*, Vol. 129: 155–163, 1966. Summarizes studies of variables operating in enhancement.

12. KALLMAN, K. D. "An Estimate of the Number of Histocompatibility Loci in the Teleost *Xiphophorus maculatus.*" *Genetics*, Vol. 50: 583–595, 1964. Numbers of loci involved in controlling the fate of fin transplants were estimated from the proportions of accepted, inbred parental grafts in F_2 and backcross generation hosts. See also *Ann. N. Y. Acad. Sci.*, Vol. 87: 10–43, 1960, for consideration of dosage and additive effects of *H* genes in this species.

13. KLEIN, G. "Lymphocytes and Antibodies in Relation to Malignant Disease," in *Ciba Found. Symp. The Thymus: Experimental and Clinical Studies,* Little, Brown & Co., Boston, pp. 348–359, 1966. Summarizes diverse tumor cell responses to host defense mechanisms.

14. RAMSEIER, H., and J. PALM. "Further Studies of Histocompatibility Loci in Rats." *Transplantation*, Vol. 5: 721–729, 1967. Inbred Lewis and DA strain rats estimated by F_2 hybrid analysis to differ by at least six histocompatibility antigens. Of these, antigens determined by the *Ag-B* locus are most effective in causing prompt allograft rejection. Lesser incompatibilities become effective only in the absence of an Ag-B disparity.

15. SNELL, G. D., and J. H. STIMPFLING. "Genetics of Tissue Transplantation," in *Biology of the Laboratory Mouse*, 2nd ed., McGraw-Hill, New York, pp. 457–491, 1966. A detailed review of the transplantation genetics of mice as known up to 1966.

16. STARK, O., and V. KREN. "Erythrocyte and Transplantation Antigens in Inbred Strains of Rats. VI. Histocompatibility-1 System and Its Alleles." *Folia Biol.* (Praha), Vol. 13: 356–360, 1967. One of a series of six articles published during this year in this journal. Numerous serologically detectable erythrocyte antigens of the $H-1 (= Ag B)$ system were tested for allelism and as transplantation antigens by skin grafting and by tumor grafting in F_2 and backcross hybrids.

SEVEN

IMMUNOLOGICAL TOLERANCE AND TRANSPLANTATION DISEASE

If an individual is exposed to an allograft or other kinds of antigens in sufficient quantity during embryonic or early postnatal life, the capacity to give an immune response to these antigens (e.g., to reject an allograft from the same donor source) is usually lacking when the individual becomes an adult. Many readers will already be aware that specific tolerance and acquired immunity represent opposite poles of immunologic responsiveness. The capacity of immunologically competent cells to distinguish "self" from "not-self" in a functional way is often fully acquired or matures near the time of birth. Thus, if an animal is exposed to an antigen before it has developed the capacity to react against it, the development of this capacity is delayed and, with continued presence of antigen, can be indefinitely postponed. In this context, tolerance may be defined as a state of essential nonreactivity of the individual at the biosynthetic level of lymphoid cells.

The roots of present understanding of immunological tolerance go back to Ray Owen's shrewd perception of persistent erythrocyte mosaicism in dizygotic twin cattle. It had been noted by the immunogenetics group at the University of Wisconsin in the early 1940s that twin cattle showed identical blood types much more often than expected on the basis of apparent identical twinning. By differential immune hemolysis tests, Owen showed that most twin cattle are not only born with, but generally retain a stable mixture of, each other's erythrocytes. Since the mixed populations of red cells were found to retain their separate antigenic identities well into adult life, it followed that red cell precursors exchanged via placental anastomoses persisted as new self-constituents in reciprocally tolerant hosts. The cattle studies, augmented by

Traub's finding of tolerance to lymphocytic choriomeningitis virus inducible in perinatal mice, led the Australian team of Burnet and Fenner to propose a general theory of immunological tolerance in 1949. Their now classic theory focused on the concept that recognition of "not-self" was an adult trait essential for immunity whereas tolerance depended on a lack of recognition of foreignness.

Properties of Immunotolerance

Although Burnet and his colleagues failed in their early attempts to induce tolerance in newborn mammals or newly hatched chicks to xenogeneic antigens, R. E. Billingham and P. B. Medawar not only extended Owen's results by successful skin grafting between cattle twins but were able, as the illustrious team of Billingham, Brent, and Medawar, to obtain allogeneic tolerance in perinatal mice by direct injection of cells from a foreign strain. During this period in the early 1950s, M. Hasek, then working in the Lysenkoist aura of "vegetative hybridization," produced specific tolerance in chickens by simply joining chick embryos across the shell in synchorial parabiosis. At hatching, such birds were not only chimeras or erythrocyte mosaics, but they also permanently accepted skin grafts from each other as well. Fraternal twin chick embryos regularly become reciprocal chimeras. Naturally occurring tolerance has also been repeatedly found in twin sheep and more rarely in dizygotic human twins. The first human example of allogeneic tolerance was rather dramatic: a woman known as Mrs. McK was shown to have in her circulation red cells descended from her co-twin brother who had died as an infant more than two decades earlier.

Immunological tolerance has been produced experimentally in diverse vertebrates ranging from teleost fishes through mammals. In general, tolerance is much more easily procured early in development than in mature individuals. We shall return to developmental requirements for tolerance toward different types of antigens in other connections. The simplistic concept of acquired tolerance as an absence of specific immune responsiveness in adults who had previous embryonal or perinatal contact with an antigen has recently been expanded to include various persistent inhibitions of the immune response, even when first exposure to antigen occurs in adult life. The general term "immunological unresponsiveness" is often used to describe any absence of a detectable response to an antigenic stimulus. Although there is an increasing trend to regard immunological tolerance as a single phenomenon, unresponsive states may be usefully divided into several categories as follows:

1. Immunotolerance typified by permanent acceptance of foreign tissue transplants which is dependent upon continued exposure to cellular alloantigens from proliferating donor cells.

2. Immunotolerance to xenogeneic proteins, polysaccharides, or simple chemical allergens, often produced as readily in adults as in juveniles, but dependent especially upon the structure, solubility, dosage, and route of inoculation of these nonreplicating sources of antigen.

3. Immunotolerance to any antigens in adults facilitated by X-ray or immunosuppressive drug administration concurrent with or soon after exposure to antigen.

Transplantation tolerance is distinctive in that chimerism attributable to a persisting population of intact donor cells appears to be required. However, the donor cells need only constitute a minor subpopulation (e.g., 5 to 10 per cent) of the individual's cells. In xenogeneic tolerance toward nonliving antigens, the tolerant or unresponsive state may often be limited in duration. Tolerance of rabbits or mice toward soluble proteins like human or bovine serum albumin usually disappears after several weeks or months unless it is reinforced by repeated injections of antigen. It was thought until recently that "overloading" with high doses of protein antigens was responsible for production of specific unresponsiveness. However, the total dosage of antigen is much less important than the absence of aggregates; complete solubility of antigen clearly favors tolerance induction. Microbial polysaccharides, such as those derived from pneumococci, may in low dosage produce life-long unresponsiveness in normal or even in already sensitized adult mice. Persistence of antigen in this instance is achieved by resistance to enzymatic degradation in the host. With simple chemicals such as picryl chloride or dinitrophenol, tolerogenesis hinges mainly on the route of adminstration; adult guinea pigs are made tolerant by either previous feeding or intravenous injection of these substances. Immunosuppressive agents nonspecifically promote acquisition of tolerance, apparently by eliminating lymphoid cells (especially, small lymphocytes) that would otherwise produce antibodies or immunity. True tolerance toward any antigen appears to be a state of essential nonreactivity of the individual at the biosynthetic level of lymphoid cells. We may now consider immunogenetic aspects of tolerance and their consequences in more detail.

Acquired Allogeneic Tolerance

Early studies of transplantation tolerance centered on the requirement for perinatal conditions reflecting immunological immaturity. It was long assumed that the same antigenic stimulus which instated tolerance in newborns would conversely induce immunity in older animals. We now realize that the "strength" or immunogenic potency of histocompatibility (H) antigens as well as their dosage are critical in determining whether tolerant states may be obtained in juveniles or adults. The capacity to reject allotransplants matures at or near the time of birth or hatching in many vertebrates. However, species and even strain differences in this respect are considerable. Cattle, sheep, and human beings are already capable of vigorous immune responses long before birth. Indeed, potential immunocompetence has been demonstrated in humans from about the 200th day of gestation (Fig. 7—1). Premature human infants are capable of

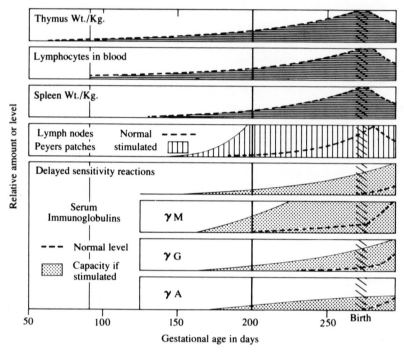

Figure 7—1.   Immunological development of human fetus.

skin allograft rejection and may show delayed hypersensitivity as well as active antibody production against various microbial antigens. Complete transition from a tolerance-type to immune-type of response against strong alloantigens is achieved in most strains of mice, rats, rabbits, and man at or within a few days after birth. Under conditions of immunosuppression or antigen "overloading," one may of course obtain tolerance in older subjects. In chickens, ducks, certain strains of rats, Syrian hamsters, and dogs, the upper age limit at which allogeneic tolerance may still be *readily* induced is seven to fourteen days after hatching or birth. By contrast, bullfrog larvae may still be made fully tolerant of otherwise strongly incompatible allografts until forty to fifty days after hatching (Fig. 7—2). Nevertheless, older larvae regularly show vigorous rejection of skin

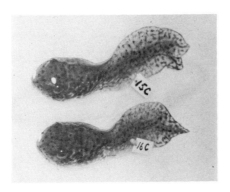

Figure 7−2. Pair of mutually tolerant larvae showing successful tailtip allografts with abnormal orientation transplanted when larvae were thirty-six days old. Single skin allografts were exchanged to test for immunologic tolerance when larvae were seventy-six days old. The margins of these fully viable grafts are barely discernible on the dorsal, central surfaces of the body behind the eyes. Photograph was taken eighty days after skin allografting. (From Hildemann and Hass, *J. Immunol.*, Vol. 83: 482, 1959. Copyright The Williams and Wilkins Co.)

allografts long before metamorphosis and the development of other adult characteristics. The only species of fish similarly investigated, a viviparous embiotocid with a five-month gestation period, rejected skin allografts made at one to three days after birth although comparable grafts were accepted by embryos. There appears to be no meaningful association between the age or stage at which immunological maturation occurs and the phylogenetic position or gestation (incubation) period of the various vertebrates for which data are available. The further qualification may be raised that the immune recognition mechanism matures at different times for disparate classes of antigens. In other words, the developing immune mechanism may respond differentially with respect to varying degrees of antigenicity or foreignness. In one series of studies at the Oak Ridge National Laboratory, Tennessee, newborn and young mice, in contrast with adult mice, showed a differential antibody response in favor of antigens from more distantly related species (sheep > rabbit > rat). It now appears that the "weaker" the histocompatibility antigen, the more easily can one procure tolerance in juveniles or even in adults.

The fetus in random breeding populations usually possesses paternal genetic characteristics which differ from those of the mother in which it is developing. Although the fetus is a natural allograft, it clearly escapes immunologic destruction. Transplantation antigens appear early in embryonic life and the mother, despite pregnancy, is able to react against these antigens. The placental trophoblast is generally thought to function as an anatomic and immunologic barrier which prevents maternal exposure to fetal antigens and rejection of the fetus by the mother. A paucity of paternal H antigens in mouse trophoblast is also consistent with the mother's tolerance toward this invasive tissue. However, apparent allogeneic tolerance to skin or tumor grafts has repeatedly been found in postpartum female mice parous by males of the strain which provided the test grafts. Moreover, tolerance toward both strong (H-2) and weak (H-Y) antigens appeared to increase with multiparity. The conceptus, rather than the semen, is the source of alloantigens eliciting the tolerance induced by parity. In other experiments, such multiparous females were shown to produce antibodies to male-strain antigens, thereby suggesting that enhancement rather than tolerance was responsible for their prolonged allograft survivals. Whether tolerance or enhancement occurs could well depend on the nature and number of antigenic disparities involved. Certainly, fetal antigens introduced into the maternal circulation initiate the altered reactivity. We already considered a prime example of this phenomenon in man in Chapter Four, namely, Rh sensitization allowed by ABO compatibility. Reconciliation of conflicting lines of evidence may lie in the reality that the placenta is an effective immunologic barrier until the very end of pregnancy when its rupture may allow fetal cells to enter the mother. Successful protection of Rh-negative women against Rh immunization by administration of anti-Rh:1 serum at the time of parturition is quite consistent with this assumption. Although passage of maternal blood lymphocytes across the placenta could well be fatal to the fetus because of graft-versus-host reactions considered later in this chapter, transplacental passage of maternal IgG antibodies is conversely an important source of protection against infectious disease for newborns of many mammalian species including humans. In this connection, the usual sparing of the fetus from deleterious consequences of the maternal immune reactions it often generates remains an intriguing problem.

Selective permeability of the placenta to certain immunoglobulins and perhaps other maternal macromolecules is presumably useful to the fetus only if it becomes tolerant to the associated maternal alloantigens. Such tolerance in most mammals is indeed evidenced by the persistence of maternal antibodies for many weeks or months after birth. Presumably, the human fetus has already been exposed to and become tolerant of maternal serum allotypes by the seventh month of gestation when its own immune responsiveness matures. Maternal cellular alloantigens apparently do not gain entrance into the embryo during the tolerance-responsive period in either mice or men since maternal grafts are normally rejected by antigenically disparate offspring.

During the 1950–1960 decade, it was generally thought that allogeneic tolerance responsiveness was an embryonic trait; juveniles were supposed to pass through a "null period" on the way to maturity when an encounter with antigen would yield neither tolerance nor immunity. With the advent of new techniques to measure perinatal responses and closer attention to immunogenetic disparity-antigen dosage relationships, we now know there is no null period. Either tolerance or immunity, or both concomitantly, may be induced in perinatal or adult life depending on the conditions. Howard and Michie, working at the University of Edinburgh in 1961, provided some of the earliest evidence that newborn mice may be immunized with preparations of the same allogeneic cells which in higher dosage will induce tolerance. More direct studies by Boraker and Hildemann at the Jackson Laboratory in Bar Harbor, Maine, revealed a well developed capacity for allograft rejection of normal and tumorous tissues at birth in mice. Transplantation immunity evoked by injection of allogeneic cells in low dosage at birth closely resembles accelerated adult rejections in terms of vigor and histopathology. However, the capacity to respond to alloantigens by humoral antibody production appears to mature more slowly than the capacity for graft rejection. Also, the temporal relationships of the appearance of antibody types after immunization of neonatal and suckling mice differ strikingly from those found in adults.

Some data are instructive in this connection. A/J (H-2^a) and C57BL/6 (H-2^b) neonatal mice which received allografts of neonatal skin reciprocally as early as the day of birth rejected such grafts vigorously with median survival times of ten to eleven days—only slightly longer than those determined for adults (Fig. 7—3). Preimmunization with 50–100×10^3 allogeneic thymocytes at birth led to accelerated rejection of test skin allografts placed four days later. Similar preimmunization effectively protected BL/6 neonates against an otherwise fatal inoculum of A/J tumor cells (Sarcoma I) injected four days later. Maturation of the allohemagglutinin response in BL/6 mice to a variety of A/J thymocyte dosages was demonstrated at about eleven days of age. In contrast, A/J mice first showed allohemagglutinin production at seventeen to twenty-three days of age and high immunogen dosage often led to unresponsiveness. Serum antibodies detected within three to four weeks of age were solely 19S-type macroglobulins whereas older mice of either strain produced 7S antibodies in addition to heavy antibodies. These antibodies induced by allogeneic antigens followed the general maturation sequence of antibody types to xenogeneic antigens described for other species. It should be noted here that concurrent 19S (IgM) and 7S (IgG) antibody production is often found in adult mammals; however, the sequence of 19S followed later by 7S production is generally characteristic of the perinatal period. While IgM is usually more easily detected in low concentration than IgG, the earlier appearance of specifically induced IgM in juveniles does not appear to be an artifact of test sensitivity. Although sensitive plaque assay techniques now reveal slight alloantibody production as early as five to seven days of age in rapidly maturing BL/6 mice, the full repertoire of adult responsiveness appears to be gradually acquired over a period of at least several weeks. The reverse requirements for tolerance responsiveness similarly change considerably as a function of the stage of development. The rate of immunological maturation

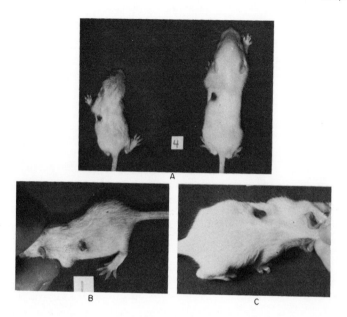

Figure 7—3.   Accelerated allograft rejection by perinatal mouse during acute transplantation disease. (A) Spleen cell-injected mouse (left) with control littermate thirteen days after injection. Experimental mouse weighed 3.45g; control weighed 6.4g. Injected animal died of acute transplantation disease two days later. (B) Close-up of experimental mouse in (A) showing totally destroyed (i.e., scabbed-over) BL/6 allograft eight days after grafting. (C) Close-up of control littermate in (A) showing fully viable BL/6 allograft nine days after grafting. Graft was subsequently rejected. (From Boraker, *UCLA Ph.D. Thesis*, 1967.)

toward H antigens varies among different mouse strains mainly as a consequence of the immunogenetic disparity between donors and recipients.

Failure to obtain allogeneic tolerance in adult animals in early studies is now attributable mostly to strong histocompatibility barriers such as *H-2* in mice, *H-1* (*Ag-B*) in rats, and *B* in chickens. Under these circumstances, a profound assault on an adult animal's immune response capacity achieved by means such as persistent antigen overloading, parabiosis, and whole-body radiation has led to partial or even substantial tolerance. It is becoming increasingly clear not only that tolerance toward weaker H antigens can be more readily achieved in adults but that tolerance responsiveness is directly proportional to effective immunogenic weakness. Female mice of the C57BL strain may easily be made tolerant of a moderately weak H-Y antigen as late as seventeen days postpartum; very high doses of male cells will produce tolerance in adult females. Parabiotic union between adult males and females may also induce a high degree of tolerance. Weakly disparate H-1 or H-3 congenic strains of mice may also become reciprocally tolerant as a consequence of adult parabiosis. With quite weak H-9 or H-12 differences in congenic mice, large skin allografts alone appear to induce prolonged tolerance in adult recipients. Relative ease of induction of adult tolerance toward weak antigens is promising in human organ transplantation as considered in the next chapter.

Since tolerated graft cells retain their antigenic identity, the tolerant state clearly reflects a systemic alteration of the host. Mice derived from pairs of conjoined, cleavage-stage embryos of different histocompatibility genotypes can remain chimeras retaining their characteristic antigenic products. These "allophenic" animals are fully and reciprocally tolerant. Notwithstanding H-2 disparities, they apparently remain free of allogeneic disease but otherwise show normal immune responses. Allogeneic tolerance is usually plural in the sense that a donor normally contains multiple antigens that are lacking in the recipient. Once established, tolerance persists so long as the foreign cells and their descendants continue to maintain a sufficient level of the relevant antigens. Less antigen appears to be required to maintain tolerance than to instate it at the outset. The latter point is nicely established with respect to chemically defined "inanimate" antigens. Although tolerance is as specific as immunity in its discrimination between one donor phenotype and another, there appears to be no distinction between one tissue and another from the same donor. This apparent lack of tissue- or organ-specific transplantation antigens is rather surprising in view of the many organ-specific antigens known to exist. Nevertheless, injection of leukocytes can confer tolerance of skin grafts, ovary, kidney, or adrenal gland. If leukocytes lacked some H antigen present in skin, for example, the observed tolerance should not obtain. Erythrocytes in general, including the nucleated red cells of chickens, do appear to be deficient in H antigens; such cells do not procure tolerance for other tissues. The question of tissue-specific H antigens is not quite settled. E. L. Triplett has shown that frog embryos deprived of their pituitary gland are later capable of rejecting their own hypophysis. In these experiments the organism and gland were grown apart from one another until the tadpoles were immunologically mature and the glands were differentiated. Perhaps the major transplantation antigens are richly represented in the structural proteins of all cell membranes save those of mature red cells. Minor or weak alloantigens peculiar to certain tissues might then tend to remain undetected except under special circumstances.

The convenient assumption that a given state of tolerance is an all-or-none phenomenon is usually an oversimplification. In many test systems, generally involving skin grafts and strong histocompatibility barriers, partial tolerance is the rule. In other words, perinatal exposure to antigens promotes prolonged, but not indefinite, survival of later skin grafts from the same donor source. Every conceivable degree of apparent tolerance has been noted in different experimental systems. The rat data from the work of Billingham and Silvers in Philadelphia, as shown in Fig. 7—4, reveals degrees of allogeneic tolerance to

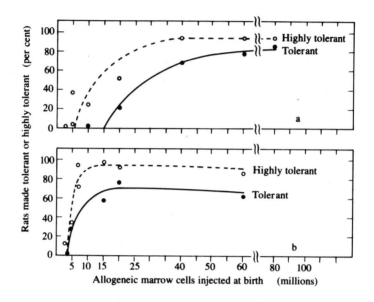

Figure 7—4.   Cell-dosage/tolerance-response curves for allogeneic bone marrow cell inocula, obtained with the B.N. → Lewis (a) and the Lewis → B.N. (b) rat strain combinations. Note the asymmetry between the tolerance responsiveness of B.N. and Lewis neonatal hosts. Highly tolerated test grafts (○) survived for fifty days or more, while tolerated test grafts (●) significantly exceeded survival times of control grafts. (Modified from Billingham and Silvers, *J. Cell. Phys.*, Vol. 60: 190, 1962.)

be markedly dependent upon the strain combination as well as cell dosage. Although the mechanism of tolerance induction, partial or complete, is still an unsolved problem, some newer evidence has heuristic value. A typical strong disparity represented by a single *H-2* allele inevitably confronts a host with a multitude of antigenic specificities (see Table 4—3). These antigens appear to act independently in tolerance induction even though they are products of the same complex locus. Here we should insert the reservation that those antigens (mainly non-H-2) which have cumulative effects in immunity (Chapter Six) might be expected to have such effects in tolerogenesis as well. Further, the multiple H-2 specificities are not equally abundant, even on the same cells. Thus, a dosage of cells sufficient to induce tolerance to most antigens may be insufficient for other antigens, thereby yielding an incompletely tolerant recipient in relation to the total "package" of antigens. Additional processes like antigen competition might possibly be involved.

A similar problem arises in conjunction with split tolerance. The studies of Leslie Brent and co-workers at University College, London, showed that A-strain mice injected at birth with (CBA × C57) hybrid cells were fully tolerant of CBA skin grafts, but only partially tolerant of C57 or even (CBA × C57) grafts. Other evidence concerning these strain combinations supports the assumption that C57 antigens are "more foreign" or immunogenic to A-strain recipients than are CBA antigens. However, this does not circumvent the problem that both sets of donor antigens are present on the same hybrid cells used to achieve chimerism and tolerance. Neither the selective survival of CBA-specific hybrid cells from conceivably heterogeneous populations nor antigenic transformation of host cells accounted for the persistence of C57 and CBA antigens on the donor cells. Indeed, maintenance of diverse tolerant states has repeatedly been shown to depend upon continuing presence of the inducing antigen. Additional hypotheses have been put forward by Brent to account for split tolerance. These are (1) a reversible suppression (or neutralization) of certain surface antigens of hybrid cells analogous to serotype transformations in ciliate protozoa (see Chapter Three), and (2) a greater vulnerability of skin grafts than hybrid spleen cells to immune destruction.

Another interesting example, in this connection, is the reported slow rejection of skin allografts between certain dizygotic cattle co-twins in spite of persistent red cell chimerism. In any event, partial or split tolerance reflects a mixed host response to multiple antigens; the host clearly responds differentially to adjacent molecular determinants and not apparently to intact cells as such, even when the latter are retained in a chimeric state. According to the tolerant cell annihilation theory (see page 222), incomplete tolerance would represent elimination of most but not all potentially reactive host cells or clones. It is not always possible to distinguish between tolerance and enhancement, which of course represent opposite host reactions, especially when weaker alloantigens are at issue.

Let us now consider abrogation of tolerance which can regularly be accomplished by an experimental device known as adoptive immunity. The required design is diagrammed in Fig. 7—5. Newborns of one inbred strain (B) inoculated with several million nucleated cells of another strain (A), under conditions ensuring reciprocal graft-host tolerance, will later accept skin grafts from the donor (A) strain without deleterious consequences. The tolerated (A) graft can be destroyed within a week by an injection of (B) lymphoid cells from an adult preimmunized with (A) cells. Inoculation of the tolerant (B) animal with *normal* rather than immune B cells will also terminate the tolerant state, but more slowly. The adoptive immunity achieved in particular by initially

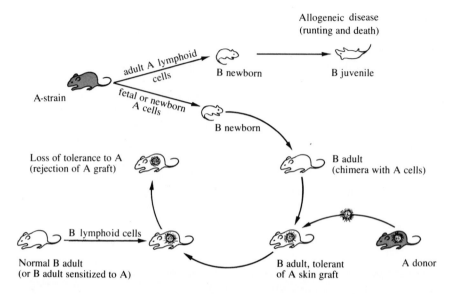

Figure 7—5. Diagram relating transplantation tolerance to allogeneic disease and abrogation of tolerance by adoptive immunity. Two antigenically disparate inbred strains are here designated as A and B. Newborn B injected with immature A cells leads to reciprocal graft-host tolerance and persistent chimerism in B adult. Such B adults will be tolerant of A skin grafts, but tolerance may be terminated adoptively by inoculation of normal or immune adult B lymphoid cells. Note requirement for cells isogenic with host to accomplish adoptive immunity. Newborn B injected with adult A lymphocytes across strong H barrier allows graft-versus-host reactions usually leading to fatal allogeneic disease.

nonimmune cells leads to the important inference that the tolerant state reflects a central failure of the immune response rather than peripheral interference with its inception or execution.

We may conclude this section by emphasizing the dependence of allogeneic tolerance on three major factors, in this order of importance: (a) the degree of immunogenetic disparity between donor and recipient, (b) the recipient's age, and (c) the antigen dosage. Since low cellular antigen dosage regularly evokes immunity whereas a five- to ten-fold higher cell dosage confers tolerance on newborn mice, one is made aware of the decisiveness of the ratio of antigen dosage to number of mature, immunocompetent cells. Once antibody formation has been initiated, tolerance becomes more difficult to induce. Strong histocompatibility differences pose formidable barriers to tolerance induction, especially in adults. Rapid systemic distribution of donor cells via the blood is thought to account for tolerogenesis following intracardiac or intravenous inoculation. By contrast, intraperitoneal inoculations in similar circumstances generally cause immunity. If tolerance induction, without deleterious consequences, were feasible in man, a child could be made tolerant to both parents; this would allow him or her to receive grafts not only from either parent, but also from any sibling, since no child should have histocompatibility genes or antigens not found in one of the parents.

Allogeneic Disease: Graft-Versus-Host Reactions

When immunologically competent cells in substantial numbers are inoculated into infant, juvenile, or even adult allogeneic animals incapable of destroying these cells, a syndrome called runt disease, homologous disease, allogeneic disease or more generally "transplantation disease" usually ensues (Fig. 7–6).

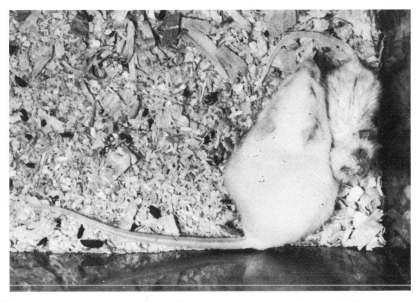

Figure 7–6. Severely runted A/J mouse and normal control littermate at forty-five days of age. The runted mouse, which died a few days later, had been inoculated by the intracardiac route at birth with about two million adult C57BL/6 small blood lymphocytes. Most such runts die at two to four weeks of age.

More severe or accelerated disease is regularly observed if lymphoid cells are obtained from specifically preimmunized donors rather than normal donors. The early initiation phase of such disease is clearly attributable to graft-versus-host

(G.v.H.) reactions. The discovery of the immunogenetic basis of transplantation disease in 1956 was independently made by Billingham and Brent in London and by Simonsen in Copenhagen, working with newborn mice and chick embryos, respectively. As in other realms of biology, early views of G.v.H. reactions have been modified and enlarged in relation to newer insights. The implications with respect to autoimmune disease, cancer, and aging are now especially interesting.

The conditions required for acute G.v.H. reactions can be put in rather precise immunogenetic terms: when two individuals or inbred strains differ with respect to one or more strong histocompatibility genes and antigens, transfer of adult (or mature) lymphoid cells from one strain to perinatal recipients of another strain (or F_1 hybrids of the two strains) commonly leads to fatal disease. There are several qualifications attached to this generalization that warrant further scrutiny. Among other experimental variables, the course and severity of allogeneic disease are substantially affected by the species-strain combination tested, by the age of the hosts, and by the type and number of donor cells. The acute forms of transplantation disease in various mammalian and avian species are associated with complex pathologic features, including inhibition of growth, emaciation, diarrhea, hepatomegaly, splenomegaly, and atrophy of lymphoid tissue.

Three essential requirements for the induction of transplantation disease may be cited: (a) the host cells must possess one or more histocompatibility antigens absent from the donor cells; (b) the donor cells must be immunologically competent or reactive; (c) the host must be incapable of rapid rejection of the donor cells. Theoretically, the least complicated situation fulfilling these requirements involves injection of adult lymphoid cells from an inbred parent strain into infant F_1 hybrids derived from the same parent strain and another inbred strain. Given the "one dominant allele—one histocompatibility antigen" rule, F_1 hybrids, regardless of their age, should be genetically incapable of reacting against parent strain cells. Actually, F_1 hybrids become increasingly resistant to allogeneic disease induction beyond the first few days after birth. If allogeneic, adult lymphoid cells are injected into embryonic or newborn recipients, the development of transplantation disease was long thought to depend upon concurrent induction of host tolerance. Medawar in his 1960 Nobel lecture argued, "a state of tolerance must obviously abet the onset and probably the progress of runt disease because if adult lymphoid cells are to attack the tissues of the animal into which they are injected they must live long enough to be able to do so." Nevertheless, convincing evidence that acute transplantation disease may develop in juveniles in conjunction with host immunity rather than tolerance is now at hand (Fig. 7–3). Although immature recipients may develop immunity rapidly in response to low dosages of donor cells, a critical immunologic attack by donor cells can evidently be consummated even more rapidly. Host-versus-graft reactions can clearly complicate interpretation of experimental results. Regardless of the test system employed, certain major variables should be considered or controlled as follows:

1. Strength of histocompatibility disparity.
2. Type(s) and numbers of donor cells inoculated.
3. Route of donor cell administration.
4. Ages of hosts.
5. Ages of donors.
6. Sex of donors and hosts.

Extensive studies with inbred and congenic lines of mice reveal that adult donor-host differences at the $H-2$ locus generally constitute a strong disparity leading either to acute graft rejection or acute transplantation disease. Conversely, weak differences associated with chronic allograft rejection may also evoke weak G.v.H. reactions which fail to produce the usual manifestations of allogeneic disease. G.v.H. reactions have been quantified by several methods. Determination of indexes sensitively reflecting G.v.H. reactions has been widely applied. The indexes are quotients representing experimental body weights or relative organ weights over the mean of the respective weights of littermate controls (Fig. 7–7). Thus, indices greater than one indicate organ enlargement

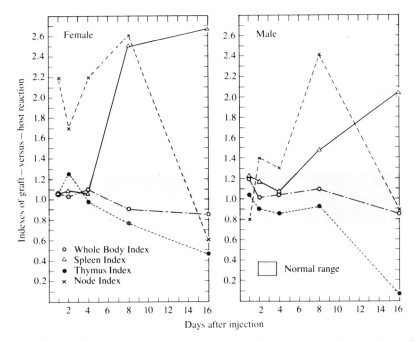

Figure 7–7.   Indexes of graft-versus host reaction at one to sixteen days after intracardiac injection of adult C57BL/6 male spleen cells into male and female (A/J ♀ × C57BL/6 ♂) F_1 newborns, respectively. (From Hildemann *et al.*, *Transplantation*, Vol. 5: 511, 1967. Copyright The Williams and Wilkins Co.)

while indices less than one indicate a body or organ weight less than that of the controls. The weight-gain assay, though less inclusive, does not require killing the experimental animals. Acute runt disease is reflected in curtailment of mean weight increases in experimental animals in relation to comparable controls. Another, more indirect method depends on measurement of phagocytic indexes. Hyperphagocytic activity in clearance of carbon particles is found during the proliferative phase of G.v.H. reactions.

Multiple histocompatibility antigens of similar strengths may have additive effects, as noted in the preceding chapter. Since conspicuous differences in the severity of infant runt disease are observed in H-2 incompatible combinations, one may suspect that other non-H-2 differences distinguishing these strains account for the wide spectrum of mortality. Relatively few studies of G.v.H. reactions involving single or multiple weak histocompatibility differences have yet been undertaken. In inbred lines of chickens, it has been demonstrated that several lines differ at one major locus determining antigens responsible for the splenomegaly component of G.v.H. reactions. This is illustrated by the comparative spleen enlargement in reciprocal backcross and F_2 embryos injected with parental adult leukocytes as shown in Fig. 7–8. Given unenlarged, control spleen weights of 25 mg. or less, one backcross (W X CW) and the F_2 each fell into two groups, one with enlarged and the other with unenlarged spleens. The proportions of embryos showing enlargement fit best the assumption of only one pair of alleles primarily responsible for the antigens leading to splenomegaly. Other evidence points to the B blood group locus as the major histocompatibility locus involved. No sex differences were discerned.

From a developmental standpoint, attention has been focused primarily on host age as a determinative variable. Although embryonic and newborn animals of numerous species are most vulnerable to transplantation disease, marked variation among species or strains is usually attributed to differences in the rate of ontogenesis of immune responsiveness. Not only mammalian fetuses, but even thirteen- to fifteen-day-old chick embryos are capable of immune responses if exposed to foreign cells at low dosage. As might be expected, donor cells capable of reacting against host cells are obtainable from young chicks or mice within a few days after birth. The ability of chicken spleen cells to evoke hepatomegaly and splenomegaly in embryo hosts was found to increase with age to a peak after twenty-one weeks of age. In mice, immunocompetent parental spleen cells in sufficient numbers to cause splenomegaly in newborn F_1 hybrid mice are readily detectable in five- to fifteen-day-old donors, depending on the strain, but heightened reactivity is obtainable from similar numbers of spleen cells derived from older donors. Both host age and donor cell age then are important variables, perhaps affecting host homeostasis as well as immune interactions.

Most allogeneic disease studies have involved inoculation of mixed populations of adult lymphoid cells. Immunocompetent cells have thus been demonstrated in

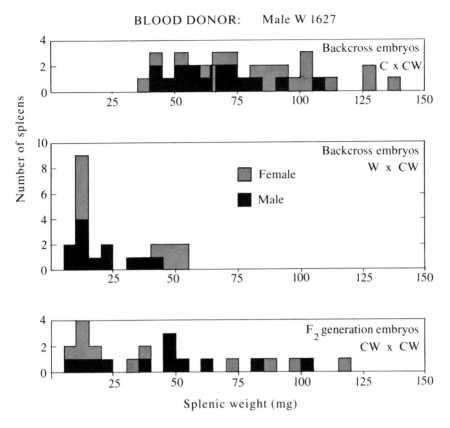

Figure 7—8. Occurrence of splenic enlargement in reciprocal backcross and F_2 hybrid chick embryos inoculated with adult parental (W-line) blood leukocytes. W × CW backcross and F_2 embryos showed distributions of enlarged and unenlarged (25 mg. or less) spleens consistent with a two allele-one major locus responsibility for splenomegaly inducing antigens. (From Jaffe and Payne, *Twelfth World's Poultry Congress Section Paper*, p. 3, 1962.)

spleen, lymph nodes, blood, bone marrow, thoracic duct lymph, skin—indeed in all tissues where lymphocytes are prevalent. Purified small lymphocytes from peripheral blood or from thoracic duct lymph are capable of producing acute runt disease in rodents. Similar small lymphocyte preparations from adult chickens consistently produce splenomegaly in embryonic hosts. Other reports implicating macrophages or large blood lymphocytes as inducers of allogeneic disease have yet to be confirmed. Our own studies reveal that small lymphocytes from adult C57BL/6 (*H-2^b*) mice promptly attack neonatal A/J (*H-2^a*) or (A/J × C57BL/6) F_1 hosts. In these combinations, the injected cells rapidly spent themselves within two days, leaving few or no descendants with the *donor* antigenic make-up. Otherwise, mixed populations of donor cells or their descendants may persist in hosts for prolonged periods, as is proven by both chromosome and antigenic markers. That purified lymphocytes disappeared so rapidly was surprising since overt symptoms of runt disease are not evident until eight days of age or later. The seemingly long latent period between the initial damage presumably done by these lymphocytes and discernible disease suggested very early changes in host lymphoid tissues. In light of compelling evidence revealing the thymus as a "master organ" regulating immunologic potential during early development, our findings were explicable if the newborn host thymus were directly attacked or if a prompt assault on peripheral lymphoid tissues indirectly led to thymic depletion.

Early "immunologic thymectomy" as a major cause of acute allogeneic disease was supported by the interdependent changes found in lymphoid tissues of neonatal hosts. Profound thymic atrophy, inversely coupled to lymph node and spleen enlargement, was confirmed in extensive experiments as the central feature of the acute disease in mice (Fig. 7–7). Relative to control animals, the normal growth of thymus and spleen was altered in opposite directions. Progressive disappearance of lymphoid cells from thymus, spleen, and lymph nodes was associated with a histiocyte conversion of these tissues. Although this process was so extensive in spleen and nodes as to produce organ weight gains, it was insufficient to offset persistent weight loss in the thymus. The influence of sex and sex-associated antigens was controlled by comparing littermate male and female recipients separately. Significant sex-associated differences were discerned among (A/J $\times$ C57BL/6) F_1 hybrids. Males were clearly more vulnerable to early death than females. Comparison of female and male F_1 littermate controls inoculated with F_1 male spleen cells revealed consistent lymph node hypertrophy after eight days as a consequence of X-linked histoincompatibility. Otherwise, this H-X disparity did not elicit acute effects. Substantial lymph node enlargement was characteristic of F_1 neonates of both sexes at twenty-four to forty-eight hours after intracardiac injection. However, significant splenic enlargement or thymic weight loss was found only after four days in response to H-2 plus non-H-2 incompatibilities. Earlier findings of undulations in thymus, spleen, and node sizes may be attributed to inadequate control of sex-associated factors and/or nonspecific stimulation. On present evidence, thymic atrophy is still attributable mostly to thymocyte depletion in attempted homeostatic restitution of rapid immunologic damage to peripheral lymphoid centers. With progressive disappearance of lymphoid cells from the thymus and peripheral tissues, both the immunologic and trophodynamic mechanisms of the host deteriorate. Many late pathologic manifestations remain poorly understood.

The organ enlargement during G.v.H. disease results mainly from *host*, rather than donor, cell multiplication. This has been shown by immunologic methods which assay the antigens present in the tissue as well as by direct chromosome cytology. An inbred mouse strain designated CBA/H-T6T6 carries a distinctive chromosomal marker in the form of a translocation which distinguishes such cells from normal diploid cells. Thus, in G.v.H. reactions involving this strain, it has been possible to demonstrate the overwhelming predominance of host cells in enlarged spleens. However, this essentially histiocytic host response appears to be a reparative reaction to injury rather than an antigraft reaction. Possible involvement of allogeneic inhibition (cf. Chapter Six) is conjectural, and in any event, cannot be universally operative. Mice derived from pairs of conjoined, cleavage-stage embryos of different histocompatibility genotypes can remain normal chimeras retaining their characteristic antigenic products. Such "allophenic" animals are usually reciprocally tolerant, remain quite free of allogeneic disease, and otherwise show normal homeostatic and immune responses.

Attempts at restoration of lethally irradiated, adult mice with allogeneic cells have generally led to many deaths at four to six weeks after irradiation. These late deaths in radiation chimeras are associated with a syndrome, often called "secondary disease," which greatly resembles allogeneic disease in nonirradiated animals. Although the time of onset and progress of the disease are variable, death within three months after irradiation is predictable in situations involving strong immunogenetic confrontations. Again, the severity of the disease depends on variables already described (page 215), in addition to the dose of irradiation. For example, 50 to 75 per cent of CBA mice fully recover from otherwise lethal radiation damage after inoculation with bone marrow from the H-2 compatible strains C3H or 101; such recovery is rare after similar treatment with more disparate A-strain, C57BL, or rat marrow. F_1 hybrid marrow is much more efficacious in rescuing irradiated F_1 hybrid mice than is marrow from either of the parent strains. Accelerated secondary disease may often be obtained if allogeneic adult spleen or lymph node cells are injected instead of, or in addition to, the bone marrow cells needed to restore hemopoiesis. Relatively fewer immunocompetent small lymphocytes are evidently present in adult bone marrow. However, in C3H-to-CBA chimeras, addition of donor lymphoid cells to the bone marrow tends to prevent the disease occurring after inoculation of bone marrow alone. Since very weak histoincompatibility exists in this strain combination, the donor lymphoid cells may be beneficial by providing immunity to certain microorganisms or their toxic products.

Given the usual genetic assumptions, irradiated F_1 hybrids treated with parental marrow should experience secondary disease while irradiated parents treated with hybrid marrow should be spared. According to H. S. Micklem and J. F. Loutit, these experiments have yielded less clear-cut results than expected but have tended to support the G.v.H. hypothesis rather than the reverse. Attempts to immunize F_1 hybrid mice against their parents have regularly failed. Antihost agglutinin production has repeatedly been found in radiation chimeras.

Persistence of fully viable donor skin grafts on xenogeneic rat → mouse chimeras during secondary disease argues against host-versus-graft reactions under the circumstances. Moreover, use of allogeneic fetal liver as a source of hemato-poietic donor cells substantially curtails secondary disease. In this situation, the immature donor cells appear to become tolerant of the host. Curiously, adult bone marrow inoculated from one parental strain into another usually leads to more severe disease than would be found in F_1 hybrid recipients. This could reflect a gene (antigen) dosage difference or greater reparative vigor in adult F_1 hybrids. Among twenty-seven inbred mouse-strain combinations tested for marrow repair of radiation injury by Uphoff and Law at the U.S. National Cancer Institute, no combination yielded good long-term survival when the strains were of different H-2 phenotypes.

Ontogenesis of Immunological Potential

The thymus is not only the first lymphocytic primordium in the maturing fetus, but it starts early to control the development of other lymphoid tissues. In birds, immune response capacity ultimately depends on both the thymus and the bursa of Fabricius, a lymphoid organ near the cloaca. A dichotomy in roles is evident: thymectomy of newly hatched chicks destroys capacity for cellular transplantation immunity whereas bursectomy greatly impairs humoral antibody production. In amphibians as in mammals, thymectomy alone early in development impairs many, but not all, immune responses thereafter. The most consistent feature of perinatal thymectomy in diverse species is a persistent, systemic deficiency of small lymphocytes. The earlier in life thymectomy is performed, the more severe is this lymphopenia. Thymectomy or bursectomy in immunologically mature juveniles or adults usually has no deleterious con-sequences, at least for a considerable period. Although the thymus appears to be a critical source of lymphocytes early in ontogeny, effective thymic function via cell-impermeable diffusion chambers has implicated a humoral control mechan-ism. Quite possibly, both cellular and humoral roles are played concurrently to different degrees during ontogeny. In the absence of antigenic stimuli, fetal lymphoid tissues mature slowly (Fig. 7–1). Precocious maturation of lymphoid tissues, as in spleen and lymph nodes, may be provoked by infection or by deliberate immunization *in utero*. Fetal lambs and fetal Rhesus monkeys are not only capable of rejecting orthotopic skin allografts at mid-gestation or even earlier, but can also produce circulating antibodies to xenogeneic antigens as found in bacteriophage ØX174 or foreign erythrocytes. Once the developing fetus is capable of a given immunologic response, a fully mature type of response may be obtainable.

A state of general tolerance responsiveness has *not* been achieved by early thymectomy. Relative tolerance responsiveness is probably achieved by the marked deficiency of immunocompetent small lymphocytes. Although mice thymectomized at birth may retain skin allografts or even rat xenografts for prolonged periods, chronic rejection is the rule. Moreover, mice, rats, or rabbits thymectomized neonatally show a diminished capacity to produce antibodies to only certain antigens. Presumably the overriding maturational role of the thymus is largely consummated long before birth. However, mice thymectomized in adult life and then heavily irradiated fail to recover the capacity of control animals to produce antibodies to sheep erythrocytes. Conversely, loss of acquired tolerance of mice to antigens such as bovine gamma globulin depends on the presence of a thymus. Adult thymectomized mice remain tolerant much longer than sham-operated controls. The thymus evidently plays a role in terminating acquired tolerance by directing the differentiation of new immunocompetent cells. Specific allogeneic tolerance can readily develop in thymectomized adult radiation chimeras. The thymus then clearly retains a potential regulatory or restorative role even in adults. However, tolerance induction does not appear to depend upon direct action of antigen on immature lymphoid stem cells differentiating within the thymus since specific tolerance is obtainable *de novo* in thymectomized adult animals. Finally, we should note that lymphoid cells from adult mice thymectomized as newborns are less able to provoke transplantation disease in allogeneic hosts than the same number and source of cells from normal mice.

Neonatally thymectomized mice develop after a month or more, a wasting syndrome with manifestations similar to those found in typical allogeneic disease. A common pathogenesis in both conditions has been suggested. However, experiments with gnotobiotic, thymectomized mice reveal that they do not develop the characteristic wasting syndrome unless subsequently exposed to microorganisms. Yet both germ-free mice and mice raised under normal laboratory conditions are equally vulnerable to allogeneic disease after neonatal injection with adult spleen cells (gnotobiotic donors in the case of gnotobiotic recipients). Transplantation disease is evidently a direct consequence of alloimmune reactions whereas postthymectomy wasting is attributable to infectious agents or their products in immunologically impaired animals. All investigators agree that generalized lymphoid tissue atrophy regularly occurs in the late stages of either disease. Nearly all deaths from acute allogeneic disease in mice occur before thirty days of age; in contrast, almost all wasting deaths following neonatal thymectomy occur after the first month of postnatal life. This conspicuous difference in timing may be interpreted as evidence that destruction of the thymus alone does not lead to the earlier deaths in transplantation disease.

Theories of Immunological Tolerance

Specific immunological recognition—which can lead to either tolerance or immunity—develops long before birth in many mammals, before hatching in birds, and before climactic metamorphosis in amphibians. Although the mechanisms of "not-self recognition" remain unknown, this concept is inherent in all theories of tolerance. Self-constituents like the potent H-2 antigens of mice are not fully manifest until the time of birth. Many different theories of tolerance have been advocated during the last several years. We shall consider three major groups:

1. Cell annihilation theory.
2. Cell blocking theories.
3. Differential maturation or transformation theories.

In the annihilation theory, tolerance depends upon specific elimination of responsive cells as a result of contact with antigen. Interaction of an antigenic determinant with a cell having a genetically determined affinity for this antigen is supposed to cause the death of the cell. This type of interaction was postulated by Burnet and by Lederberg to occur especially during early ontogeny. According to this view, there are no tolerant cells in an individual, but only cells capable of immune responses. Autoimmune responses are normally absent because all potentially responsive clones have been destroyed during embryonic development. Cessation of tolerance or appearance of autoimmunity is ascribed to mutation or differentiation of the "forbidden" cell clones. Thoracic duct lymphocytes from specifically tolerant rats are unable to achieve G.v.H. reactions in rats of the tolerance-inducing donor type. Presumably this means that lymphocytes are the key cells affected by tolerance induction. N. A. Mitchison, who favors the annihilation theory, supposes that more direct access of antigen (e.g., small doses of highly soluble proteins) to specific receptors on lymphocytes implements tolerogenesis whereas immunization conversely involves a step of complexity (e.g., macrophage processing of antigen). In other words, the manner of presentation of antigen to lymphocytes may determine whether the outcome is tolerance or immunity. These extensions of the annihilation theory could account for tolerant states in mature animals or even unresponsiveness induced in previously sensitized animals; however, the various degrees of incomplete tolerance are not straightforwardly accommodated by this theory. Of course, entrapment of antigen and processing by macrophages of the reticuloendothelial system as a precondition for induction of immunity rather than tolerance can be fitted into most current theories of tolerance.

The blocking theories assume that antigen hits a critical receptor of lymphocytes and either prevents the maturation of potential immunocytes or turns off the synthesis of specific antibodies. In both instances, tolerant cells are invoked which are supposed to remain unresponsive so long as antigenic determinants maintain the blocking effect. A blocking of cellular differentiation is assumed in the stem cell theory. The essence of this conception is that stem cells respond to antigen by becoming tolerant while mature cells in the same individual are conversely triggered toward immune responses. This would account for the ease of tolerance induction in embryos or neonates in which stem cells are much more numerous than mature cells. Exposure of embryos to potential antigens is supposed to establish complete tolerance provided sufficient antigen reaches all reactive stem cells, thereby preventing their further differentiation. Tolerance in adults would represent the replacement of immunocompetent mature cells by a nonreactive population. On this basis, some mature cells should begin an immune response which might or might not be detectable in the continued presence of antigen. Without further recruitment, such cells could either expend themselves or be destroyed by "allergic injury" on persistent exposure to antigen. An alternative theory assumes an essentially homogeneous population of antigen-responsive cells. Thus, given cells should become either tolerant or immune depending on the nature of the encounter with antigen rather than the stage of maturation of the cell. One could then expect to find both tolerant and antibody-forming cells at the same time in an individual as in states of partial tolerance.

More recent theories tend to accept the notion of a dual response to an injection of antigen: some cells become tolerant (or are eliminated) and other cells become immune (or transform into reactive immunocytes). In other words, antigen can either prime or paralyze depending on the status of the cells encountered. Three levels or successive stages of cell maturation (X-Y-Z) are frequently assumed, with numerous possible variations, as follows:

$$\underset{\text{(stem cell)}}{\text{X-cell}} \xrightarrow{1° \text{ Ag}} \underset{\substack{\text{(primed cells and}\\ \text{memory cells)}}}{\text{Y-cell}} \xrightarrow{2° \text{ Ag}} \underset{\substack{\text{(terminal Ab}\\ \text{producer)}}}{\text{Z-cell}}$$

Here, $1°$ Ag and $2°$ Ag are meant to symbolize initial exposure and renewed contact with an antigen, respectively. Tranformation of X-cells to Y-cells may be either blocked or promoted in embryos or adults depending on the quality and quantity of antigen encountered. Even if reactive Y-cells are produced in moderate numbers, further contact with sufficient antigen could elicit terminal differentiation (Z-cells) with subsequent tolerance, or proliferation with increased antibody production. Proponents of this theory tend to view tolerance as a favorable balance between relatively few "immune" cells and many "unresponsive" cells. Two major states of antigen-induced unresponsiveness have been described in this connection. The first, tolerance or paralysis, may be defined as complete inhibition of immune responsiveness in "virgin" animals while the second, immune exhaustion, refers to a state of unresponsiveness following an earlier period of significant antibody production. A population of memory cells in immunologically experienced animals appears to become exhausted by a supraoptimal dose of antigen. In contrast to the cell-blocking theories, the differential maturation or transformation theories involve more realistic attempts to cope with the known complexity of immune responses. Thus, memory and major differences in primary versus secondary responsiveness are taken into account.

Perhaps the most critical question bearing on the major theories outlined is whether or not specifically tolerant cells really exist. In other words, is tolerance a condition of the entire organism or of a population of lymphoid cells? Among the more imaginative theories beyond the scope of our concern, one postulates that tolerance is established by elimination of "antibody viruses" (each containing nucleic acid coding for a specific antibody) encountering an antigen which can combine with their coat-protein antibody in an environment where "viral" replication cannot be initiated.

Immunogenetic Concepts of Cancer and Aging

Those essentially autoimmune diseases, like acquired hemolytic anemia, which involve tissues naturally exposed to circulating lymphocytes could result from reactions of mutant or aberrant lymphoid cells against normal tissue macromolecules. For such lymphoid cells to react against self-constituents (loss of tolerance), a loss or mutation of a histocompatibility gene in a clone of lymphoid cells may be required. Association of subtle, chronic reactions with weak antigenic disparities or with more resistant adult hosts has been suggested as a theoretical mechanism in development of cancer and of aging. Certain autoimmune diseases in man show clinical features analogous to transplantation disease as produced in experimental animals. The lesions of disorders such as systemic lupus erythematosus, acquired hemolytic anemia, scleroderma, and rheumatoid arthritis have pathological counterparts in experimental transplantation disease, especially in the more chronic disease in adult animals. Cutaneous lesions evoked in adult rats and hematologic abnormalities produced in adult mice in conjunction with G.v.H. reactions have been considered as models of similar human disease thought to have an autoimmune basis. In our study of strong histocompatibility differences that led to acute runt disease in juvenile hosts, no histologic evidence for processes resembling the human disorders was discerned, such as connective tissue changes like those encountered in "collagen diseases" in the heart, kidney, joints, or elsewhere. These changes might require a more chronic disease process which could depend in turn upon a less vulnerable victim or weaker incompatibility.

Albert Tyler of the California Institute of Technology proposed that spontaneous cancer arises from single cells that suffer loss or inactivation of *H* genes. These cells are assumed to react against normal cells possessing the relevant antigen(s) as in G.v.H. reactions. At heterozygous loci, only one allele would need to be lost or inactivated whereas loss or mutation of both alleles at homozygous loci (e.g., in inbred strains) would be required.

The precancer cell is supposed to respond to the proliferative stimulus of the newly foreign "host" antigen with the result that normal cells are gradually destroyed and replaced by neoplastic cells. If this hypothesis were valid, one would expect that animals which escape acute transplantation disease should later show a consistently higher incidence of tumors. Roy Walford of the University of California, Los Angeles, advanced a similar theory of aging. In this context, aging is supposed to result primarily from prolonged histoincompatibility reactions among immunologically diversifying cells within an individual. Chronic "autoimmune" reactions pathogenetically associated with the aging process could be a consequence of spontaneous somatic mutation of "weak" *H* genes in immunocompetent cells. In essence then, both theories invoke immunogenetic mutation leading to subsequent deleterious reactions among somatic cell populations. Certain lines of experimental evidence lend support to these theories.

Chronic immunopathologic reactions typical of transplantation disease were evident in parabiotic Syrian hamsters showing only weak histocompatibility differences. Also, amyloidosis essentially identical to the senile type was found in chronologically young to middle-aged animals in parabiosis. Apparently then, the major disease of aging in hamsters is substantially accelerated in the face of weak parabiotic incompatibility. Newborn mice injected with adult spleen cells from a congenic strain reflecting weak incompatibility ($H\text{-}1^b \rightarrow H\text{-}1^a$) did not manifest acute disease but did show significant life shortening compared with control animals inoculated with isogenic spleen cells ($H\text{-}1^a \rightarrow H\text{-}1^a$). Moreover, the experimental groups showed a higher incidence of lymphomas during mid-adult life which also appeared much earlier than in control animals. Both C3H mouse strains studied normally manifest only a very low incidence of lymphoma or leukemia. Experiments with other inbred strains of mice differing at both *H-2* and non-*H-2* loci also reveal that malignant lymphomas may be produced in conjunction with chronic transplantation disease. In one study, six-week-old male (C57BL/6 × DBA/2) F_1 mice were given four weekly injections each of about 80 million male C57BL/6 spleen cells. The long-term survivors of this immunologic assault developed lymphoid neoplasms of host origin which resembled Hodgkin's disease and lymphosarcoma. Provocative findings of this type, though not sufficient to allow conclusive interpretation, suggest escalation from an immunologic to a neoplastic disease.

The ubiquitous manifestations of allogeneic disease as an experimental "model" have obviously complicated determination of sequential cause-and-effect relationships. The early phase of initiation of deleterious reactions in terms of immunogenetic disparities and lymphoid tissue changes is now much better understood than later phases yielding overt disease. Very much less may be confidently deduced about chronic processes necessarily involving a large part of the total life span.

KEY REFERENCES

1. BILLINGHAM, R. E., and W. K. SILVERS. "Some Factors That Determine the Ability of Cellular Inocula to Induce Tolerance of Tissue Homografts." *J. Cell. and Comp. Physiol.*, Suppl. 1, Vol. 60: 183–200, 1962. Diverse evidence is presented that histologic origin and dosage of donor inoculum in conjunction with age and sex of hosts are important factors in induction of tolerance.

2. BRENT, L., and T. H. COURTENAY. "On the Induction of Split Tolerance," in *Mechanisms of Immunological Tolerance*. Czech. Acad. Sci., Prague, pp. 113–121, 1962. Split tolerance is evaluated as a function of chimerism in terms of possible phenotypic transformations and differential persistence of graft cells.

3. DE WECK, A. L., and J. R. FREY. "Immunotolerance to Simple Chemicals." *Monogr. in Allergy*, Vol. 1, Amer. Elsevier Publ. Co., New York, 1966. Types of immunological unresponsiveness are nicely reviewed, especially in relation to possible mechanisms of tolerance.

4. HILDEMANN, W. H. "Mechanisms and Ontogenetic Implications of Transplantation (Allogeneic) Disease," in *Ontogeny of Immunity*, Univ. of Florida Press, Chap. 14, pp. 112–121, 1967. A recent review of major variables and immunogenetic mechanisms thought to be involved in diverse forms of allogeneic disease.

5. ———, W. E. RATHBUN, and R. L. WALFORD. "Early Manifestations of Acute Transplantation (Allogeneic) Disease in Mice." *Transplantation*, Vol. 5: 504–513, 1967. Genetic and developmental aspects of transplantation disease were evaluated in relation to early changes in host lymphoid tissues.

6. JAFFE, W. P., and L. N. PAYNE. "The Genetic Basis for Graft-Against-Host Reaction Between Inbred Lines of Fowls. Differences Between Reaseheath C and I Inbred Lines." *Immunology*, Vol. 5: 399–413, 1962. An instructive analysis of the genetic determination of antigens causing reactions leading to splenic enlargement.

7. KALISS, N., and M. K. DAGG. "Immune Response Engendered in Mice by Multiparity." *Transplantation*, Vol. 2: 416–425, 1964. Immunologic aspects of pregnancy are evaluated in relation to tolerance, enhancement, or immunity induced in multiparous females mated interstrain.

8. LENGEROVA, A., and V. MATOUSEK. "Strength of Histocompatibility Barriers and Induction of Immunological Tolerance." *Folia Biol.* (Praha), Vol. 12: 319–334, 1966. A quantitative study of tolerance induction in genetically defined strains of mice in relation to strong and weak histocompatibility barriers.

9. MICKLEM, H. S., and J. F. LOUTIT. *Tissue Grafting and Radiation.* Academic Press, New York, 1966. Chapter 6 deals especially with radiation chimerism and secondary (allogeneic) disease.

10. MILLER, J. F. A. P., and D. OSOBA. "Current Concepts of the Immunological Function of the Thymus." *Physiol. Rev.,* Vol. 47: 437–520, 1967. Sections on immunological tolerance, immunological deficiency diseases, autoimmunity, and neoplasia are especially pertinent from an immunogenetic standpoint.

11. MINTZ, B., and W. K. SILVERS. " 'Intrinsic' Immunological Tolerance in Allophenic Mice." *Science,* Vol. 158: 1484–1487, 1967. Mice derived from pairs of conjoined, cleavage-stage embryos of different histocompatibility genotypes can remain chimeras retaining their characteristic antigenic products. These "allophenic" animals are fully and reciprocally tolerant, remain free of allogeneic disease, but otherwise show normal immune responses.

12. MITCHISON, N. A., "Immunological Tolerance," in *Symp. on Tissue and Organ Transplantation,* suppl. to *J. Clin. Path.,* Vol. 20: 451–455, 1967. Newer conceptions of tolerogenesis are presented with emphasis on possible roles of macrophages and lymphocytes.

13. OWEN, R. D. "Immunogenetic Bases of Transplant Tolerance and Rejection," in *Mechanisms of Immunological Tolerance.* Czech. Acad. Sci., Prague, pp. 133–142, 1962. Histocompatibility genetics studies of natural populations at genetic equilibrium yield results which depend upon allele frequencies in the population. The relative specificities of tolerance and immunity are compared at several levels of gene frequency.

14. STERZL, J., and A. M. SILVERSTEIN. "Developmental Aspects of Immunity," in *Advances in Immunology,* Academic Press, New York, Vol. 6, pp. 337–459, 1967. This is a thorough and nearly comprehensive review of the ontogeny of immune reactivities.

15. TYLER, A. "A Developmental Immunogenetic Analysis of Cancer," in *Henry Ford Hospital International Symposium: Biological Interactions in Normal and Neoplastic Growth,* Little, Brown & Co., Boston. pp. 533–571, 1962. Many studies are reviewed in relation to cancer as a type of allogeneic disease.

16. WALFORD, R. L. "Further Considerations Towards an Immunologic Theory of Aging." *Exp. Geront.,* Vol. 1: 67–76, 1964. A concise review of evidence bearing on immunogenetic aspects of aging.

EIGHT

HISTOCOMPATIBILITY TYPING AND CIRCUMVENTION OF ALLOIMMUNE REACTIONS

We may well begin by considering what are the purposes of tissue typing. Current preoccupation with human histocompatibility typing for matching compatible donors and recipients of kidney allografts reflects a half decade of intensely productive interaction between immunogeneticists and surgeons. To be sure, a need for accurate tissue typing has long been recognized in the more usual situation of whole blood transfusions. Indeed, blood grouping by standardized serological techniques now allows identification or characterization of individuals to a remarkable extent. Other human applications range from establishing correct parent-offspring relationships and recognition of mono-zygotic-versus-fraternal twins to identification of blood stains in criminal cases. However, not all cellular alloantigens persist in mature red cells, and this is a decisive limitation of blood group serology. Additional typing of antigens restricted to nucleated cells or their products has proved to be highly desirable for various reasons. Besides organ allotransplantation, these include therapeutic skin grafts for extensive burns, endocrine grafts to restore needed hormones, and bone marrow grafts for repair of severe radiation injury. In this chapter, we shall examine tissue typing methods and especially leukocyte typing in man. Given the likely prospect of incomplete matching for organ allografts in the foreseeable future, circumvention of alloimmune reactions also deserves special consideration.

Tissue Typing Methods: Their Significance and Limitations

The clinical goal of tissue typing, however accomplished, is to match potential donors and recipients for major or relatively strong histocompatibility antigens. With inbred strains and especially congenic lines, identification of *H* alleles and their relative strengths can be readily accomplished as described previously. In heterogeneous human populations, by contrast, both mono-specific antiserums and target cells of known antigenic phenotype are often difficult to obtain. Until recently, serologic typing of human leukocytes or platelets has depended mostly on antiserums containing many specificities as a result of their chance production in patients following multiple transfusions or repeated pregnancies. Differential absorptions of such antiserums has not proved conveniently feasible, mainly for lack of appropriate absorbing cells (or antigens) in sufficient quantity.

Early attempts at clinical allotransplantation suggested that red cell antigens were not important because matching for most blood groups (alone) did not allow prolonged survival in many instances. This kind of evidence turned out to be misleading, and we now know that the ABO as well as the P antigens affect graft survival. Studies by Dausset and Rapaport in Paris clearly demonstrated that AB erythrocyte antigens can also act as strong transplantation antigens. As illustrated in Table 8–1, volunteers sensitized by four successive injections of purified ABO-incompatible erythrocytes regularly showed accelerated rejection of skin grafts from other AB-incompatible donors compared with grafts from compatible (O) donors. Since leukocytes also carry AB antigens, one might raise the question, in light of the poor immunogenic potency of red cells in other transplantation situations, whether buffy coat contamination of these preparations could account for the results. Additional group (O) recipients pretreated with intradermal injections of water-soluble (A) substance isolated from hog stomach subsequently showed very rapid rejection of grafts from A donors while concurrent grafts from (O) donors showed slow first-set type reactions. Since red cells carry (A) as a glycolipid while gastric (A) occurs in glycoprotein, A as a transplantation antigen must represent a carbohydrate determinant—probably *N*-acetylglucosamine (cf. Chapter Four). Ceppellini and co-workers in Italy have further shown $A_1 \rightarrow O$ incompatibility is very strong in comparison, for example, to $A_2 \rightarrow O$. Data given in Fig 8–1 clearly show that genetic disparities in addition to ABO incompatibility affect skin allograft survival times in normal recipients. $P_1 : P_2$ incompatibility may exert a significant effect. Other blood group systems, including those of no importance for transfusion, should be further evaluated in this connection. Weaker antigens may of course escape detection if any strong disparities supervene. Antigenic polymorphisms of human serum β-lipoproteins, also apparently associated with leukocyte *H* loci, have similarly been found to influence skin graft survival times.

Table 8–1 Response to Skin Homografts After Sensitization with Four Successive Injections of ABO-Incompatible Erythrocytes (Modified from Dausset and Rapaport, Ann. N.Y. Acad. Sci., Vol. 129: 410, 1966)

Route of Administration	Blood Group of Recipients	Blood Group of Donor Erythrocytes	Fate of Skin Homografts from Other Donors Applied to the Sensitized Recipients (Days)					
			Skin Grafts from Compatible (O) Donors			Skin Grafts from Other Incompatible (AB) Donors		
			1	2	3	1	2	3
Intradermal	1) O, Rh+	A_2B	11	11	11	6	7	6
	2) O, Rh+	A_2B	11	10	15	6	8	5
			Mean = 11.1 days			Mean = 6.3 days		
Intravenous	1) O, Rh–	A_2B	10	6	7	White Mixed Graft	White Graft	White 4–5
	2) O, Rh+	A_2B	10	6	7	White Mixed Graft	White Graft	White 4–5
			Mean = 7.7 days					

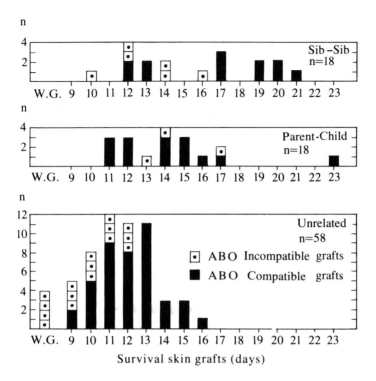

Figure 8–1.   Distribution of skin graft survival times for the three genetically different classes of donors. Black squares: ABO-compatible grafts. White, dotted squares: ABO-incompatible grafts. WG: white grafts reflecting strong $A_1 \rightarrow O$ incompatibility. (After Ceppellini *et al., Ann. N.Y. Acad. Sci.,* Vol. 129: 432, 1966.)

Although human blood platelets contain transplantation antigens as evidenced by capacity to sensitize recipients against skin grafts from platelet donors, only recipients of large quantities of platelets ($> 10^{11}$) have rejected donor grafts at an accelerated rate. Much more work needs to be done in this area before definitive conclusions can be made. Blood platelet antigens have been tentatively implicated in the rejection of human kidney allografts, possibly as a consequence of antigens known to be shared in common with leukocytes and skin. In experimental animals, pretreatment with allogeneic thrombocytes has thus far given opposing or equivocal results in terms of skin allograft survivals. However, there is no doubt about the existence of numerous alloantigens on platelets. Two specific platelet antigen systems in humans have been detected with serums from certain polytransfused patients that contain IgM antibodies demonstrable by saline agglutination. These are the Ko and Zw groups, each with two known codominant alleles yielding distinctive antigens present on platelets, but not on leukocytes or erythrocytes. The *Ko* and *Zw* loci are neither sex-linked nor closely linked to known red cell or serum group loci. Complement fixation has also proved useful as a sensitive technique for measuring platelet alloantibodies. The platelet H antigens revealed by test skin grafting have shown no correlation with the platelet groups Ko^a, Ko^b or Zw^a, Zw^b just described. Although platelets are not endowed with the full spectrum of transplantation antigens, they are easily obtained and they do possess important HL-A antigens which are detectable by complement fixation.

Other tests for compatible donor selection have been described and evaluated in some detail. We have yet to consider the third-man test, the normal lymphocyte transfer reaction, mixed lymphocyte cultures, and the "mainstream" of lymphocyte typing by serology. The chief advantages and limitations of the six-tissue typing methods in relation to allograft donor selection are summarized in Table 8–2. In the "third-party test," compatibility between prospective donor-recipient pairs is assessed by the incidence of cross-reactions induced by skin grafts from these subjects in an unrelated third person. Operationally, recipients are sensitized with skin grafts from one individual, for example, a person needing a kidney allograft; after rejection, recipients are grafted with skin from one or more prospective donors. If the second graft(s) shows accelerated rejection, one may conclude (optimistically) that the two successive donors shared one or more strong antigens absent from the test recipient. However, if the second graft shows a typical first-set rejection time, the two donors may be regarded as antigenically disparate. The "third man" test sequence is diagrammed in Fig. 8–2. This test then provides an estimate of the likeness or similarity of two individuals in terms of their H-antigen profiles. It does not detect differences between them. The test has the advantage of avoiding possible preimmunization of a prospective organ allograft recipient and the disadvantage of a test-host who might or might not share important antigens with the test-donors. The closer the antigenic correspondence of the third-party recipients to the original immunizing donor (i.e., future recipient), the greater is the discriminatory efficacy of this test. Although the test may prove worthwhile within a family, it is not promising for screening of unrelated individuals. Indeed, equivocal results have been obtained under the latter circumstances.

The normal lymphocyte transfer (NLT) test offers an alternate approach to the problem of tissue typing in vivo. This method involves the induction of localized, cutaneous graft-versus-host reactions by injected blood lymphocytes. As originally applied to guinea pigs by Brent and Medawar, a good correlation was obtained between the delayed inflammatory reaction evoked by intradermally injected lymphocytes from a potential recipient in various donors and the survival times of subsequent skin allografts from those donors to the chosen recipient. However, differentiation between relatively weak reactions posed some problems. This test has been applied by Gray and Russell at Harvard

Table 8–2.   Tissue Typing Methods in Relation to Allograft Donor Selection

Method	Chief Advantages and Limitations
Erythrocyte typing	Antigens already well characterized by standardized serological techniques. Many important transplantation antigens are absent from or poorly represented on red cells. At least some red cell antigens appear irrelevant.
Platelet typing	Platelets are easily obtained, handled, and tested. Although certain alloantigens, including transplantation antigens, are present on platelets, other important antigens appear to be absent or sparsely present.
Third-man test	Potentially useful in families with similar H-antigen profiles, but not promising for screening of unrelated individuals. Discriminatory power of test increases, the closer the antigenic correspondence of the third-party recipient to he first donor (i.e., future organ allograft recipient).
Normal lymphocyte transfer reaction	Can identify strongly incompatible donor-recipient combinations, but appears unsuitable for mass screening of unrelated persons. Test may be difficult to interpret objectively.
Mixed lymphocyte culture reaction	Usually detects stronger histoincompatibilities and may even reveal certain antigens not readily detectable by serological tests. This method is unable to detect weak antigenic disparities and could not select the best match from among random pairs of individuals.
Leukocyte (lymphocyte) typing	Most useful procedure for large-scale selection among unrelated individuals. Capable of detecting both strong and weak H antigens in potential donors, whether living or cadaver. Monospecific antiserums for numerous antigens are not yet available or are difficult to obtain. Some and perhaps many lymphocyte antigens do not appear to function as transplantation antigens

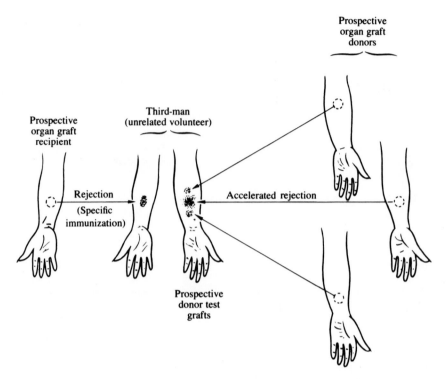

Figure 8–2. "Third-man" test sequence. Skin allograft from prospective organ graft recipient is placed on unrelated volunteer (third man). After this graft is rejected (about fourteen days), skin allografts from prospective organ donors are placed on the third man. Accelerated rejection then identifies the most promising organ donor(s).

Medical School to studies of skin allograft survival in man. The method is illustrated in Fig. 8–3. The sensitivity of the technique in selection of the least compatible donor from a panel was examined by attempting to predict from the intensity (size and induration) of the skin reactions the sequence of rejection of later skin grafts from cell recipients to cell donors. In other instances, human kidney donors have been selected on the basis of the NLT test, and subsequent graft survival was evaluated from this standpoint. The delayed reaction as manifest after forty-eight hours was scored as the best indicator of the genetic disparity between donor and recipient. Subjects with the least or smallest skin reactions were considered to be most compatible with the future recipient. The sensitivity of the test in humans was not impressive in relation to reciprocal skin graft survival times. Although the NLT test can identify strongly incompatible donor-recipient combinations, the narrow range of graft rejections in the absence

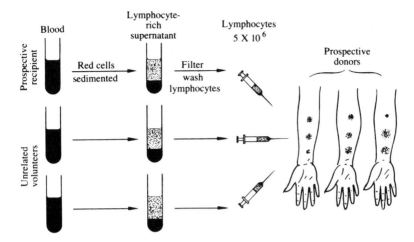

Figure 8–3. Normal lymphocyte transfer test. Blood lymphocytes from the prospective recipient and from unrelated volunteers are injected intradermally into prospective organ donors. Reactions after forty-eight hours are judged in relation to inflammatory reactions produced by unrelated (healthy) lymphocytes. The individual with the least reaction from the prospective recipient's lymphocytes is selected as organ donor.

of immunosuppression would tend to preclude detection of weaker histocompatibility barriers as might well be found among related individuals. More detailed experiments by Ceppellini and co-workers showed that NLT reactions are also dependent on the dose of lymphocytes injected. The percentage of positive reactions was higher at all cell doses for unrelated than for related individuals. The NLT test appears unsuitable for mass screening of unrelated persons and is, of course, inapplicable to potential cadaver donors. Also, lymphocytes from certain patients, such as those with uremia, may produce misleading weak reactions in prospective donors. Finally the intensity and timing of cutaneous alloimmune reactions in adults may involve host-versus-graft as well as graft-versus-host components.

An analogous test worthy of note makes use of irradiated hamsters which retain for a time the capacity to show vigorous delayed-type skin reactions, despite their own immunologic neutralization. Some thirty hours after irradiation at high dosage (1500 rads), an adult Syrian hamster is given intradermal injections of lymphocytes from a prospective allograft recipient and prospective donors, both separately and in mixtures. Antigenically disparate lymphocyte mixtures generally produce large, inflammatory skin reactions. Theoretically, the most promising donor should provoke the least reaction after contact with the prospective recipient's lymphocytes.

Determination of histoincompatibility by mixed leukocyte cultures (MLC) hinges on the initial observation that mixtures of blood leukocytes from two genetically unrelated individuals provided reciprocal stimulation, evidenced especially by enlargement and mitosis of lymphocytes. A correlation between the degree of stimulation and the extent of cross-reactions of skin from the two individuals placed on a third unrelated person was discerned early on. Inability to distinguish two-way from one-way stimulation of potential donor and recipient lymphocytes was an initial disadvantage. The desired evaluation of one-way stimulation has been achieved by pretreating the cells of one individual with irradiation or mytomycin C. If potential donor lymphocytes are treated before culture, they retain the capacity to stimulate recipient lymphocytes, even though their own ability to transform and divide is effectively inhibited. In effect, treated cells cannot respond by incorporating thymidine (i.e., DNA synthesis), but they can still stimulate untreated allogeneic cells to do so. The survival of human skin allografts between siblings matched by one-way stimulation is revealing. MLC incompatible grafts survived eleven to thirteen days while MLC compatible grafts persisted for fifteen to thirty-six days. The MLC test does appear to have predictive value in assessing the duration of both skin and kidney allograft survival. This test is diagrammatically outlined in Fig. 8–4.

Human MLC data are consistent with the assumption that reactivity is determined by the genotype at one "strong" locus with many alleles. In any family, only four different alleles may be represented, and a maximum of four genotypes can therefore occur in siblings. Hence, about one-fourth of sibling donors should fail to stimulate each other as a result of identity at this locus. However, cells from unrelated individuals should stimulate each other more frequently with increasing numbers of alleles in the test population. Expected proportions of nonstimulators among sibs versus unrelated individuals for different numbers of loci and alleles are set out in Table 8–3. Equal allele frequencies and no gene-product interactions are assumed. Among 209 sibling pairs in twenty-nine families surveyed by Fritz Bach and Bernard Amos, 29 per cent did not stimulate. All 282 mixtures of lymphocytes from unrelated pairs, on the other hand, were reactive. Within 95 per cent confidence limits, the combined data best fit the expectation of one locus with fifteen or more alleles. These results correlated well with those of leukocyte typing by cytotoxic antiserums in family studies. However, some antigens revealed by MLC tests were not detected by the antiserums employed. Beyond inability to detect weaker incompatibilities, the MLC test could not be expected to detect the best match from among random pairs of individuals. Given initial selection by leukocyte typing, however, MLC reactions might reveal disparities not detectable serologically.

In rats, differences at the major *Ag-B* histocompatibility locus have regularly

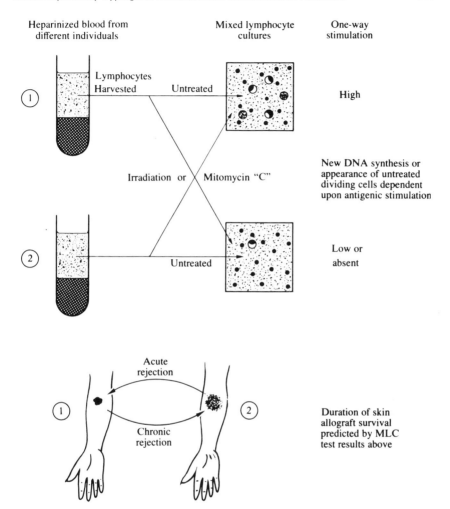

Figure 8—4.   Mixed lymphocyte culture (MLC) test. Irradiated or mytomycin C treated lymphocytes cannot incorporate thymidine (DNA) synthesis), but may stimulate untreated allogeneic lymphocytes to do so (e.g., 2 stimulates 1) if treated cells possess strong antigen(s) missing from untreated cells. MLC stimulation is predictive of acute allograft rejection in the same direction whereas absence of stimulation predicts chronic rejection.

been correlated with both MLC reactivity and acute allograft rejection. The MLC tests in one study were performed with blood lymphocytes from heterogeneous but genetically defined backcross populations. The overall experimental design is instructive. Inbred strains of DA and Lewis rats are $Ag-B^4$ and $Ag-B^1$,

Table 8–3. Expected Percentages of Nonreacting Mixtures in MLC Tests When One-Way Stimulation Was Used (From Bach and Amos, *Science,* Vol. 156: 1507, 1967. Copyright 1967 by the American Association for the Advancement of Science.)

Alleles (No. per Locus)	Genetic Relationship	
	Sib-Sib	Unrelated
One locus		
1	100	100
2	78	63
3	61	33
10	35	3.7
15	32	1.7
20	30	0.96
30	28	0.43
∞	25	0.00
Two loci		
2	61	39
3	37	11
4	27	4
5	21	1.8
6	18	0.94
Three loci		
2	47	24
3	22	3.6
4	14	0.8
Four loci		
2	37	15
3	14	1.2

respectively. (DA × Lewis) F_1 hybrid rats were backcrossed to Lewis animals. Half the progeny should be heterozygous $Ag\text{-}B^1/Ag\text{-}B^4$ and the remainder should be homozygous $Ag\text{-}B^1/Ag\text{-}B^1$. Although the offspring possessed a complete set of Lewis H genes, they varied with respect to DA genes received from the F_1 hybrid parent. Discriminatory MLC reactions between Lewis and backcross lymphocytes then were attributable to unidirectional responses of Lewis cells to DA antigens of cells from certain backcross progeny. Ideally, the intensity of particular reactions should be proportional to the degree of histoincompatibility. Comparisons were made for lymphocyte stimulation (uptake of tritiated thymidine), skin allograft survival times, and matching of Ag-B antigens. Ag-B incompatible individuals as determined by hemagglutination tests gave positive MLC tests as well as acute skin graft rejections on Lewis recipients. Ag-B compatible pairs failed to react in MLC tests, but otherwise showed graft rejections on Lewis animals ranging from acute to prolonged chronic (8 to > 100 days). As in humans, the MLC reactions detected only strong histoincompatibility. However, certain strong non-Ag-B disparities, perhaps attributable to cumulative effects of otherwise weak antigens, were not identified by MLC testing. Ag-B compatible animals were also found to be more susceptible to alloimmune immunosuppression by cyclophosphamide. This raises the possibility that MLC reactions could be useful in excluding potential combinations refractory to moderate immunosuppressive therapy.

Leukocyte Typing

Since transplantation or histocompatibility antigens are contained in structural lipoproteins which are probably the same in all nucleated cells of any individual, much effort is being devoted to blood leukocyte typing in man. The goal is to match particular donors and recipients, whether from the same family or unrelated, especially for major or strong transplantation antigens. Given reliably rapid typing techniques, cadaver donors of organ transplants might well be used in most instances. Indeed, cadaver donors are obviously required for unpaired organs. An overview of leukocyte immunogenetics in man together with various serological typing methods was given in Chapter Four (pages 115–118).

The two techniques of leukoagglutination and especially lymphocyte cytotoxicity by alloantibodies in conjunction with rabbit complement have thus far proved most promising and reproducible. Antibodies distinguishing human leukocyte and platelet alloantigens have been obtained by immunization of anthropoid apes with human cells, but such antibodies have not been elicited in monkeys or mammals other than primates. The most useful lymphocytotoxic antiserums have been alloimmune—selectively produced in humans after skin allografting and/or intradermal leukocyte injections. Given preliminary typing, donor-recipient pairs may be selected for deliberate immunization on the basis of one or few disparities with consequent promise of evoking nearly monospecific antibodies. At this writing, at least three independent genetic loci or systems determining leukocyte antigens in man have been firmly identified. As late as 1966, population studies (of unrelated individuals) undertaken mainly with multispecific antiserums yielded equivocal results in terms of both the number and interdependence of the antigens detected. Recent emphasis on family studies involving both parents plus multiple offspring tested with monospecific antiserums has allowed a spectacular clarification of the whole picture. Moreover, prospective rather than retrospective leukocyte typing is now increasingly promising in relation to organ allografting. A resume of known leukocyte and histocompatibility alloantigen systems in man is given in Table 8–4.

By far the most apparent and perhaps the major histocompatibility antigen system in man is now designated HL-A (HL = Human Leukocyte). Some nine different groups of investigators more or less concurrently detected the twelve to fourteen antigens of this system in recent years, most often with multispecific reagents, and assigned their own letter or numerical symbols accordingly. Extensive cross-testing with potent monospecific antiserums, at the Torino Histocompatibility Workshop in 1967, especially of families, revealed most of the known leukocyte antigens to be indeed attributable to a single genetic locus. As in the *Rh* system, one cannot confidently distinguish between multiple alleles or cistrons of one locus, and subloci or polycistrons of a complex locus (typical of bacteria and viruses). However, there are clearly interdependent combinations of antigens in certain phenogroups. Thus, Dausset's antigen 1 occurs only in conjunction with antigen 2 while antigens 4 and 5 may occur alone or together, but only in the presence of antigen 3. Dausset and co-workers had earlier discerned this locus with its multiple antigenic products, four or five of which were postulated to function as strong transplantation antigens on the basis of test skin graft survival times following preimmunization with typed leukocytes. Morton Simonsen also supposed a single major histocompatibility locus in man, but with only three decisive alleles on the basis of kidney transplant registry data involving immunosuppressed recipients. Family studies now reveal at least forty alleles or phenogroups associated with the *HL-A* locus. However, the relative strength or efficacy of these antigens as transplantation antigens remains in doubt since all relevant kidney allograft recipients have received substantial immunosuppressive treatments which may have masked the true degree of donor-recipient incompatibility.

The leukocyte typing evidence of Terasaki in relation to kidney allograft survivals points toward transplantation antigens of HL-A origin which are intermediate or individually weak in strength. In other words, numerous mismatches confirmed with various antiserums did *not* usually lead to early renal allograft rejections. Nevertheless, multiple mismatches were positively correlated with poorer clinical outcomes, even though no individual antigenic mismatch provided a bad clinical prognosis. A single mismatch was recorded by Terasaki when a donor's cells reacted positively and a recipient's cells negatively with a given antiserum. If strong H-2 type transplantation antigens were involved in many HL-A phenogroups, it is probable that the actual prolonged survivals obtained could not have been achieved with the moderate immunosuppression employed. However, the key assumption invoking differential effectiveness of immunosuppression cannot be readily confirmed in patients for obvious reasons. It could be evaluated with considerable confidence in genetically defined strains of rats now available. Several important questions are still at issue. Given similar

Table 8-4. Leukocyte and Histocompatibility Antigen Systems in Man (circa 1969)

Locus or System	Previous Designations	No. of Alleles or Phenogroups (Minimum)	No. of Alloantigens Detected	Characteristics of System
HL-A*	Hu-1 LA "4"	40	12–14	Most leukocyte antigens detected serologically are determined by genes at this probably complex locus. This locus appears analogous to H-1 (rather than H-2) in mice since its antigenic products show a whole spectrum of "strengths" in terms of histoincompatibility.
HL-B	"5"	2	2	The two known leukocyte antigens associated with this locus are distinctive in that they do not appear to function as histocompatibility antigens. However, they could be very weak transplantation antigens.
ABO	same	4	3†	This major blood group locus and its products represent a major histocompatibility barrier. The allelic combination is important since A₁ is a very strong antigen in group O, moderate in group B, and weak or compatible in an A₂ recipient.
Thompson‡	—	2	1	This provisionally designated locus has been found by Walford as a lymphocyte antigen in both population and family studies. Evidence for its distinctiveness is illustrated in Fig. 8–5.

*For details of new nomenclature for factors of the HL-A system and previous designations, see Bull. World Health Org., Vol. 39: 483–486, 1968.

‡One of a small group of recently discovered antigenic specificities (others are tentatively designated TO[1](NA 1) and 9a) that appear to be inherited independently of the three well established systems. Certain blood group systems such as P may also be significant for histocompatibility.

†Only the antigenic products of the A₁, A₂, and B alleles have been studied in this connection.

immunosuppressive regimens, most human kidney allotransplants which cease to function do so within the first three months. Does this situation reflect stronger antigenic disparities, including augmentative effects of multiple weak H antigens, or critical technical-therapeutic shortcomings? Alternatively, many acute rejections are attributed by Terasaki to presensitized recipients who possess cytotoxic antibodies prior to grafting. Of 218 prospective recipients tested, 23 per cent of the men and 46 per cent of the women had antibodies to HL-A leukocyte antigens. In numerous instances, cytotoxic antibodies in the women's serums reacted with their husband's cells and could be attributed to earlier pregnancy. Other women and the men with such antibodies were probably immunized by transfusions since normal males and nulliparous females not transfused lacked naturally occurring cytotoxins. To what extent preimmunization nullifies immunosuppression also remains to be determined with respect to different HL-A phenogroup incompatibilities.

The *HL-B* system, formerly known as *Group 5,* has been well studied in the Netherlands by J. J. van Rood and co-workers. The two known leukocyte antigens, readily detected by leukoagglutination tests, are governed by two alleles at this locus inherited independently of *HL-A.* Expected and observed frequencies of HL-B phenotypes in a group of 500 random individuals are shown in Table 8—5. On the assumption· of two alleles (5^a and 5^b) yielding three

Table 8—5. Expected and Observed Frequencies of the Phenotypes of HL-B (Group 5) in a Group of 500 Random Donors as Determined by Leukoagglutination (Modified from van Rood and van Leeuwen, *In Histocompatibility Testing,* Division of Medical Sciences, National Academy of Sciences-National Research Council, Washington, D.C., 1965)

Observed	Numbers	Fraction of Total
5(a+b−)	18	0.036
5(a+b+)	145	0.290
5(a−b+)	337	0.674
	Total 500	
	Gene freq. $5a$ = 0.18	
	Gene freq. $5b$ = 0.82	

Expected	Numbers
5(a+b−) = 0.18^2 × 500	16.4
5(a+b+) = 2 × 0.18 × 0.82 × 500	148.2
5(a−b+) = 0.82^2 × 500	335.4
X^2 = 0.239	0.70 > p > 0.50

phenotypes in Hardy-Weinberg equilibrium ($p^2 + 2pq + q^2 = 1$), good agreement between observed and expected frequencies was obtained. Typing of an additional 272 persons also led to gene frequency estimates of about 0.19 for 5^a and 0.81 for 5^b. Moreover, some 129 children of thirty matings were studied; no exceptions to the three postulated phenotypes in the children were observed in relation to parental phenotypes. The specificities of the typing serums used were also checked by cross-absorption. Additional data on this system involving both unrelated individuals and families are in accord with these earlier findings (see reference 7). As emphasized in Chapter Four, suitable cross-absorption tests serve to prove that critical typing reagents recognize only one antigen. Of course, even under these circumstances, a new antiserum might reveal an additional antigen which previously remained undetected in a system.

To test the efficacy of HL-B antigens as transplantation antigens, future test-graft recipients were immunized by an intradermal injection of leukocytes from a disparate donor and were challenged two weeks later with skin allografts from two other donors. Thus, 5a-negative recipients were preimmunized with 5a-positive leukocytes. To control unintentional immunization with other antigens, the two skin graft donors in this situation were 5a-positive and 5a-negative, respectively. A similar experimental design has been used for other alloantigens, including ABO, as considered earlier in this chapter. In the example cited, 5a-positive skin grafts survived fifteen or more days on specifically preimmunized recipients. Such prolonged survival suggests that this antigen is either ineffective or only weakly effective as a transplantation antigen. Nevertheless, one should bear in mind the congenic mouse studies, detailed in Chapter Six, which emphasize the potential additive effects of otherwise weak immunogens.

Thompson is a provisionally designated system found by Roy Walford. It has been detected as a lymphocyte antigen in both population and family studies. *Thompson* is one of a small group of recently discovered antigenic specificities that appear to be inherited independently of the three well-established systems (i.e., *HL-A*, *HL-B*, and *ABO*). Evidence for its distinctiveness is illustrated by the family study in Fig. 8–5 showing independent segregation of *Thompson* and the *HL-A* system. The possible role of *Thompson* as a transplantation antigen remains to be evaluated. Preliminary data suggests that β-lipoprotein serum allotypes also influence graft survival in man. When donor and recipient were of different *Lp* type, test skin allografts were rejected significantly earlier than when they were of the same type, even with exclusion of ABO incompatibility. *Lp* types may be genetically associated with leukocyte antigens, analogous to the *Ss* gene included in the *H-2* complex in mice.

Leukocyte antigens in Rhesus monkeys have been shown to function as transplantation antigens. Repeated skin grafting followed by intravenous injection of donor blood has given potent alloimmune serums active in

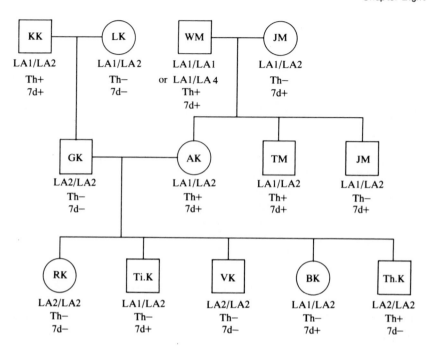

Figure 8–5.   Family study showing independent segregation of the LC-2A (Thompson) specificity and the *HL-A* (*LA*) system. The results for RK and VK are consistent with those of Ti.K, BK, and Th.K except on the basis of independent segregation or crossing-over. Note that 7d shows no evidence of segregating independently of the *LA* system. (After Walford *et al.*, *Histocompatibility Testing 1967*, Munksgaard, Copenhagen, p. 229, 1967.)

leukoagglutination and lymphocytotoxicity. Reactions of hyperimmunized monkeys to skin allografts were compared with their serum antibody activities according to the design illustrated in Fig. 8–6. Ten monkeys were tested with a total of thirty-two skin allografts. In most instances, accelerated allograft destruction occurred in recipients who also had high titers of agglutinating and cytotoxic antibodies for the donor's leukocytes. This type of experiment does not of course indicate whether one or several alloantigens was responsible for the observed results. Cross-absorption or selective absorption analysis of the antiserums is additionally required. Two major leukocyte antigens of Rhesus monkeys have been identified in recent work. Other model systems for defining leukocyte-transplantation antigen relationships are now being explored in rats, guinea pigs, and dogs.

IMMUNIZE
MONKEY X   TEST SERUM X

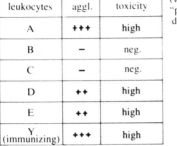

leukocytes	aggl.	toxicity
A	+++	high
B	–	neg.
C	–	neg.
D	++	high
E	++	high
Y (immunizing)	+++	high

skin graft and/or
leukocytes i.d.
from monkey Y

TRANSPLANT
MONKEY X

(with skin from serologically
"positive" and "negative"
donors)

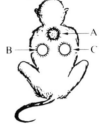

Figure 8–6. "Correlation" test for leukocyte and transplantation antigens in Rhesus monkeys. (Modified from Balner and Dersjant, in *Histocompatibility Testing 1965, Munksgaard, Copenhagen, p. 108, 1966.)*

Probabilities of Achieving Compatibility

Just how important is genetic relationship with respect to human allograft survival times? As shown in Table 8–6, nearly 80 per cent of kidneys transplanted between identical twins were still fully viable after three years in stark contrast to only 15 per cent survivals between unrelated persons by this time. Not surprisingly, grafts from brothers or sisters fared better than those from mothers or fathers in the absence of precise histocompatibility typing, which has only recently become feasible. If one considers a larger body of data, wherein related (parent, sib, and other blood relatives) and unrelated kidney

Table 8–6. Survival of Human Kidney Transplants Among More than 600 Recipients from 1964 to 1967*

Donor Source	No. of Transplants	Percentage of Kidneys Functioning		
		4–6 Months	1 Year	2–3 Years
Identical twins	41	89	80	77
Sibling	172	61	58	53
Parent	323	59	52	43
Living– Unrelated	108	35	18	15

*This simplified tabulation does *not* take into account histocompatibility matching or differences in immunosuppressive therapy.

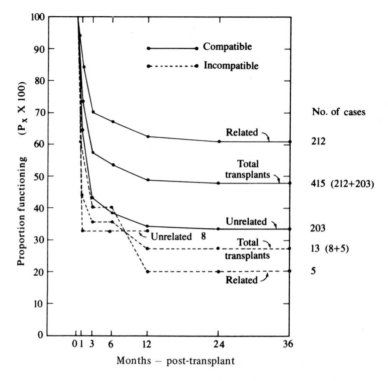

Figure 8–7.   Estimated proportion of transplants functioning (P_x) according to compatibility of ABO blood group and genetic relationship of kidney donor. Note: Proportion of transplants expected to function up to 1,3, . . . ,36 months post-transplant. (After Gleason and Murray, *Transplantation,* Vol. 5: 348, 1967. Copyright The Williams and Wilkins Co.)

donors are compared (Fig. 8–7), about 60 per cent of grafts from unrelated donors survived for three years whereas only about 35 per cent from unrelated donors were retained. In this comparison, both groups were ABO-compatible. The higher incidence of prolonged survivals from unrelated donors in these more recent and comprehensive data probably reflects improvement in both prospective typing and in immunosuppressive techniques. During the period 1965–1968, kidneys from related donors showed 65±6 per cent survivals at one year while cadaver donors gave only 39±4 per cent survivals after the same interval.

Despite obvious gaps and uncertainties in our knowledge of histocompatibility variables, it is still instructive to estimate probabilities of achieving compatibility in relation to different numbers of *H* loci, alleles, and antigens. Incisive mathematical approaches also require information on allele frequencies, gene dosage effects, and even gene-product interactions which are poorly known. Probabilities of compatibility of allografts in various donor-recipient combinations were considered in Chapter Six on the simplifying assumption that all alleles are antigenically effective on a one-to-one basis and no immunosuppression is involved. To avoid unmanageable complexity, one assumes histocompatibility loci in general to be autosomal, multiallelic, codominant, and noninteracting. Although the relative frequencies of alleles often vary widely, equal frequencies are usually assumed in the absence of actual data. Actually, for each locus and any number of alleles, the lowest probability of compatibility is obtained when the alleles are equally frequent in a population. Even if our concern were restricted, for example, to four genetic loci specifying a total of thirty alleles and antigens, less than one graft per thousand between random pairs might be expected to be indefinitely successful. Obviously, controlled immunosuppression has greatly improved the probabilities. If one supposes only the *HL-A* locus to be critical in the face of immunosuppression and of ABO-compatibility, the immunogenetic model constructed by Serra and O'Mathuna is revealing (Fig. 8–8). Genetic compatibility has a higher probability between siblings than between parents and children and is higher between the latter than between unrelated individuals. These authors adopt the more restrictive assumption that every *H* gene present in the donor must also be

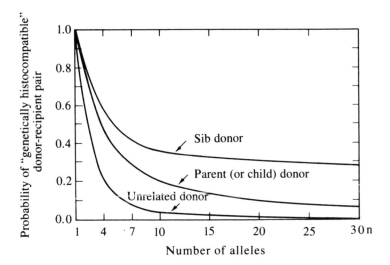

Figure 8–8. Graphs of the variation of the probability of a genetically histocompatible donor-recipient pair on the number of alleles, in the hypothesis of one locus and equal frequencies of the alleles. With forty alleles already known at the *HL-A* locus, prospective typing of unrelated donors is seen to be critical. (After Serra and O'Mathuna, *Ann. Human Genet.,* Vol. 30: 106, 1966.)

present in the recipient to assure compatibility. With forty alleles of very unequal frequencies already known at the *HL-A* locus, prospective typing of unrelated donors is seen to be critical for avoidance of multiple mismatches.

Just how critical can tissue typing be, especially among unrelated members of a population? Walford has vigorously argued for use of monospecific reagents to facilitate grafting from positive to positive (or negative to negative) for each antigenic specificity. Allograft survival prospects in relation to the four possible tissue typing patterns of antigen positive and negative donors and recipients are summarized in Table 8—7. The positive donor—negative recipient is obviously a

Table 8—7. Survival Prospects of Allografts on the Basis of Tissue Typing Patterns (After Walford *et al., Histocompatibility Testing 1965,* Munksgaard, Copenhagen, p.90, 1966)

Reaction with Antiserum of Cells of		Survival Prospects Assuming	
Donor	Recipient	Antiserum Is Monospecific	Antiserum Is Multispecific
+	+	Best possible situation as indicating identity at corresponding allelic sites.	Of decreasing predictive value with increasing multispecificity.
−	+	Poor assuming most or all alleles at the locus are strong. No definite information otherwise.	Of increasing predictive value with increasing multispecificity, assuming existence of weak or "null" alleles at some sites.
+	−	Poorest possible prospect.	Poor prospect.
−	−	No definite information unless number of alleles is small.	Same as − + situation given above.

poor prospect in relation to any previously identified histocompatibility antigen. However, grafting from negative donors to positive recipients may also be unwise unless the apparent donor "negativity" is referable to "weak" or "null" alleles. Observed differences in kidney allograft survival have not proved impressive in relation to the two categories of positive donors—negative recipients and vice versa whereas donor-recipient pairs typed as identical have been much more successful. The importance of relative interallelic disparities in this connection has already been emphasized in reference to extensive studies with congenic lines of mice in Chapter Six. In humans, we already know that A_1 is a strong alloantigen in a group O, moderate in a group B, and weak or practically nonimmunogenic in a group A_2 recipient. Until much more is known about interallelic "strengths" of incompatibility, additive effects and gene-product interactions in man, meaningful probability estimates will better be served by actual statistics than by simplified theoretical calculations.

Circumvention of Alloimmune Reactions

Most of the prolonged allograft survivals obtained in patients could not be achieved without drug-induced suppression of the immune response. More than anything else, such immunosuppression has allowed circumvention of numerous antigenic barriers revealed by tissue typing. The most efficacious combination of drugs currently in clinical use is a purine analog, Imuran (or Azathioprine, both Burroughs Wellcome & Co.), prednisone (a steroid), and actinomycin C (inhibiting DNA-dependent RNA synthesis). Unfortunately, these classes of drugs have two major disadvantages: they are toxic to the patient and they inhibit immune responsiveness nonspecifically, thereby making the patient vulnerable to a variety of infectious agents. Excessive immunosuppression has predictably led to many deaths from infectious diseases. Although detailed consideration of possible mechanisms of action of immunosuppressive drugs is provocative, it is sufficient to indicate that all components of the allograft reaction are potential targets. Corticosteroids generally inhibit phagocytosis and antigen uptake; lymphocyte depletion is also consistently found. Nucleic acid and protein synthesis may be inhibited by a variety of so-called antimetabolites which compete with natural metabolites for appropriate enzyme sites. Radiation, alkylating agents and certain antibiotics principally affect end stages of nucleic acid synthesis and assembly of proteins. Many nucleic acid analogs actually replace the natural purine or pyrimidine bases during synthesis. However, inhibition of cell proliferation does not account for all drug effects, and cell destruction, especially of sensitive lymphocytes, commonly occurs.

Immunosuppressive activity and systemic toxicity are not always parallel probably because the former reflects mainly lymphocyte suppression. However, the nearer the dose of chemical agents to toxic levels, the more pronounced in general is the effect on immune responses. Also, agents tend to be most effectively suppressive when administered during the latent and early logarithmic phases of antibody responses. Synergistic drug combinations have the advantage of blocking different steps or pathways. Since some initial induction of allograft immunity is usually found, one needs to be able to block effector sequences which are still poorly understood. M. C. Berenbaum of the St. Mary's Hospital Medical School, London, has called attention to the promising combined use of immunosuppressive and "protective" agents. For example, cysteine and glutathione reduce radiation deaths without concomitant sparing of immunocompetent cells. Massive doses of the folic acid antagonist, methotrexate, were given to guinea pigs bearing skin allografts without overt toxicity, provided folinic acid was also administered. By such counteraction of the toxic effect of an antimetabolite with the natural metabolite, very prolonged allograft survival was obtained by Berenbaum.

Alloimmune suppression by means of whole-body irradiation, thymectomy, splenectomy, and thoracic duct drainage have all been tried experimentally and clinically. These otherwise partially effective procedures have been largely abandoned either because of deleterious consequences or failure to improve results already achieved by reversible drug therapy. Local irradiation given to the thymus, spleen, kidney allograft site, or to a combination of these areas appears to have some beneficial effect on continuing transplant function. Data from the 1967 Kidney Transplant Registry suggest postoperative azathioprine, postoperative steroids, actinomycin, and postoperative local irradiation as the best known regimen with either related or unrelated donor-recipient combinations. Lymphocyte depletion by chronic thoracic duct drainage may be regarded as a nontoxic and acceptable adjunct to the preferential regimen cited. Very recent work suggests that certain purinethiols produce increased skin allograft survival in H-2 disparate mice without concurrent inhibition of other serum antibody responses. This raises hope that more nearly specific chemosuppressants of allograft responsiveness may be forthcoming.

Much research has recently focused on antilymphocyte serums as powerful and less "nonspecific" immunosuppressive agents. Xenogeneic antilymphocyte serums (ALS) are clearly capable of attenuating immunological responses—even to repeat allografts or xenografts. Allogeneic skin graft survival in mice involving strong H-2 differences can be prolonged to an impressive degree by repeated injections of recipients with rabbit ALS. Repeated administration of horse antihuman-lymphocyte globulin has apparently improved the usual functioning of at least one series of human renal allografts without excessive risk of anaphylactic reactions, serum sickness, or infectious disease. Human subjects given a purified 7S gamma globulin fraction of a rabbit antihuman lymphocyte serum by Paul Russell and co-workers showed transient lymphopenia associated with modest prolongation of skin allograft survival and inhibition of positive delayed-type skin reactions to microbial antigens. In certain animal experiments, these antiserums actually appear to wipe out preexisting immunity while in others prolonged allograft survival appears merely to be consequent upon lymphocyte depletion by ALS. There is now qualified enthusiasm for clinical use of ALS, especially purified IgG preparations, even though the theoretical risks and uncertainties attending repetitive inoculation of foreign serum protein cannot be lightly dismissed. The whole array of alloantigens concerned with histocompatibility may be targets of the antibodies contained in most ALS reagents. Effective serums are not demonstrably lymphocyte-specific, and their lymphocyte cytotoxicity is not predictive of ability to prolong allograft survival.

When the mode of action of ALS with known antibody specificity is better understood, its appropriate assay and use should become less controversial.

Adult Tolerance and Radiation Immunogenetics

Beyond the ultimate, but remote prospect of complete matching of allograft donors and recipients, prolonged or permanent allograft survival may well continue to depend on a combination of factors. According to current thinking, these include limiting mismatches to weak antigens, moderate immunosuppression to prevent subacute or chronic rejection, and gradual induction of host tolerance so immunosuppression can eventually be terminated. The induction of host tolerance in adults generally appears to be favored by weak antigens in contrast to strong ones, especially under the conditions of high dosage inherent in transplants of large organs like the kidney or liver. Tolerant states to skin allografts have been obtained in adult mice in several different ways. Besides procedures involving substantial chemosuppression, at least partly specific approaches have included: (a) prolonged parabiosis or daily injections of donor-strain spleen cells for several weeks, (b) sublethal irradiation and injection of donor-strain spleen cells in high dosage, and (c) irradiation at lethal dosage levels followed by injection of donor-type hematopoietic cells. These procedures all have in common protracted exposure of recipients to cellular antigens in high dosage. Development of transplantation disease as a consequence of graft-versus-host reactions has proved to be a considerable hazard following inoculation of large numbers of immunocompetent cells, even in adult experimental animals. Transplants of whole organs like kidney, liver, or heart should largely avoid this hazard because only modest numbers of donor small lymphocytes would be included in the transplant. The quick benefits of whole-body irradiation are far outweighed by potentially irreparable damage produced in most patients.

Adult thymectomized mice restored with isogeneic bone marrow following heavy irradiation exhibit a longlasting impairment of primary responsiveness to allogeneic skin grafts. Under certain conditions, drug-induced immunosuppression in mice can be effectively potentiated by previous adult thymectomy. But permanent immunologic "crippling" following thymectomy is too undesirable to be justified, even in less vulnerable adults. Since recovery of immune responsiveness in adult rodents given high doses of radiation and bone marrow therapy depends on the presence of the thymus, it is clear that this "master organ" is necessary for reconstitution of immunologic capacity.

In addition to promising provision of new organs for worn-out ones, much "nuclear age" attention has been devoted to the immunogenetic determinants of the ability of cellular inoculums to repopulate and save lethally irradiated recipients. The most fundamental considerations have already been noted in previous chapters. If there is a major incompatibility between the usual adult bone marrow inoculum and the irradiated host, allogeneic disease leading to death of the host is the expected outcome. The "rules of transplantation" (Chapters Six and Seven) nicely obtain in the attempted repair of radiation injury. Inoculation of parental strain marrow into irradiated F_1 hybrid mice commonly leads to deleterious graft-versus-host reactions whereas F_1 marrow is compatible and affords protection under the same conditions. However, growth of parent-strain marrow grafts in irradiated F_1 hosts can be greatly augmented by introduction of parental lymphoid cells into the F_1 host before irradiation. Presumably, parental spleen or lymph node cells destroy and replace host cells in this situation, thereby promoting a predominantly donor-type chimerism following irradiation. Conspicuous differences in the relative abilities of parental marrows to repopulate F_1 hybrid mice are not fully explicable at the present time. For example, (C57BL $\times$ 101) F_1 recipients of C57BL marrow survive less well than similar recipients of 101 marrow. R. A. Popp, working at the Oak Ridge National Laboratory, Tennessee, demonstrated the heritability of factors governing regression of C57BL marrow grafts in such F_1 recipients as follows. Survivals of F_1 recipients of F_2 marrow of phenotypes H-2 b/k, H-2 b/b, and H-2 k/k were 94.8, 83.5, and 81.0 per cent, respectively; these differences are correlated with H-2 incompatibility. Yet differences in survival of F_1 recipients of C57BL compared with 101 marrow (31.4 and 70.4 per cent, respectively) are not solely referable to the H-2 b/b versus H-2 k/k types of the donors since survival of F_1 recipients of F_2 marrow of the same homozygous genotypes showed no such disparity.

Extensive results from allogeneic marrow inoculation after midlethal irradiation in various donor-host combinations of inbred mice and F_1 hybrids have been obtained by Delta Uphoff at the U. S. National Cancer Institute. She has classified the effects as follows: (a) an uncommon early lethal effect associated with prompt host-versus-graft rejection; (b) no beneficial or deleterious effect, largely associated with strong immunogenetic disparities and early graft rejection; (c) initial protection followed by late deaths, involving both H-2 and non-H-2 associated graft-versus-host reactions; and (d) lasting protection, always afforded by marrow of the same H-2 phenotype as the irradiated host. Use of the fetal hematopoietic tissue, such as fetal liver cells in mice, has minimized or circumvented graft-versus-host reactions, presumably because reciprocal tolerance is more readily achieved. One perceives then that the repair of radiation injury even in genetically defined mice involves complex interactions which are not yet fully predictable.

The Future of Immunogenetics

At the most basic level, the interdisciplinary fields of immunogenetics are still in their infancy. The practical scope of antigen typing of microorganisms, red cells, and tissue cells has become extensive. The usefulness of such information in animal husbandry and medicine is increasingly obvious. Yet detailed understanding of gene-antigen-antibody relationships is emerging quite slowly. We are now entering a period when simpler generalizations are having to be restructured or at least substantially modified. Elof Carlson has quite properly emphasized that Occam's razor—accepting the simplest sufficient hypothesis—is usually not a valid instrument for the resolution of contending models or explanations. The "one dominant allele → one antigen" conception of C. C. Little and J. B. S. Haldane must be qualified in several respects. These include multiple nonallelic genes acting sequentially in the synthesis of antigenic macromolecules, gene-product interactions typified by Lewis B in man, and correspondence between phenogroups and probable subunits inherent in classical alleles. All would now acknowledge the chemical complexity of Mendelian genes: if the average gene size is related to a polypeptide of 100 amino acids and if the codon is a triplet, the nucleotide pairs required would be 300. From this standpoint then, multiple alleles may be tentatively regarded as a series of different combinations of intercalary nucleotide determinants or as clusters of mutons (recons?) of the same functional unit (cistron). Here one should note that the case for occurrence of operons in metazoan species rests mainly on analogy to bacteria and viruses. The term *pseudoallele*(s) remains objectionable in most immunogenetic contexts because it implies proof of additional "true" allelic or strictly alternative relationships within a complex locus. Pseudoallelism has also fallen into conceptual disfavor with the ascendance of the more attractive molecular model of fine structure. Current productive controversy will no doubt continue concerning the organization (i.e., fine structure) of genetic information in complex loci of mammals vis-a-vis oligosaccharide or amino acid products detected as antigens. Continuing dissection of the multicomponent *H-2* locus in mice by Shreffler, Snell, and Stimpfling is most revealing at present, but not necessarily typical even of loci that specify cellular alloantigens. I would emphasize the newer realization that antigens are not immediate gene products but are generally determined at a distance from the nucleus (e.g., in cell membranes) by enzymes synthesized in cytoplasmic polysomes.

The significance of individual antigens should increase to the extent that determinants now represented only by letter or numerical symbols are chemically characterized and related to larger biosynthetic sequences as in the H-ABO-Lewis alloantigens. Nevertheless, definitive typing of individuals or populations and mating tests of inheritance do not depend on knowing the chemistry of the antigens used as "markers." The simplistic idea of a "one antigen → one antibody specificity" relation has only been reluctantly deserted by many immunogeneticists. One can now hardly evade the finding that even repeatedly purified antibodies raised against simple haptenic determinants represent a population of molecules with considerable cross-reactive specificities.

In other words, not all antibodies are uniquely complementary to the antigenic determinants that evoked them. This consideration of course involves a fundamental limitation in the specificity of immune responses. The assignment of antigenic symbols and their subsequent interpretation should entail a recognition that antigen units as such may represent larger or smaller molecules or portions thereof definable ultimately only in relation to a certain population of antibodies. Inheritance of specific immune response capacities has received the least investigative attention and may well offer the greatest scope for pioneering studies. The most incisively revealing findings in this area should come with congenic lines of animals, especially those with nonoverlapping responses to well-defined antigens.

Although the field of serum allotypes is relatively new, major insights concerning the structure and genetic specification of immunoglobulins have emerged on the basis of allotypic markers. Their further significance, in addition to being good genetic markers, will probably be in relation to immunologic diseases of diverse etiology. It would be premature to suggest any direct cause-and-effect relationship between given allotypes and particular aberrations. However, there is already some evidence of certain antibody specificities being preferentially associated with certain allotypes, even though known allotype positions on H or L chains do not appear to be included in antibody combining sites. Immunoglobulin allotypes may also have more pertinence to placental transfer of antibodies and to maternal-fetal incompatibility than is now realized.

Increasing understanding of the molecular and cellular dynamics of immunological tolerance will have an important bearing on virtually all areas of immunogenetics. The governance and regulation of antibody production obviously hinges on whatever receptors tend to promote or prevent instigation of specific tolerance. Although transplantation disease may occur in the absence of specific host tolerance of the attacking cells, this problem does not appear to be serious in connection with human organ transplantation. To the extent that experimental allogeneic disease is a valid model of certain autoimmune diseases, cancer, and aging, its further elucidation, especially in relation to chronic and weak incompatibilities, should clearly be encouraged.

We are now entering a period in which rapid advances in clinical transplantation are being made on the basis of more than two decades of intensive basic research in immunogenetics and transplantation immunology. More than 600 men and women with incurable renal disease are presently being kept alive by borrowed kidneys. Witness also the recent liver and heart transplants which will no doubt be extended even to other human organs in the near future. Additional progress may be envisaged along these frontiers: (a) refinement of histocompatibility typing to improve selection of donors whose tissues are more nearly compatible to recipients; (b) development of approaches, such as antigen loading or use of antilymphocyte serum, which facilitate induction of tolerance under conditions of minimal general immunosuppression; (c) identification and use of less toxic immunosuppressive drugs on a more selective basis to avoid clobbering the overall immune response capacity. Given histocompatibility typing for strong antigens, it may be hoped that moderate chemosuppression alone will implement induction of acquired tolerance toward many weak antigens and thereby allow indefinite survival of diverse tissue grafts.

Techniques of organ and tissue preservation are still rather primitive. Yet one may foresee widespread organ banks in the future, where kidneys, livers, hearts, lungs, and other tissues from accident victims of known leukocyte types will be preserved frozen until required. With successful transplantation the rule rather than the exception, moral and legal problems of organ procurement will have to be faced in a new light.

KEY REFERENCES

1. *Advance in Transplantation.* Munksgaard, Copenhagen, 1968. Proceedings of the First International Congress of the Transplantation Society, Paris, June, 1967. The sections on methods of immunosuppression and organ transplantation are especially relevent to this chapter.

2. BACH, F. H., and D. B. AMOS. "Hu-1: Histocompatibility Locus in Man." *Science*, Vol. 156: 1506–1508, 1967. Both MLC tests and lymphocyte typing shown to be predictive of skin allograft survival times referable to HL-A disparities.

3. BERENBAUM, M. C. "Immunosuppressive Agents." *Brit. Med. Bull.*, Vol. 21: 140–146, 1965. Reviews modes of action of diverse immunosuppressive drugs with special attention to immunosuppressive therapy in relation to allograft incompatibility.

4. CEPPELLINI, R., E. S. CURTONI, P. L. MATTIUZ, G. LEIGHEB, M. VISETTI, and A. COLOMBI. "Survival of Test Skin Grafts in Man: Effect of Genetic Relationship and of Blood Groups Incompatibility." *Ann. N. Y. Acad. Sci.*, Vol. 129: 421–445, 1966. Reporting that not only ABO but also the P and perhaps other blood group antigens affect allograft survival.

5. Conference on Transplantation, Santa Barbara. *Transplantation*, Vol. 5 (Part 2): 775–1245, 1967. Sections on determination of histocompatibility and abrogation of the immune response by irradiation therapy, lymphocyte depletion, and drug therapy are especially relevant to this chapter.

6. DAUSSET, J., and F. T. RAPAPORT. "The Role of Blood Group Antigens in Human Histocompatibility." *Ann. N. Y. Acad. Sci.*, Vol. 129: 408–420, 1966. Data show that AB erythrocyte antigens and certain platelet and leukocyte antigens function as transplantation antigens.

7. *Histocompatibility Testing.* Publ. 1229, Natl. Acad. Sci., Washington, D.C., 1965; *Histocompatibility Testing 1965.* Munksgaard, Copenhagen, 1966. These two sequential monographs rather thoroughly cover early work,

especially on human tissue typing, with special emphasis in diverse techniques and their limitations.

8. *Histocompatibility Testing 1967.* Munksgaard, Copenhagen, 1967. This conference and workshop emphasizes and analyzes the substantial recent progress in human leukocyte typing.

9. *Human Transplantation.* Ed. F. T. Rapaport and J. Dausset, Grune & Stratton, New York and London, 1968. A substantial progress report by a variety of experts and divided into five sections: introduction to human transplantation, organ transplantation, experimental approaches designed to attenuate human allograft responses, and a miscellany designated as immunobiological horizons.

10. MICKLEM, H. S., and J. F. LOUTIT. *Tissue Grafting and Radiation.* Academic Press, New York and London, 1966. Chapters 3, 4, and 8 deal comprehensively with radiation in relation to transplantation immunity, radiation chimerism, and surgical replacement of tissues.

11. POPP, R. A., "Inheritance of Factors Affecting the Ability of Bone Marrow of (C57BL $\times$ 101) F_2 Mice to Establish Permanent Grafts in Irradiated F_1 Mice." *J. Nat. Cancer. Inst.,* Vol. 33: 7–14, 1964. Points up immunogenetic complexities in establishment and persistence of bone marrow grafts.

12. SERRA, A., and D. O'MATHUNA. "A Theoretical Approach to the Study of Genetic Parameters of Histocompatibility in Man." *Ann. Human Genet.,* Vol. 30: 97–118, 1966. Mathematical models of histocompatibility in man are analyzed in relation to number of loci, number of alleles at each locus, and relative frequency of alleles. See also Ceppellini, Chapter 6, reference 3.

13. SILVERS, W. K., D. B. WILSON, and J. PALM. "Mixed Leukocyte Reactions and Histocompatibility in Rats." *Science,* Vol. 155: 703–704, 1967. Differences at important *Ag-B* locus found to be associated with positive, one-way MLC reactions and with prompt rejection of skin allografts.

14. UPHOFF, D. E. "Genetic Factors Influencing Irradiation Protection by Bone Marrow." *J. Nat. Cancer Inst.,* Vol. 30: 1115–1151, 1963. Two of a series of papers relating the repair of radiation injury to allogeneic marrows in genetically defined donor-recipient combinations.

15. WALFORD, R. L., E. SHANBROM, G. M. TROUP, E. ZELLER, and B. ACKERMAN. "Lymphocyte Grouping with Defined Antisera," in *Histocompatibility Testing 1967,* Munksgaard, Copenhagen, pp. 221–229, 1967. Criteria of monospecificity based on absorption analysis; a critique of panel testing and parallel serum testing to establish identity of specificities; and a consideration of certain problems of chi-square testing are set forth.

INDEX